Essential Clinical
Neuroanatomy

Essential Clinical Neuroanatomy

Thomas H. Champney
Professor
Miller School of Medicine
University of Miami
Miami, Florida, USA

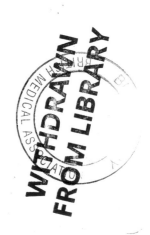

WILEY Blackwell

This edition first published 2016 © 2016 by John Wiley & Sons, Ltd.

Registered Office
John Wiley & Sons, Ltd, The Atrium, Southern Gate, Chichester, West Sussex,
PO19 8SQ, UK

Editorial Offices
9600 Garsington Road, Oxford, OX4 2DQ, UK
The Atrium, Southern Gate, Chichester, West Sussex, PO19 8SQ, UK
111 River Street, Hoboken, NJ 07030-5774, USA

For details of our global editorial offices, for customer services and for information about how to
apply for permission to reuse the copyright material in this book please see our website at
www.wiley.com/wiley-blackwell

Library of Congress Cataloging-in-Publication Data

Champney, Thomas, author.
Essential clinical neuroanatomy / Thomas Champney.
  p. ; cm.
  Includes bibliographical references and index.
  ISBN 978-1-118-43993-7 (pbk.)
I. Title.
[DNLM: 1. Nervous System–anatomy & histology.   WL 101]
  QM451
  611′.8–dc23
                                                    2014046419

A catalogue record for this book is available from the British Library.

Wiley also publishes its books in a variety of electronic formats. Some content that appears in print
may not be available in electronic books.

Cover image: © Science Photo Library/Pasieka
Cover design by Visual Philosophy

Set in 10/12pt Adobe Garamond Pro by SPi Global, Pondicherry, India
Printed and bound in Singapore by Markono Print Media Pte Ltd

1   2016

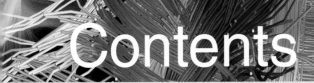

Contents

Preface

Essential Clinical Neuroanatomy is the first neuroanatomy text that consistently illustrates and discusses the anatomy of the central nervous system from the clinical perspective. All of the illustrations are provided in the clinical view (using the axial radiologic standard of computed tomography and magnetic resonance imaging). This provides consistency throughout the text and throughout the career of the reader. In addition, the neural pathways are color coded for easier recognition and recall with green indicating sensory components, red indicating voluntary motor components, and purple indicating involuntary (autonomic) components. The clinically relevant neuroanatomy is highlighted, with case studies, clinically-oriented study questions, and clinical boxes of interest. Anatomic details that do not have direct clinical relevance are de-emphasized.

The text is divided into two main sections: the first eleven chapters provide the neuroanatomy of the central nervous system, while the last seven chapters provide descriptions of the sensory, motor, and integration systems within the central nervous system. Each chapter begins with objectives and an outline of the material to be covered. Within each chapter, highlighted clinical boxes are presented, while case studies and clinically relevant multiple choice questions are found at the end of each chapter. Each chapter contains a list of additional readings that include more detail-oriented textbooks, as well as current review articles.

This text is designed for those in the health sciences who require a basic introduction to clinical neuroanatomy. This can include allied health students, first-year medical students, dental students, and neuroscience students. Because of its essential nature, it can be useful for those reviewing neuroanatomy for major licensing or competency examinations.

Thomas H. Champney

Acknowledgments

The development and production of *Essential Clinical Neuroanatomy* utilized the skills and strengths of numerous individuals. First, Dr Ron Clark, my predecessor at the University of Miami, generously provided access to his photographic files, his illustrations, and his notes. The foundation of the book is built on his many years of teaching neuroanatomy. Second, all of the clinical imaging (radiographs, computed tomographs, magnetic resonance images) were graciously provided by Dr Charif Sidani, a neuroradiologist associated with the University of Miami. He provided many hours of help in recommending and selecting images for use in the text.

The editorial staff at Wiley Blackwell were extremely helpful in all phases of this project. Specifically, Elizabeth Johnston, Karen Moore, and Nick Morgan were professional and highly organized. In addition, the excellent illustrations by Jane Fallows and Roger Hulley are an integral part of this project. Any anatomy text is only as good as its illustrations. All of these individuals made the daunting task of this project much more manageable.

Finally, I express my gratitude to all of the students who have provided feedback on the neuroanatomy lectures that are at the center of this text. Their comments and critiques on the lecture material provided the focus for teaching the essentials of clinical neuroanatomy.

Thomas H. Champney

About the companion website

Don't forget to visit the companion website for this book:

 www.wileyessential.com/neuroanatomy

There you will find valuable material designed to enhance your learning, including:

- More multiple-choice questions for self-testing

- Interactive flashcards with on/off label functionality

- PowerPoint figures from the book for downloading

Scan this QR code to visit the companion website:

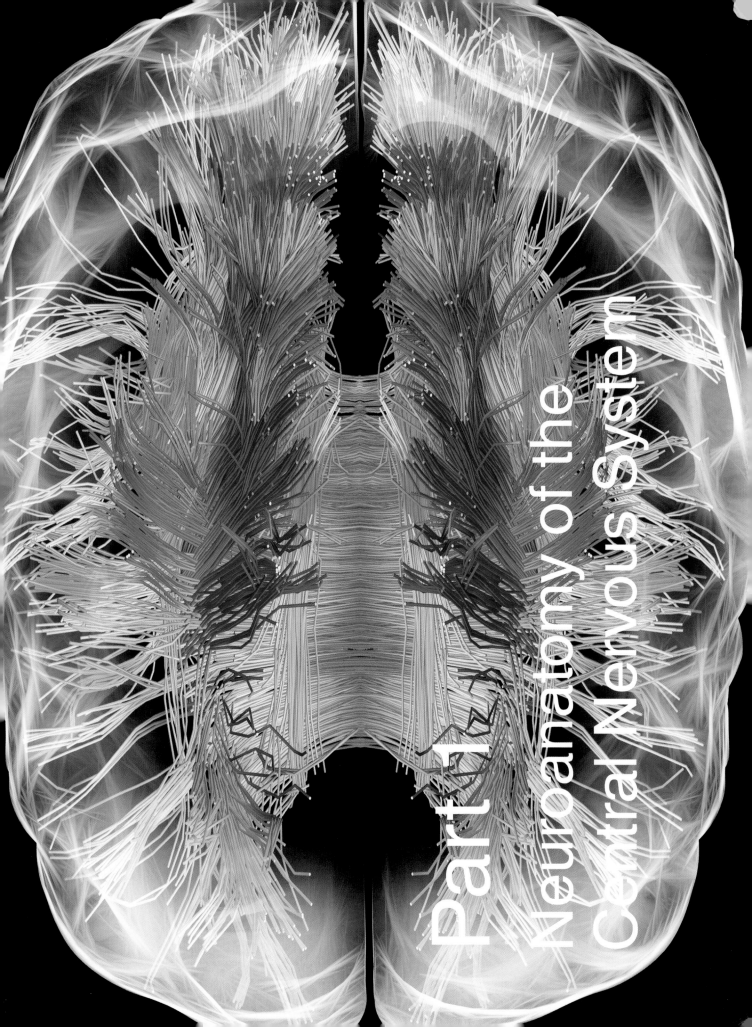

Part 1

Neuroanatomy of the Central Nervous System

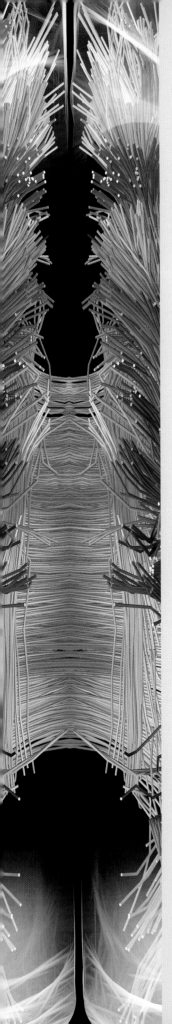

CHAPTER 1

Overview of the nervous system

Learning objectives

1. Describe the basic subdivisions of the human nervous system.
2. Understand basic neuroanatomical terminology.
3. Identify the major structures on the external surface of the gross brain.
4. Identify the major structures on the midsagittal surface of the brain.
5. Identify the cranial nerves.

Anatomic
1. Central nervous system (CNS)
   a) Brain and spinal cord
   b) Collection of nerve cell bodies = nucleus
2. Peripheral nervous system (PNS)
   a) Peripheral nerves
   b) Collection of nerve cell bodies = ganglia

Functional
1. Sensory (afferent)
   a) General – touch
   b) Special senses – sight, sound, taste, smell, balance
2. Motor (efferent)
   a) Voluntary (somatic) – skeletal muscle
   b) Involuntary (autonomic) – smooth and cardiac muscle
      i. Parasympathetic – craniosacral (III, VII, IX, X, S2–S4)
      ii. Sympathetic – thoracolumbar (T1–L2)
3. Integrative – interneurons within the CNS

Neurons
1. Highly specialized, excitable cells
2. Morphologic diversity

Glia – supporting cells
1. Schwann cells (neurolemmocytes) – myelin producing
2. Oligodendrocytes – myelin producing

Essential Clinical Neuroanatomy, First Edition. Thomas H. Champney.
© 2016 John Wiley & Sons, Ltd. Published 2016 by John Wiley & Sons, Ltd.
Companion website: www.wileyessential.com/neuroanatomy

3. Astrocytes – nutritional support
4. Microglia – macrophages (immune support)

Neurons 8

Cellular structure
1. Dendrites
2. Axon
   a) Axon hillock
   b) Terminal arborization/terminal boutons
   c) Synapse/synaptic vesicles
   d) Anterograde/retrograde flow
3. Soma (perikaryon, cell body)
   a) Nucleus/nucleolus
   b) Nissl bodies (rough endoplasmic reticulum and polyribosomes)
   c) Lipofuscin
4. Cell membrane (plasmalemma, neurolemma)
5. Types: unipolar, bipolar, multipolar, pseudounipolar

Glia – central nervous system 9

Oligodendrocytes – myelin production; one oligodendrocyte for many axons

Astrocytes – support cells, glial fibrillary acid protein (GFAP), end feet
1. Fibrous astrocytes – white matter
2. Protoplasmic astrocytes – gray matter

Microglia – macrophage-like, scavenging cells

Ependymal cells – columnar, ciliated cells lining the ventricles

Central nervous system 9

Gray matter
1. Nerve cell bodies (nuclei)
2. Dendrites and axons
3. Glia

White matter
1. Nerve fibers (axons) – myelinated
2. Glia

Brain neuroanatomy 11

Orientation of the brain – 90 degree rotation at midbrain flexure
1. Superior – inferior
2. Anterior – posterior
3. Dorsal – ventral
4. Rostral – caudal

Planes of the brain
1. Sagittal plane
   a) Midsagittal
   b) Parasagittal
2. Horizontal plane (transverse, axial)
3. Frontal plane (coronal)

Views of the brain
1. Superior
   a) Interhemispheric fissure (sagittal)
   b) Precentral gyrus (primary motor)
   c) Central sulcus
   d) Postcentral gyrus (primary somatosensory)
2. Inferior
   a) Interhemispheric fissure (sagittal)
   b) Lateral fissure (Sylvian)
   c) Midbrain – cerebral peduncles
   d) Pons
   e) Medulla oblongata – pyramids, inferior olives
   f) Cerebellum
   g) Olfactory bulb and tract
   h) Optic chiasm and tract
   i) Infundibulum (pituitary stalk)
   j) Mammillary bodies
   k) Cranial nerves (12)
      i. Olfactory nerve (I)
      ii. Optic nerve (II)
      iii. Occulomotor nerve (III)
      iv. Trochlear nerve (IV)
      v. Trigeminal nerve (V)
      vi. Abducens nerve (VI)
      vii. Facial nerve (VII)
      viii. Vestibulocochlear nerve (VIII)
      ix. Glossopharyngeal nerve (IX)
      x. Vagus nerve (X)
      xi. Spinal accessory nerve (XI)
      xii. Hypoglossal nerve (XII)
3. Lateral
   a) Lateral fissure (Sylvian)
   b) Brain stem (midbrain, pons, and medulla)
   c) Cerebellum
   d) Central sulcus
   e) Precentral gyrus (primary motor)
   f) Postcentral gyrus (primary sensory)
   g) Lobes of the brain
      i. Frontal lobe
      ii. Parietal lobe
      iii. Occipital lobe (vision)
      iv. Temporal lobe (auditory)
   h) Insular cortex
   i) Superior temporal gyrus (auditory)
4. Midsagittal
   a) Frontal cortex
   b) Parietal cortex

Introduction

The nervous system is a remarkable communication system that can send a message from one part of the body to the brain, react to that message, and produce a response within seconds. The goal of this chapter is to introduce the components and organization of the nervous system. This may be a review for some, but it will set a foundation on which the remainder of the text can be built.

Nervous system organization

The nervous system can be described in two ways: anatomically or functionally. Anatomically, the nervous system is divided into a central component (**brain** and **spinal cord**) and a peripheral component (**cranial nerves** and **peripheral nerves**). The central component, called the **central nervous system (CNS)**, is made of groups of neuronal cell bodies (called **nuclei**), their dendritic and axonal processes, as well as many supporting cells (**glia**). The peripheral component, called the **peripheral nervous system (PNS)**, is composed primarily of axonal neural processes, but there are also small collections of neuronal cell bodies (called **ganglia**) and only one type of supporting cell (**Schwann cells** or neurolemmacytes) (Figure 1.1). It should be borne in mind that a collection of neural cell bodies has a different name depending on its anatomical location: ganglia in the PNS and nuclei in the CNS. These nuclei are collections of cell bodies and should not be confused with cellular nuclei that contain chromosomes. Also, to complicate matters, there are some nuclei in the central nervous system that are referred to as the basal ganglia. This is not the best nomenclature and can be confusing.

Functionally, the nervous system is divided into three components: a **sensory** (**afferent**, input) component; an **integrative**, decision-making component; and a **motor** (**efferent**, output) component (Figure 1.1). The sensory portion contains peripheral receptors that respond to numerous factors (e.g. touch, vibration, pain, chemical compounds (taste, smell),

light (vision), sound (hearing), and position sense (balance)). These receptors interact with peripheral axons that propagate the signal towards the central nervous system. The majority of these neurons have their cell bodies in the periphery (in ganglia) and send a process into the central nervous system carrying the signal. Within the central nervous system, these processes can take a number of paths. They can ascend to inform the brain (cortex and cerebellum) of the information and they can also synapse in the spinal cord to produce reflexes. This information can be relayed by other neurons to numerous portions of the central nervous system, where the information can be **integrated** with other inputs and a **motor output** can be executed. As a simple example, you could place your hand on a hot stove and feel the heat and pain associated with the stove. You would then rapidly remove your hand by a reflex arc with the muscles in the hand, forearm, and arm. This will actually occur within the spinal cord and before you have any conscious awareness of the pain. If you want to continue to "cook" your hand, you can voluntarily override the reflex arc and force

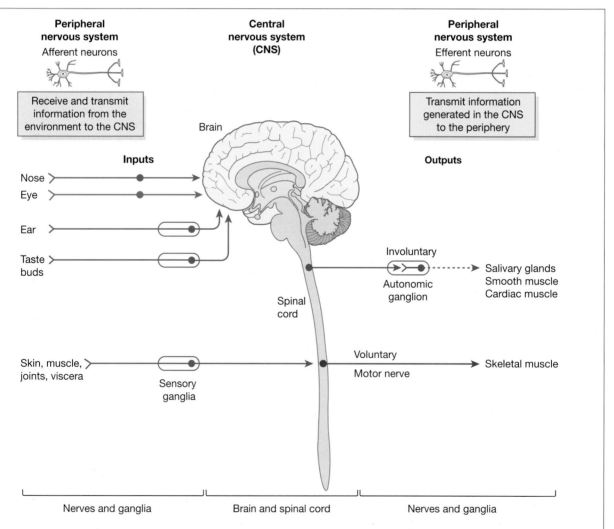

Figure 1.1 A diagrammatic representation of the central and peripheral nervous system with a collection of central cell bodies referred to as a nucleus (plural: nuclei), while a collection of peripheral cell bodies is referred to as a ganglion (plural: ganglia).

Clinical box 1.1

The autonomic nervous system is particularly important in clinical medicine since dysfunction of the heart, lungs, and digestive systems can be linked to autonomic nerves. Physicians modify a patient's autonomic nerve function by prescribing drugs that stimulate or inhibit the firing of these nerves or their receptors. For example, individuals with heart problems can be prescribed "beta blockers" which are drugs that interact at the beta adrenergic receptors in the heart modifying the autonomic tone to the heart. It is, therefore, quite important to know the organization and distribution of the autonomic nervous system.

Both of the subdivisions of the autonomic nervous system (the parasympathetic and sympathetic systems) are a two neuron chain in which acetylcholine is released at the preganglionic synapse. In the parasympathetic nervous system, acetylcholine is also released at the postganglionic synapse with the target organ, while in the sympathetic system, norepinephrine is released at the postganglionic synapse (except for sweat glands which also use acetylcholine). Therefore, cholinergic compounds can interact at both systems, while noradrenergic compounds only affect sympathetic function.

For further details on this system, consult a basic anatomy textbook (Moore, *et al*., 2014), as well as a neuropharmacology textbook (Stahl, 2013).

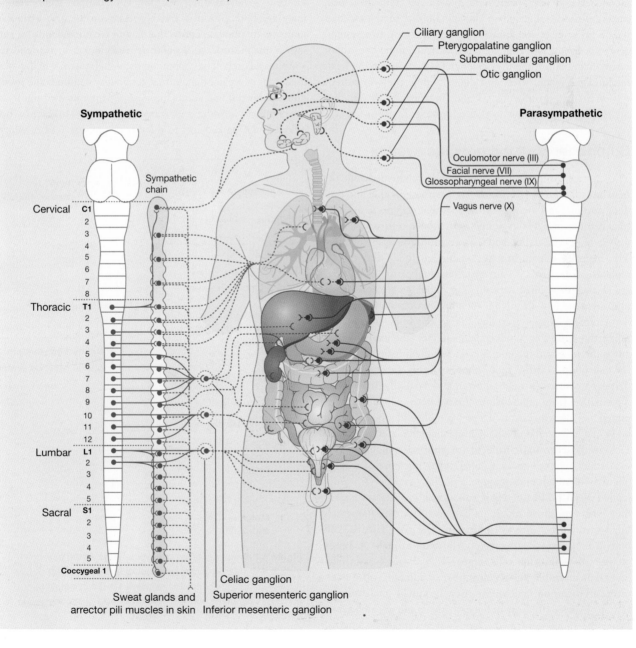

your hand to stay on the stove. This is using the integrative function of the brain to direct a willful activity.

With the previous discussion, the output used skeletal muscles to move an extremity. This is called a **voluntary** (**somatic**) motor response. There is also an **involuntary** (**autonomic** or visceral) motor response that drives smooth muscle and cardiac muscle. For example, you can see a portion of your favorite food, hot and ready for you to eat, and you will begin to salivate and your stomach may make sounds. These are involuntary smooth muscle actions as you prepare to eat. The **autonomic motor system** is further subdivided into two components: a **parasympathetic** and a **sympathetic** portion. The parasympathetic portion has its central neuronal cell bodies located in the brain stem or in a small portion of the sacral spinal cord (the second through fourth sacral nerves). The sympathetic system has its central neuronal cell bodies located in the spinal cord in the thoracic region and upper two lumbar segments. These two systems generally produce opposite effects, with the parasympathetic system stimulating the digestive system and decreasing heart rate and respiration (rest and digest), while the sympathetic system activates numerous systems (increases heart rate, respiration, and blood flow to skeletal muscle: flight or fright).

Components of the nervous system

The cells in the nervous system can be subdivided into the **neurons** that react to stimuli, interact with each other and produce outputs, and the supporting cells that make sure the neurons can do their job. Neurons are excitable cells with a high degree of specialization and a large morphological diversity. The majority of neurons are unable to divide and cannot replenish themselves if damaged. The supporting cells (**glia**) are smaller than most neurons, can divide to replenish their numbers, and have numerous roles in neuronal support.

A typical neuron contains a large cell body (**soma**) and numerous processes. One of the processes (the **axon**) is usually quite long and is the main conduit for information from the cell body to other cells. The remaining processes (**dendrites**) are usually much shorter and typically they bring information from other cells to the cell body, where it is summated for determination if the axon should fire. The cell body of a neuron has distinguishing characteristics including: 1) a large **euchromatic nucleus** (meaning it is highly active) sometimes referred to as a "bird's eye" nucleus; 2) a large quantity of rough endoplasmic reticulum and polyribosomes (called **Nissl bodies** or **Nissl substance** which stain a dark blue with typical histologic stains); and 3) accumulated cellular waste in the form of **lipofuscin**. The axon exits the cell body from a clear staining region (the **axon hillock**) and ends at synapses with other cells (Figure 1.2). A single axon may branch at its end to supply a number of adjacent cells (a terminal arborization) and within these terminals small **vesicles** can be observed. Because of the extreme length of some axons (from the spinal cord to the foot – over a meter in length),

there are mechanisms which allow for transport of materials to and from one end of the axon to the other. Flow from the cell body to the terminals is termed **anterograde axoplasmic transport**, while flow from the terminal to the cell body is termed **retrograde axoplasmic transport**. As mentioned previously, the neuron is an excitable cell and this excitation is maintained and modified by the specific characteristics of the neuronal cell membrane (the plasmalemma or neurolemma). The membrane has numerous ion channels and ion pumps that can maintain an ionic gradient across the membrane, producing the excitability.

A typical neuron is described as a large cell body and nucleus with numerous small dendrites and one very long axon. This is a **multipolar neuron**, which is found in many parts of the nervous system (Figure 1.2). There are, however, a number of other morphologically distinct neurons. For example, in the retina, there are both unipolar and bipolar neurons. The **unipolar neurons** are photoreceptors that do not have any dendrites and only a small axon. The **bipolar neurons** have a single dendrite and a single axon. The chapter on the visual system will describe these cells in greater detail. Another unique neuron is the **pseudounipolar cell** that acts as the main cell for sensory input from the periphery into the central nervous system. This neuron has its cell body "parked" off to the side of the single axon, which

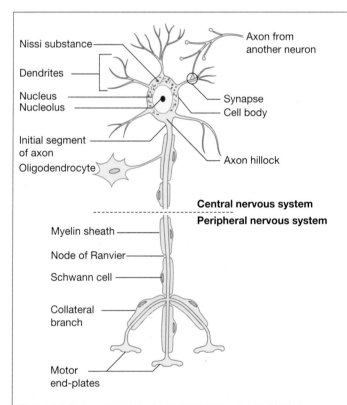

Figure 1.2 A representation of a typical large motor, multipolar neuron with a large euchromatic nucleus and prominent nucleolus, dark staining Nissl substance in the cytoplasm, numerous dendrites, and a long axon extending into the periphery.

has a peripheral projection and a central projection. This allows for rapid input of sensory information from the periphery to the central nervous system without the need to summate or interpret the information at the cell body.

The glial supporting cells are found in both the peripheral and central nervous systems. In the peripheral nervous system, the **Schwann cell** (neurolemmacyte) protects the axons as they are distributed throughout the body. In some cases the Schwann cells simply enclose the axons in their cell membrane, providing nutritional and mechanical support. These are termed **unmyelinated axons** and there may be many of this type of axon supported by one Schwann cell. In other cases, a single Schwann cell will support only one portion of an axon and it will wrap its cell membrane around the axon numerous times, insulating the axon. This is termed a **myelinated axon**. Since one Schwann cell only myelinates a small portion of an axon, other Schwann cells are required to myelinate the remaining length of the axon. Where the myelin layers of the adjacent Schwann cells meet, there is a small gap between the cells, a **node of Ranvier**. While this myelin sheath insulates and protects the axon, it also modifies the ionic flow across the axon cell membrane, producing a stronger, faster, and more reliable axonal signal (saltatory conduction). Therefore, myelinated nerves are faster than their unmyelinated counterparts.

In the central nervous system, there are other glial cells that provide support. The myelin producing cells in the central nervous system are the **oligodendrocytes**. They produce myelin sheaths for a number of axons in the area. The ability to myelinate neurons has important clinical aspects, since there are diseases, such as multiple sclerosis, that can affect myelination and neural function. Another glial cell within the central nervous system is the **astrocyte**. The astrocyte is a supporting cell that provides nutrition for neurons, modifies neurotransmitter uptake, and, importantly, has foot processes that surround the blood vessels in the brain, producing a special immunologically privileged area: the **blood-brain barrier**. There are two types of astrocytes; the fibrous astrocyte associated with white matter and the protoplasmic astrocyte associated with gray matter.

Astrocytes can be immunohistochemically identified by the presence of a particular intermediate filament: **glial fibrillary acidic protein (GFAP)**. This protein can also be used in clinical diagnosis of central nervous system tumors. If GFAP is present in a tumor, it means that the tumor was originally derived from astrocytes. Another glial cell within the central nervous system is the **microglia**. These are small macrophage-like cells that act as a local immune response agent, phagocytosing foreign materials. The microglia can be identified using similar immunologic techniques that would identify macrophages in the periphery. An additional supporting cell within the central nervous system is the **ependymal cell**. This is an epithelial, simple columnar, ciliated cell that lines the ventricular system. Modified versions of these cells are responsible for the production of cerebrospinal fluid.

Central nervous system structure

When examining the central nervous system, it is apparent that there are two distinct regions. Historically, these regions were named by their color. One region looked white and was called the **white matter**. This is due to the highly myelinated nerve fibers present in this region. Myelin is made of numerous wrappings of cell membrane and therefore contains large quantities of cholesterol, phospholipids, and other lipid-based compounds. This produces the white appearance of the white matter. The other region of the central nervous system contains both myelinated fibers and neuronal cell bodies. This area is, therefore, less white and is referred to as **gray matter**. Therefore, the gray matter contains neuronal cell bodies, axons, and glia, while the white matter contains only axons and their supporting glial cells (Figure 1.3).

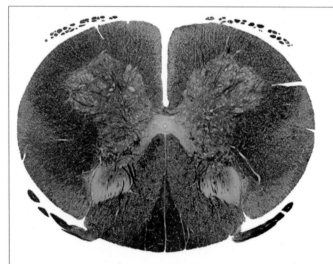

Figure 1.3 A typical cross section of the spinal cord, stained to indicate the presence of myelin, with the outer white matter (containing axons and glia) more densely stained and the inner gray matter (containing neuronal cell bodies, axons, and glia) less densely stained. Note the clinical orientation, with the posterior aspect of the spinal cord at the bottom of the image.

Clinical box 1.2

There are numerous diseases associated with improper glial cell function. **Multiple sclerosis** is an autoimmune disease in which a patient develops antibodies to their own myelin sheaths. The antibodies damage the myelin sheath covering the axon and disrupt the neuronal firing. There are different types of multiple sclerosis, depending on the severity and progression of the disease. There is also an interesting global distribution of the disease, with more cases found in countries further away from the equator and more cases in industrialized nations. The reason for this distribution is not known.

Clinical box 1.3

There are numerous methods utilized to view the components of the central nervous system. Clinically, the use of plain films, computed tomography (CT), magnetic resonance imaging (MRI), and ultrasound are used routinely to visualize a patient's brain or spinal cord. Chapter 18 on Imaging Essentials provides details on these and other techniques that are used clinically. However, the resolution of these techniques is presently not detailed enough to provide good differentiation of the nuclei and tracts within the central nervous system, so neuroanatomists still rely on specific histologic methods to visualize the components of the nervous system.

The simplest visualization of the nervous system is with the naked eye. Fresh tissue sections of the brain and spinal cord can be viewed with white matter and gray matter easily distinguishable. Structures such as the substantia nigra in the midbrain are easily observed in fresh tissue.

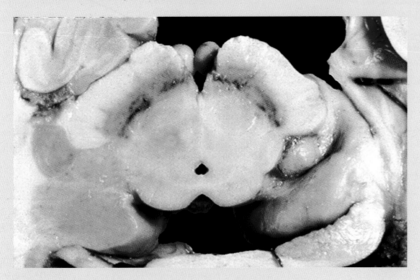
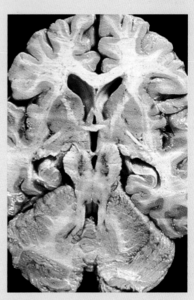

These are fresh tissue sections of the midbrain and surrounding cortical tissues without any staining or treatment. Note the two dark regions in the upper middle portion of the field (the substantia nigra). These areas are normally dark due to the presence of neuromelanin in the cells. The white matter and gray matter can also be observed, although the gray matter actually has a brown coloration in fresh tissue.

Similar sections of midbrain and cortex can be histologically processed to indicate the presence of myelin (a myelin stain). This is a typical presentation that highlights the tracts and nuclei of the central nervous system.

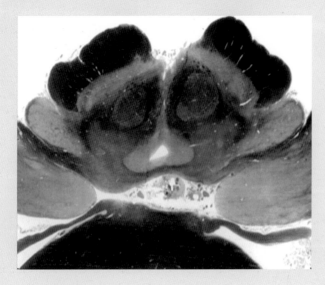
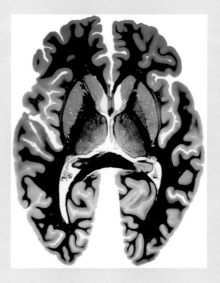

These are myelin stained sections of the midbrain and cortex. Note that the dark staining regions are the tracts of myelinated axons (white matter), while the light staining regions are the nuclei (gray matter). The lighter staining gray matter is variable in density, depending on the quantity of cell bodies present and whether myelinated axons pass by or through the area. In this presentation, the substantia nigra is light staining due to the presence of many cell bodies, with the neuromelanin not visualized.

There are also special histologic stains and techniques that can be used to further identify specific types of neurons. For example, a typical hematoxylin and eosin stain can be used to identify the nucleus in a neuronal cell body, while immunocytochemistry and fluorescence microscopy can be used to identify individual types of cells.

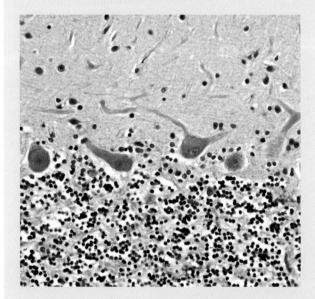 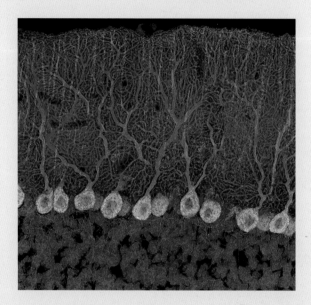

Source: Science Photo Library/Dr Gladden Willis; Science Photo Library/Thomas Deerinck.

These are histologic slides of the cerebellum with a standard hematoxylin and eosin presentation on the left and a histofluorescence presentation on the right. Note the ability to distinguish individual cells with both techniques.

When examining figures, it is important to determine the type of presentation used, since it can be confusing when comparing a fresh tissue section with a myelin stained section (compare the first four figures in this box). As clinical imaging develops in the future, it may be possible to use these non-invasive techniques to visualize all of the neuroanatomical tracts and nuclei without the need to use other histologic methods.

Within the spinal cord, the white matter is found on the periphery of the spinal cord and the gray matter is found centrally. The gray matter forms a central "butterfly" shaped appearance, while the white matter fills in these spaces around the butterfly (Figure 1.3). In the brain, however, the white matter is found centrally and the gray matter is found peripherally. Notice that this is opposite of the arrangement in the spinal cord and the mechanism of this transition will be described at a later point.

Central nervous system orientation

When examining the central nervous system, remember that the nervous system developed as a long tube with a central canal (see Chapter 3 for further details). The end of the neural tube closest to the nose is the **rostral** end, while the end of the neural tube closest to the legs is the **caudal** end. The region of the tube nearest the back is the **posterior** portion (**dorsal**), while the area nearest the abdomen is the **anterior** portion (**ventral**).

During embryologic development, this tube becomes more complex at the rostral (nasal) end, due to the extensive development of the cerebrum, cerebellum, and the brain stem. With this complex development, the brain rotates **90 degrees anteriorly**. This also positions the eyes, nose, and mouth on the anterior (ventral) portion of the body as opposed to the rostral end. This means that there is a change in orientation at the midbrain, causing an anterior rotation termed the **midbrain flexure**. Therefore, what was anterior (ventral) now becomes inferior and what was posterior (dorsal) now becomes superior (Figure 1.4). This rotation can be confusing and needs to be kept in mind when discussing the orientation of cerebral structures.

When viewing the brain, it is important to keep in mind the various planes that can be viewed, especially with the advent of computed tomography (CT) and magnetic

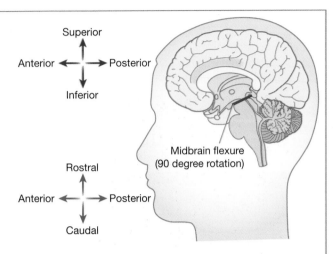

Figure 1.4 A drawing of the midbrain flexure indicating the brain rotation of 90 degrees anteriorly during development. This produces a shift in describing positions in the brain compared to the spinal cord.

resonance imaging (MRI). If a cross section of the body occurs, this would section the spinal cord, the brain stem, and various levels of the cerebrum in a **horizontal (transverse) plane**. If a sagittal section of the body is continued into the brain, this produces two hemispheres of the brain with a section through the interhemispheric fissure **(sagittal plane)**. Parallel cuts in this orientation are **parasagittal** sections. The third dimension for viewing sections of the brain is a **frontal (coronal) plane**. This plane is perpendicular to a sagittal plane and can be thought of as the patient walking into a door (Figure 1.5).

When viewing cross sections of the brain or spinal cord, the orientation of the cross section must be determined. This is especially important in the spinal cord, due to a difference between the **clinical view** and the **anatomic view**. Historically, anatomists oriented a cross section of the spinal cord with the posterior (dorsal) surface of the spinal cord at the top of the field and the anterior (ventral) surface at the bottom. Neuroanatomists have used this orientation for decades. With the development of cross-sectional radiology, radiologists set the standard orientation with the patient lying on his back being viewed from his

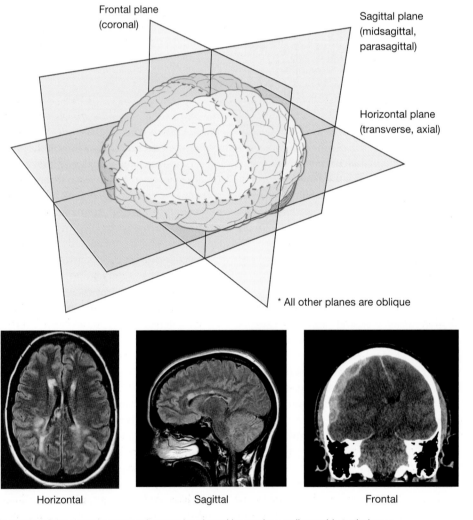

Figure 1.5 Anatomic planes of the nervous system that can be viewed by modern radiographic techniques.

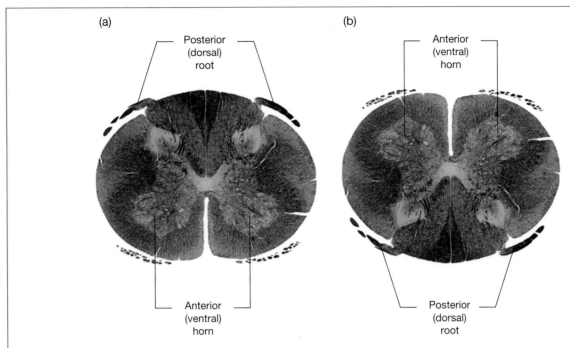

(a)

Posterior
(dorsal)
root

Anterior
(ventral)
horn

(b)

Anterior
(ventral)
horn

Posterior
(dorsal)
root

Figure 1.6 Anatomical (a) versus clinical (b) view of the spinal cord. The clinical view is the view that is used with CT, MRI, and other imaging systems and is described as the patient lying on their back (supine) in bed with the clinician viewing them from the foot of the bed (inferiorly). This view (b) will be consistently used throughout this text, since it is the clinically relevant, standard view. The anatomical view may still be used in older textbooks and atlases.

feet. In this orientation, the posterior (dorsal) surface of the spinal cord would be at the bottom of the field, while the anterior (ventral) surface of the spinal cord would be at the top of the field (opposite from the anatomic view). This has caused confusion in the past when examining cross sections of the spinal cord. In this text, the clinical view (CT view) will be used in order to maintain consistency and clinical relevance. However, other neuroanatomy texts may use the anatomic view and this requires the appropriate adjustment (Figure 1.6).

Views of the brain

When viewing the whole brain anatomically, it can be seen from three distinct views – **superior** (dorsal), **inferior** (ventral), and **lateral**. An additional view, a **sagittal midline view**, can be described that involves cutting the brain in half through the interhemispheric fissure in the sagittal plane.

In the superior view of the brain, the lobes of the cortex can be identified, along with the **interhemispheric fissure**. Midway along the superior surface of the brain, a primary sulcus can be found, the **central sulcus**. On either side of the central sulcus reside two primary gyri: the **precentral gyrus**, which is the primary motor gyrus, and the **postcentral gyrus**, which is the primary somatosensory gyrus.

On the lateral surface of the brain, the most prominent feature is the **lateral (Sylvian) fissure**. Above the fissure are the frontal and parietal lobes of the cortex, while below the fissure the temporal lobe of the cortex is found. Posterior to the fissure,

the occipital cortex can be seen. It is also possible to identify the **central sulcus** and the **precentral** and **postcentral gyri**. If the lateral fissure is spread open, a portion of cerebral cortex (the **insular cortex**) is observed within the fissure (Figure 1.7).

In the inferior view of the brain, the lobes of the cortex can also be identified, along with portions of the interhemispheric fissure and the **lateral (Sylvian) fissure**. In addition, the midbrain with the cerebral peduncles, the pons with the middle cerebellar peduncles, and the medulla oblongata with the pyramids, can be observed. The base of the brain and the brain stem also contain the roots of the twelve cranial nerves, including the **olfactory bulbs** and the **optic nerves and chiasm**. Caudal to the optic chiasm is the **infundibulum** (pituitary stalk) and the **mammillary bodies**. In this area the primary blood supply to the brain is also found – the **cerebral arterial circle** (of Willis). It is important to be able to identify all of these components on the inferior surface of the brain (Figure 1.8).

On a midsagittal view of the brain, portions of the lobes of the cerebral cortex can also be identified. A large white arc of myelinated nerve fibers can be observed and is known as the **corpus callosum**. Superior to the corpus callosum is the **cingulate gyrus**. Inferior to the corpus callosum is the **septum pellucidum** separating the two **lateral ventricles**. Inferior to the septum pellucidum is the **diencephalon** with the **thalamus**, **hypothalamus**, and **pineal gland** easily identifiable. In addition, the midbrain, pons, medulla, and cerebellum can be observed in sagittal section (Figure 1.9).

Figure 1.7 A lateral view of the brain highlighting the major sulci and gyri, including the lateral fissure (Sylvian), the central sulcus, and the precentral and postcentral gyri. The lobes of the brain can also be observed: the frontal lobe, parietal lobe, temporal lobe, and occipital lobe.

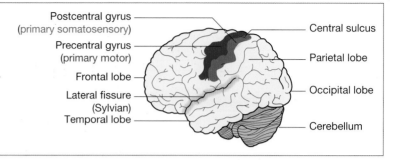

Figure 1.8 A ventral view of the brain highlighting the interhemispheric fissure, the lateral fissure (Sylvian), the brain stem with the prominent pons, the roots of the cranial nerves, and the cerebellum. The frontal and temporal lobes of the brain can also be observed.

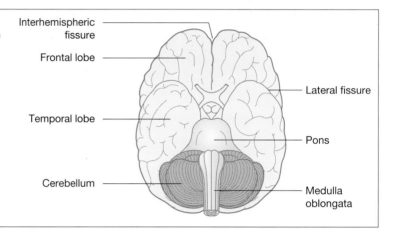

Figure 1.9 A midsagittal section of the brain highlighting the diencephalon, with the thalamus, the brain stem with the prominent pons, and the cerebellum. The frontal, parietal, and occipital lobes of the brain can also be observed.

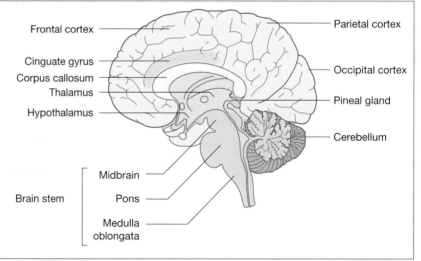

Central nervous system subdivisions

The central nervous system can be subdivided anatomically. Beginning caudally (or inferiorly), the **spinal cord** is found inside the vertebral column and extends from the base of the cranium to the second or third lumbar vertebrae. The spinal cord continues into the cranium as the **brain stem**. The brain stem is subdivided into three specific regions based on the relationship to the **pons**. The structure caudal to the pons is the **medulla** or, more specifically, the **medulla oblongata**. The structure rostral to the pons is the **midbrain**. Extending from the midbrain is the **diencephalon**, comprised of the hypothalamus, thalamus, and epithalamus. The diencephalon extends into the remainder of the skull as the **telencephalon**, principally made up of the large cerebral cortex. A unique structure located posterior to the brain stem and at the caudal end of the cortex is the **cerebellum** (Figure 1.9).

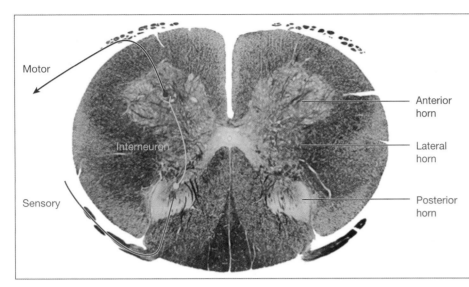

Motor

Interneuron

Sensory

Anterior horn

Lateral horn

Posterior horn

Figure 1.10 The regions of the spinal cord including the posterior (dorsal) horn, lateral horn, and anterior (ventral) horn, with their general functions indicated (posterior horn = sensory = green; lateral horn = autonomic motor function = purple; anterior horn = somatic motor function = red). These colors will be used throughout the text to indicate the functional attributes associated with the labeled structures.

Spinal cord

As an introduction to the overall structure of the central nervous system, each region will be described briefly. The **spinal cord** when viewed in cross section consists of an outer portion termed the **white matter** and an inner "butterfly-shaped" region termed the **gray matter**. These were named based on their coloration in fresh tissue; the white matter containing only nerve fibers (many that are myelinated) and the gray matter containing nerve cell bodies along with nerve fibers, as mentioned previously. The gray matter can be subdivided into a posterior (dorsal) region termed the **posterior (dorsal) horn** and an anterior (ventral) region termed the **anterior (ventral) horn**. Generally, each of these horns is responsible for a separate function; the posterior horn is responsible for incoming sensory activity and the anterior horn is responsible for outgoing motor activity. In some regions of the spinal cord, there is a small **lateral horn** which contains nerve cell bodies of the autonomic nervous system. Within the spinal cord, incoming sensory nerves can be linked to outgoing motor nerves by small **interneurons**, providing basic reflex actions (Figure 1.10).

The spinal cord is composed of 31 spinal segments, producing 31 spinal nerves and subdivided by the region of the vertebral column where each nerve exits. The first eight segments are in the neck and are termed the **cervical nerves** (C1–C8). The second region of the spinal cord is the thoracic section, containing 12 segments (**thoracic nerves**) (T1–T12). The third region of the spinal cord is the lumbar section, containing five segments (**lumbar nerves**) (L1–L5). The fourth region of the spinal cord is the sacral section, containing five segments (**sacral nerves**) (S1–S5). The fifth and final region of the spinal cord is the coccygeal section, containing just one segment (Cy1) (see chapter 4 for more details).

Brain stem

The upper cervical level of the spinal cord enters the cranium through the foramen magnum and expands to form the brain stem. The sensory fibers ascending in the spinal cord continue into the

brain stem by passing through the **medulla oblongata**, then into the **pons**, and further into the **midbrain** (the three subdivisions of the brain stem), before reaching the **diencephalon**. Likewise, fibers descend from the diencephalon through the midbrain, pons, and medulla before reaching the spinal cord. The pathways taken by these fibers and the nuclei present in these regions can be quite complex and will be discussed in greater detail in subsequent chapters.

Diencephalon

The diencephalon contains a major relay region of the central nervous system, the **thalamus**. Virtually all information that is sent to the cerebral cortex passes through the thalamus. The diencephalon also contains regions that maintain an individual's homeostasis, the metabolic and hormonal balance throughout the body. These regions include the **hypothalamus** (that communicates with the pituitary gland) and the **epithalamus** (with its associated **pineal gland**) (Figure 1.9).

Telencephalon

The telencephalon is a large region that makes up the majority of the neural structures within the skull. The telencephalon includes the **cerebral cortex** with its subdivided lobes: the **frontal lobe**, the **parietal lobe**, the **occipital lobe**, the **temporal lobe**, and the **insular cortex**. Generally, these lobes have specific functions associated with them, although each lobe has integrative aspects. For example, the temporal lobe is associated with hearing, while the occipital lobe is associated with vision. The parietal lobe has a major role in receiving primary sensory input, as well as directing primary motor output. The frontal lobe is associated with personality and decision-making capacity (Figures 1.7, 1.8, 1.9).

The cerebral cortex, when examined microscopically, displays six cellular layers. Each of these layers contain variable quantities of neurons and can be morphologically distinct. The telencephalon also includes centrally located structures such as the **basal ganglia** and the components of the **limbic system**. All of these structures will be discussed in more detail in subsequent chapters.

Cerebellum

The cerebellum is a small "brain" of its own that receives input from virtually all sources of the nervous system, but most notably the vestibular system. It processes these inputs and provides balance, localization, and motor control information to the central nervous system. The cerebellum has a simpler cortical structure than the cerebral cortex, with only three layers: the molecular layer, Purkinje cell layer, and the granule cell layer (see chapter 10 for more details).

Cranial nerves

Just as there are spinal nerves which exit from specific spinal segments, there are twelve nerves which enter or exit the skull. These nerves are termed **cranial nerves** and are denoted by a Roman numeral (I–XII). A brief description of each cranial nerve follows, with greater detail in subsequent chapters. These cranial nerves can be observed leaving the inferior surface of the brain and are considered part of the peripheral nervous system at this point. The cranial nerve cell bodies (nuclei) and the portion of their axons within the brain or brain stem are considered part of the central nervous system.

Cranial nerve one is the **olfactory nerve (I)** and it relays the sense of smell to the central nervous system. The second cranial nerve is the **optic nerve (II)** and it relays vision to the central nervous system. The third cranial nerve is the **oculomotor nerve (III)** and it supplies five small optic muscles within the orbit which move the eye and raise the eyelid. The oculomotor nerve also contains parasympathetic neurons which innervate muscles that constrict the pupil and modify the shape of the lens. The fourth cranial nerve is the **trochlear nerve (IV)** and it supplies one optic muscle, the superior oblique muscle. The fifth cranial nerve is the **trigeminal nerve (V)**, with three major branches (ophthalmic, maxillary, and mandibular). The trigeminal nerve (V) relays general sensation from the face to the central nervous system as well as supplying motor activity to the muscles of mastication and four other small muscles. The sixth cranial nerve is the **abducens nerve (VI)** and it controls one optic muscle, the lateral rectus muscle.

The seventh cranial nerve is the **facial nerve (VII)** and it supplies the muscles of facial expression, as well as supplying parasympathetic innervation to the lacrimal gland, the nasal cavity, the submandibular gland, and the sublingual gland. The facial nerve (VII) also relays the sense of taste from the anterior tongue to the central nervous system. The eighth cranial nerve is the **vestibulocochlear nerve (VIII)** and it relays the sense of hearing and balance to the central nervous system. The ninth cranial nerve is the **glossopharyngeal nerve (IX)** and it relays general sensation from the pharynx and the posterior tongue to the central nervous system. The glossopharyngeal nerve (IX) also supplies one pharyngeal muscle. The tenth cranial nerve is the **vagus nerve (X)** and it has a multitude of functions. The vagus nerve (X) relays general sensation from the larynx as well as visceral sensation from the heart, lungs, and gastrointestinal

system to the central nervous system. This nerve also provides the skeletal muscles of the larynx and pharynx as well as parasympathetic innervation to the heart, lungs, and gastrointestinal system. The eleventh cranial nerve is the **spinal accessory nerve (XI)** and it does not arise from the brain stem. It arises from the upper five cervical segments, ascends through the foramen magnum and exits the skull through the jugular foramen to supply the sternocleidomastoid and trapezius muscles. The twelfth cranial nerve is the **hypoglossal nerve (XII)** and it supplies the majority of muscles in the tongue.

Caveats

It is important to highlight a few nomenclature issues that arise when studying neuroanatomy. One such issue is the use of the terms dorsal and ventral instead of posterior and anterior. Posterior and anterior are the more appropriate anatomical terms. Historically neuroanatomists have, however, used the terms dorsal and ventral in place of posterior and anterior. Some more recent texts have switched to the proper anatomical terminology and have replaced the term dorsal with posterior and the term ventral with anterior.

Another important nomenclature issue is the use of the terms **ipsilateral** and **contralateral**. These terms are used to describe the location of symptoms in a patient compared to the location of the nervous system lesion that produces the symptoms. For example, if a lesion were to occur on the left side of the nervous system and the symptoms were displayed on the left side, then this would be an **ipsilateral** effect. On the other hand, if a lesion were to occur on the left side of the nervous system and the symptoms were displayed on the right side of the body, then this would be a **contralateral** effect. This allows clinicians to refer to the location of a lesion in relation to the side of the symptoms without resorting to a right or left determination.

The final caveat to be described was mentioned previously, but is important to reiterate. This is the difference between an **anatomical** cross-sectional view (with the posterior (dorsal) surface at the top of the field) compared with a **clinical** cross-sectional view (with the posterior (dorsal) surface at the bottom of the field). In order to maintain consistency and to present relevant clinical information, the **clinical view** will be utilized throughout the text.

Clinical considerations

One take home message from this chapter is that specific areas of the brain are responsible for specific functions. Therefore, a patient's symptoms can be critical in determining the location and extent of a neural lesion. Throughout this text, numerous cases will be presented in which specific neural lesions have occurred. While real estate agents may use the slogan "location, location, location", neuroanatomists use a variation on that slogan – **"lesion, lesion, lesion"**. These lesions could be due to vascular damage (ischemia or stroke) or they can be due to traumatic injury. In either case, it is especially important to understand the neuroanatomical location of specific structures and their functional attributes. With this knowledge, a clinician can pinpoint a lesion based on the presentation of symptoms in the patient. In addition, it is important to understand which neural structures are located in close proximity to other structures, since a lesion may impact multiple structures in a small area. This is referred to as the "**neighborhood effect**", since structures in the neighborhood can be damaged by a small localized lesion.

Case 1

Mrs Daniela Jones is a 46-year-old mother of three, with a catering business. While preparing meals, she notices a tingling in her hands and chalks it up to overuse. A few weeks later, she becomes quite fatigued and has muscle weakness in both her lower limbs. Again, she believes this is due to the stress of her job and her hectic schedule. After a few days' bed rest, the symptoms go away and she returns to her job. One month later, she has a spell of dizziness and vertigo, as well as a loss of sensation from her right arm. This concerns her and she schedules an appointment with her physician, Dr Jill Jameson. When she sees her physician, two weeks later, all of the symptoms have been resolved.

Dr Jameson, after taking a detailed history, and hearing Daniela describe the neural signs and frequency of problems, decides to schedule Daniela for further tests. First, she is scheduled for a magnetic resonance image (MRI) (see Chapter 18) and the results of the MRI suggest that small plaques are found in various white matter regions of the brain (Figure 1.11). With this information, Daniela is then scheduled for a lumbar puncture (see Chapter 2) to gather a small amount of cerebrospinal fluid.

The fluid is tested for the presence of oligoclonal bands of IgG – an inflammation marker. When this test is positive, Dr Jameson meets with Daniela and suggests that she may have **multiple sclerosis**, an inflammatory, autoimmune disease that targets the neuronal myelin sheaths in the central nervous system. Recall that myelin is produced in the central nervous system by oligodendrocytes and in the peripheral nervous system by Schwann cells. With a reduction in myelination of random nerves, a variety of neural symptoms can occur.

While there is no cure for multiple sclerosis, Daniela is given guidance on managing the disease. This includes avoiding stress (which can reduce the ability to fight inflammation), as well as avoiding inflammation provoking events. She is given oral corticosteroids to use during an event (which may help lower the severity of the attack) and is told of other pharmacologic treatments that may be available if the number and severity of events increases. She is asked to monitor her experiences, so that a time course for the progression of the disease can be determined. If she is lucky, she can live a reasonably full life without serious complications from her multiple sclerosis.

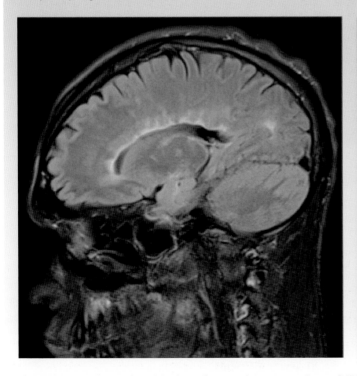
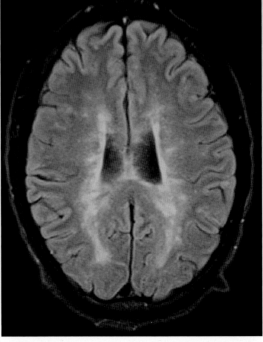

Figure 1.11 A sagittal and axial (horizontal) magnetic resonance image (MRI) of a patient with multiple sclerosis. Note the hyperintensity near the ventricles and the small plaques located in white matter regions.

Case 2

Mr Timothy Woods is a 78-year-old retired truck driver who lives with his wife in a small single family home. His wife notices that Timothy will forget where he placed small items like the car keys and that he becomes easily frustrated with simple memory tasks like remembering phone numbers or addresses. During his yearly physical examination, his physician, Dr Bill Adams, performs a simple neurological exam and notices that Timothy has some memory impairment. Upon further questioning with Timothy and his wife, Dr Adams suspects that Timothy may have symptoms of **age-related cognitive decline** (Figure 1.12).

Dr Adams attempts to determine if there is a systemic reason for Timothy's cognitive decline, including drugs that he may be taking, any vascular disorders (blood pressure or atherosclerosis), or lifestyle issues (smoking, vitamin deficiencies). While Timothy does not appear to have a systemic reason for his decline, Dr Adams encourages him to increase his exercise (by a daily brisk walk), to take a daily vitamin supplement, and to engage in daily mental activity (crossword puzzle). While there is still debate about the effectiveness of these life style changes, many individuals can experience slight improvements or a reduction in the cognitive decline (perhaps due to a placebo effect). With these modest changes, both Timothy and his wife notice that his memory, while not perfect, does improve slightly. If his memory were to continue to decline, Timothy could utilize pharmacologic treatments that can improve or prevent further memory loss.

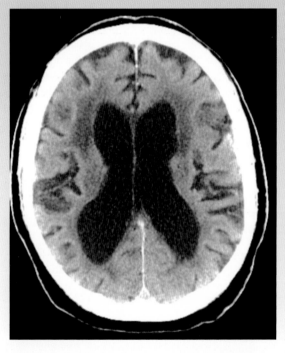 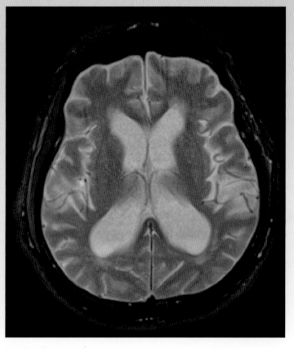

Figure 1.12 An axial (horizontal) computer tomograph (CT) and magnetic resonance image (MRI) of the same elderly patient with age-related cognitive decline. Note the enlarged ventricles and atrophy of the cortex (larger than normal sulci) in the brain.

Study questions

1. When examining a CT of a patient with a spinal cord lesion, and the symptoms occur on the same side as the lesion, the _____ surface would be at the top of the field and the lesion would produce _____ effects.
a) posterior (dorsal), ipsilateral
b) posterior (dorsal), contralateral
c) anterior (ventral), ipsilateral
d) anterior (ventral), contralateral

2. In order to determine where a patient has had a small cerebral cortical stroke, it is important to equate structure with function. If a patient presents with a primary motor deficit, then a stroke could have occurred in the:
a) precentral gyrus
b) postcentral gyrus

c) cingulate gyrus

d) superior temporal gyrus

e) calcarine gyrus

3. If a patient presents with multiple sclerosis (a central myelination disorder), which of the following cells would be primarily involved?

a) Schwann cells

b) astrocytes

c) ependymal cells

d) microglia

e) oligodendrocytes

4. The diencephalon contains the hypothalamus, the thalamus, and the:

a) cingulate gyrus

b) pineal gland

c) midbrain

d) pituitary gland

e) cerebellum

5. Create a table listing the twelve cranial nerves with their name and number, then list whether they have a sensory role, motor role, or carry both functions, describe how they leave the skull, and, if lesioned, the general symptoms that would be present.

For more self-assessment questions, visit the companion website at
www.wileyessential.com/neuroanatomy

FURTHER READING

For additional information on the general overview of neuroanatomy, the following textbooks may be helpful:

Blumenfeld H. 2002. *Neuroanatomy Through Clinical Cases*. Sinauer Associates, Sunderland, Massachusetts.

Felten DL, Shetty A. 2009. *Netter's Atlas of Neuroscience*, 2nd edition. Saunders Elsevier, Philadelphia, Pennsylvania.

Haines DE. 2012. *Neuroanatomy: An Atlas of Structures, Sections and Systems*, 8th edition. Lippincott Williams & Wilkin, Baltimore, Maryland.

Moore KL, Dalley AF, Agur AMR. 2014. *Moore Clinically Oriented Anatomy*, 7th edition. Lippincott, Williams & Wilkins, Philadelphia, Pennsylvania.

Patestas MA, Gartner LP. 2006. *A Textbook of Neuroanatomy*. Blackwell Publishing, Malden, Massachusetts.

Stahl SM. 2013. *Stahl's Essential Psychopharmacology*, 4th edition. Cambridge University Press, Cambridge, England.

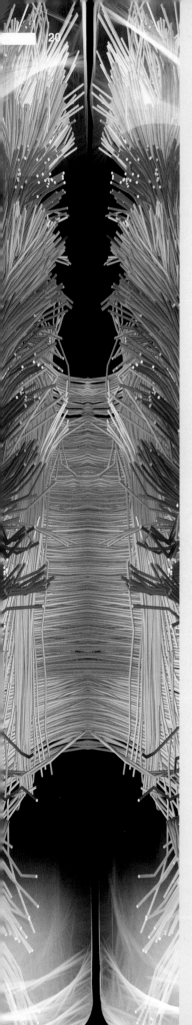

CHAPTER 2
Blood vessels, meninges, and ventricles

Learning objectives

1. Identify the main blood vessels on the external surface of the brain.
2. Identify the main blood vessels on the sagittal surface of the brain.
3. Identify the main blood vessels in the cerebral arterial circle (of Willis).
4. Describe the components of the blood–brain barrier.
5. Identify the components of the ventricular system.
6. Discuss the embryological development of the ventricular system.
7. Describe the location of the choroid plexus.
8. Trace the flow of cerebrospinal fluid within the ventricular system and subarachnoid space.

Essential Clinical Neuroanatomy, First Edition. Thomas H. Champney.
© 2016 John Wiley & Sons, Ltd. Published 2016 by John Wiley & Sons, Ltd.
Companion website: www.wileyessential.com/neuroanatomy

Introduction

The brain is encased in a solid bony cranium and requires both structural and nutritional support to function appropriately. Structurally, the brain has connective tissue coverings that protect it and create a space for the brain to "float" in a supportive fluid. These coverings (meninges) also provide structural components for the venous drainage of the brain, as well as producing a separation of the various regions of the brain.

Cranial meninges

There are connective tissue layers that surround the brain and the spinal cord and provide protection to these fragile tissues. The first of three layers, the **dura mater** ("tough mother"), is a thick, dense irregular connective tissue layer that is furthest away from the neural tissue. It has a portion that tightly adheres to the bones of the cranial cavity, forming an inner periosteal lining. It also has a portion that follows the outer surface of the brain and this portion creates folds that segregate the two

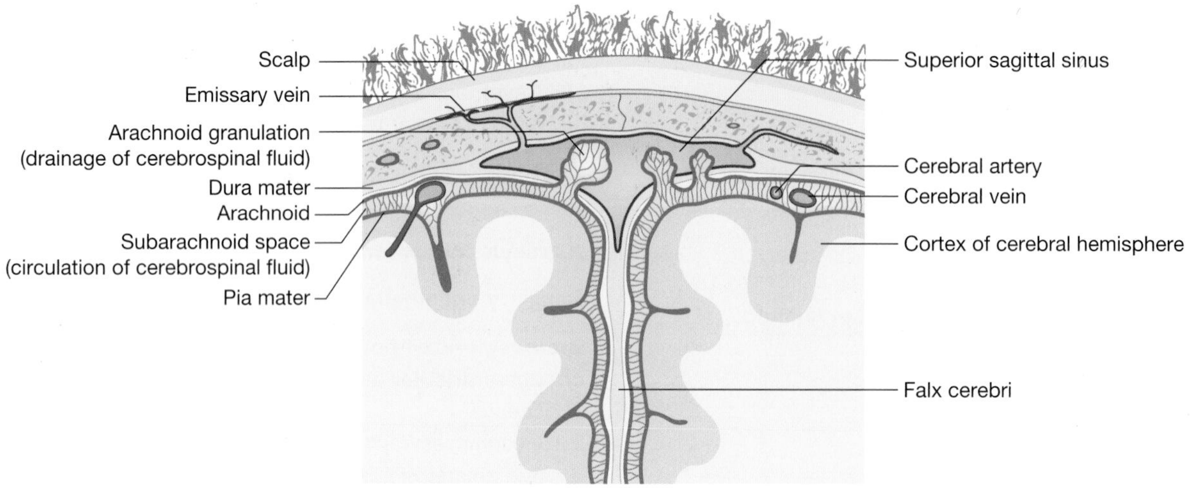

Figure 2.1 A frontal view of the brain and skull indicating the dura mater, the formation of the falx cerebri, and the superior sagittal sinus with the associated arachnoid granulations. Note that the cerebrospinal fluid circulates in the subarachnoid space and is drained into the dural venous sinuses through the arachnoid granulations.

Clinical box 2.1

While the dura mater in the cranium is tightly adherent to the bones of the cranium, the dura mater in the vertebral column is not attached to the vertebrae. Therefore, the dura mater around the spinal cord is like a loose bag and there is a space between it and the surrounding bone (**epidural space**). This space is usually filled with fat and small venous blood vessels. This can be useful clinically, because anesthetic can be injected into this space, where it will bathe the spinal nerves in that region, anesthetizing them. This is used quite commonly during childbirth. On the other hand, there is no true epidural space in the cranium – only a potential space. If the **middle meningeal artery** is broken due to trauma, this potential space between the dura mater and the cranium can fill with blood, producing an **epidural hematoma**. Between the dura mater and the arachnoid mater there is another potential space – the **subdural space**. This space can be filled with blood after trauma of cerebral veins, producing a **subdural hematoma**. The cerebral arteries pass through the **subarachnoid space**, before giving off smaller branches that penetrate the brain. If these rupture, a **subarachnoid hematoma** (hemorrhage) can occur.

cerebral hemispheres (the **falx cerebri**) as well as segregating the cerebrum from the cerebellum (the **tentorium cerebelli**). Where these two portions of the dura mater separate, they form a triangular space between them. This space is occupied by structures that will drain the blood from the brain, the **dural venous sinuses**. For example, the inner lining of the dura splits to form the falx cerebri, while the outer lining continues to

follow the bony cranial cavity, creating a triangular space that is filled with the **superior sagittal sinus** (Figure 2.1). Likewise, the inner lining of the dura splits off to form the tentorium cerebelli and the outer layer follows the bone, with the resulting space being filled by the **transverse sinus**. Notice how a number of the dural venous sinuses are formed by spaces between the two linings of the dura mater (Figure 2.2).

Deep to the dura mater, there is a layer of connective tissue which has fibers that cross between the dura mater and the brain surface. These fibers look like spider webs and are named **arachnoid mater**. Fluid flows around the fibers of the arachnoid mater keeping the brain "floating" in a fluid filled space. This is the **cerebrospinal fluid**. If a clinician wants to sample cerebrospinal fluid, the needle used would have to pass through a number of layers, including both the dura mater and the outer layer of the arachnoid mater. The cerebral arteries that supply the brain pass through the **subarachnoid space** before giving off smaller branches that penetrate the brain.

Deep to the arachnoid mater and immediately adjacent to the brain surface is a thin layer of connective tissue, the **pia mater** ("soft mother"). The pia mater provides support for the outer surface of the brain (Figure 2.3).

Cranial ventricular system

As mentioned previously, there is a specialized fluid system that circulates around the central nervous system, providing structural and nutritional support for the brain and spinal cord. This fluid is an acellular, modified filtrate of the blood called **cerebrospinal fluid**. It is produced in the central portion of the brain from specialized groups of **ependymal cells** called **choroid plexus** (Wolburg and Paulus, 2010). It flows through a central system of spaces (**ventricles**) and eventually flows into the **subarachnoid space**. The fluid then circulates around the outside of the entire central nervous

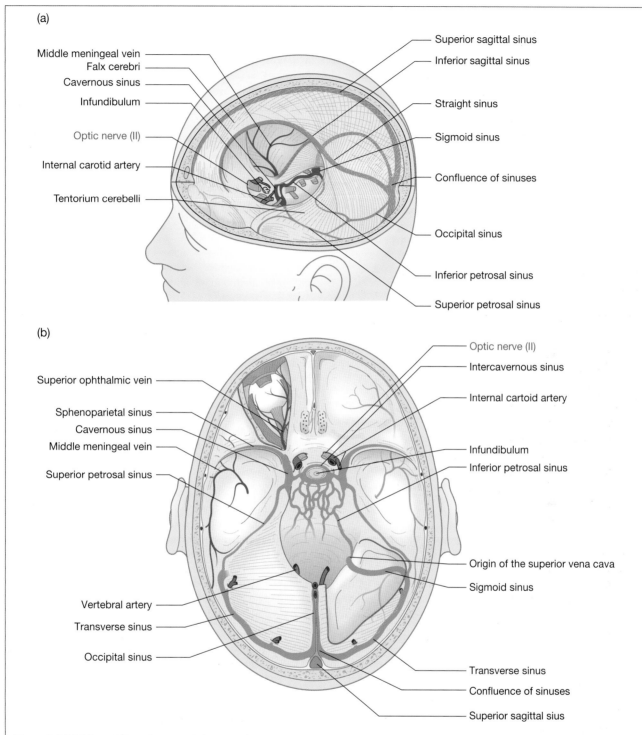

Figure 2.2 (a) A lateral view of the interior of the skull with the brain removed. Note the dura mater fold that separates the two hemispheres of the brain (falx cerebri). In the superior border of the falx cerebri is the superior sagittal sinus, while the inferior sagittal sinus is in the inferior border. The inferior sagittal sinus ends at the straight sinus, which is found in the dura folds created by the separation of the cerebellum from the cortex (tentorium cerebelli). (b) A superior view of the interior of the skull with the brain removed. Note the dura mater coverings on the interior of the skull that form the transverse sinuses, the petrosal sinuses, and the cavernous sinuses.

system (the brain and the spinal cord), providing a fluid environment that cushions the nervous tissue and reduces its apparent weight (buoyancy). The brain "floats" in this fluid, reducing gravitational compression on the base of the brain and limiting torsion due to acceleration. The cerebrospinal fluid drains from the ventricular system through small tufts of **arachnoid mater** that project into the **dural venous sinuses** – the **arachnoid granulations** – found primarily in the superior sagittal sinus (Figures 2.1 and 2.3). The production of cerebrospinal fluid (~500 ml per day) is matched by its drainage, to keep a constant amount of fluid (~150 ml) within the cranial ventricular system. If too much fluid is produced or if its drainage is prevented, then increased amounts of fluid collect in the system and this increases the intracranial pressure, producing detrimental effects (hydrocephalus).

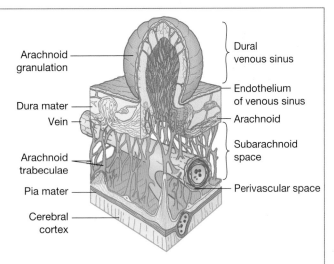

Figure 2.3 An expanded view of the cranial meninges. Notice the outer dura mater and the middle arachnoid mater, with the cerebrospinal fluid in the subarachnoid space draining through the arachnoid granulations into the dural venous sinus. The inner pia mater lines the brain.

A more detailed description of the flow of cerebrospinal fluid begins in the central portion of the telencephalon of the brain in two large **lateral ventricles**. The choroid plexus in these ventricles produces cerebrospinal fluid that flows through the ventricles into a singular, midline **third ventricle**. The lateral ventricles are connected to the third ventricle by two **interventricular foramen** (of Monro). From the third ventricle, cerebrospinal fluid flows through the **cerebral aqueduct** (of Sylvius) into the **fourth ventricle**, a diamond-shaped ventricle in the brain stem just deep to the cerebellum. The cerebrospinal fluid can flow in two directions from the fourth ventricle: it can continue in the central portion of the brain stem and spinal cord, flowing in the **central canal**, or it can flow out of the central system into the laterally placed **subarachnoid space**. To gain access to the subarachnoid space, the fluid passes through one of three foramina: two laterally placed foramina (of Luschka) and one medially placed foramen (of Magendie). The cerebrospinal fluid in the subarachnoid space then flows around the entire brain and spinal cord, collecting in large spaces (**suabarachnoid cisterns**) and it is finally reabsorbed into the venous system through the **arachnoid granulations** (Figure 2.4). One particular subarachnoid cistern of interest is the **lumbar cistern** at the distal end of the dura mater, where the spinal cord is absent and only spinal nerve rootlets are present. This will be the site of a **lumbar puncture** or **spinal tap**.

Arterial supply

The brain, like all organs of the body, needs arterial supply to provide oxygen and nutrients to its tissues, as well as venous drainage to remove carbon dioxide and waste products. As you

Clinical box 2.2

A few hundred years ago, it was believed that the cranial ventricular system contained the essence of the soul. Early investigators would pour hot wax into the system, remove the surrounding brain tissue and produce wax ventricular casts. Plastic versions of these casts provide a three-dimensional view of the ventricular system. Any mechanism that increases the amount of cerebrospinal fluid in the ventricular system can lead to **hydrocephalus**, a dangerous condition that can be life threatening.

Ventricular cast

Lateral view

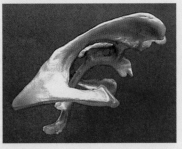

Anterior view

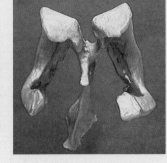

Posterior view

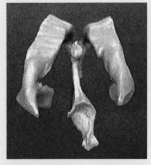

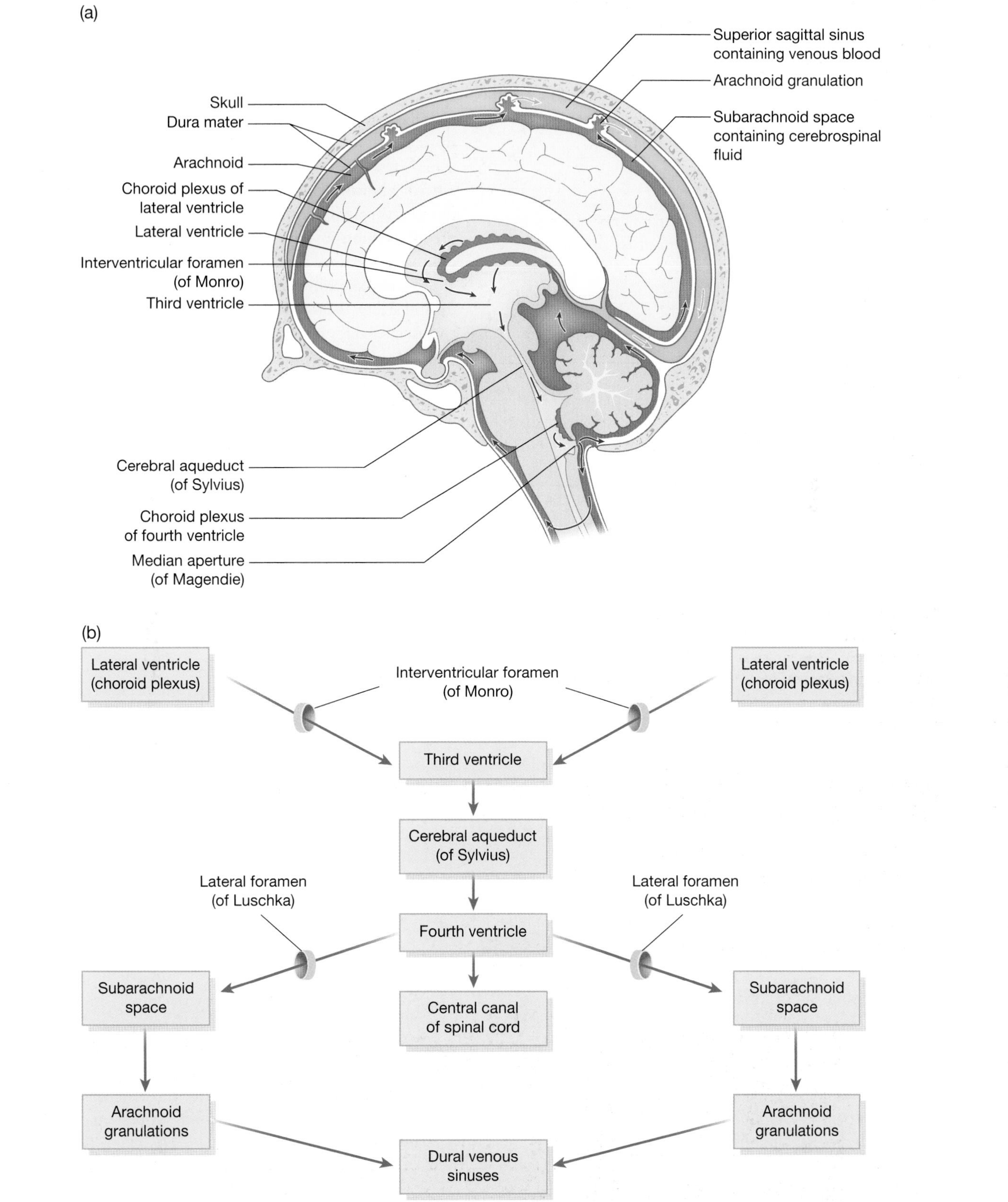

(a)

Skull
Dura mater
Arachnoid
Choroid plexus of lateral ventricle
Lateral ventricle
Interventricular foramen (of Monro)
Third ventricle

Superior sagittal sinus containing venous blood
Arachnoid granulation
Subarachnoid space containing cerebrospinal fluid

Cerebral aqueduct (of Sylvius)
Choroid plexus of fourth ventricle
Median aperture (of Magendie)

(b)

Lateral ventricle (choroid plexus)

Interventricular foramen (of Monro)

Lateral ventricle (choroid plexus)

Third ventricle

Cerebral aqueduct (of Sylvius)

Lateral foramen (of Luschka)

Lateral foramen (of Luschka)

Fourth ventricle

Subarachnoid space

Central canal of spinal cord

Subarachnoid space

Arachnoid granulations

Arachnoid granulations

Dural venous sinuses

Figure 2.4 (a) A midline view of the brain, the skull, and the dural venous sinuses, indicating the flow of cerebrospinal fluid from the lateral ventricles through the ventricular and cistern system to drain through the arachnoid granulations into the dural venous sinuses. (b) A diagrammatic rendition of the flow of cerebrospinal fluid through the ventricles and cisterns.

may know, the brain is especially vulnerable to disruptions in its blood supply, because of its high and continuous requirements for oxygen and glucose. Therefore, the brain has multiple ways to ensure that it receives adequate blood supply, most notably two main arterial sources: the vertebral system and the carotid system.

The carotid arterial system

The common carotid artery arises from the brachiocephalic artery on the right and from the arch of the aorta on the left, and ascends through the neck in parallel with the internal jugular vein and vagus nerve (X). At about the sixth cervical vertebra, the common carotid artery divides into an external

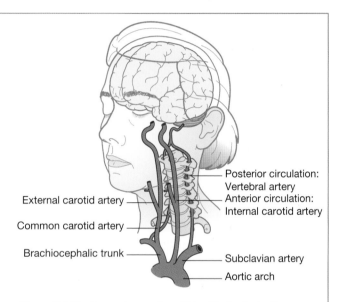

External carotid artery

Common carotid artery

Brachiocephalic trunk

Posterior circulation:
Vertebral artery
Anterior circulation:
Internal carotid artery

Subclavian artery

Aortic arch

Figure 2.5 The two main supplies of blood to the brain: the anterior internal carotid supply and the posterior vertebral artery supply. These arteries or their branches meet at the base of the brain to form the cerebral arterial circle (of Willis).

Clinical box 2.3

Branches of the **ophthalmic artery** (from the internal carotid artery) anastomose with branches of the **facial artery** or **superficial temporal artery** (both from the external carotid artery), providing a mechanism for blood to continue to supply the brain if blood flow in the internal carotid artery becomes restricted. This can be relevant when the internal carotid becomes slowly blocked (e.g. by arteriosclerosis). It is not as effective when a rapid blockage of the artery occurs (e.g. by a thrombus (clot)). Notice that the restriction could take place anywhere between the branching of the carotids and the internal carotid branch of the ophthalmic artery.

and **internal carotid artery**. The **external carotid artery** supplies the face and neck (Figure 2.5). The internal carotid artery continues through the neck, enters the skull through the carotid canal, takes a tortuous "S" shape through the cavernous sinus and gives off its first branch, the **ophthalmic artery**. This artery passes into the orbit through the optic canal with the **optic nerve (II)** and supplies the orbital contents as well as the skin on the forehead and the bridge of the nose. It also gives off a small branch – the central retinal artery – that supplies the retina and can be visualized with an ophthalmoscope. This provides a non-invasive way of examining the quality of the ophthalmic arterial supply.

Once the ophthalmic artery branches off the internal carotid artery, the internal carotid continues for a short distance and then divides into its terminal branches: the anterior cerebral and middle cerebral arteries. The **anterior cerebral artery** passes superior to the corpus callosum (a connection between the two cerebral hemispheres) and supplies the frontal portion of the ipsilateral cerebral hemisphere (recall that this means the same side of that half of the brain). This artery supplies the portion of the hemisphere along the midline. The anterior cerebral artery from the left internal carotid artery anastomoses with the anterior cerebral artery from the right internal carotid artery by way of an **anterior communicating branch**. This provides a connection between the two internal carotid arteries, so that if one were compromised the other could continue to supply the remainder of the brain. The **middle cerebral artery** courses up the lateral surface of the brain and supplies a large portion of the temporal, parietal, and frontal lobes of the ipsilateral cerebral hemisphere. Two important branches arise from the middle cerebral artery; one is the **posterior communicating artery**, which provides an anastomosis with the vertebral artery system. The other branch is the **lenticulostriate artery** (or small series of arteries) that supplies specific structures within the brain (basal ganglia) and can be clinically relevant for stroke victims (Figure 2.6).

When examining the accompanying illustrations, it is easy to see that the anterior and middle cerebral arteries supply approximately two-thirds of the brain (Figures 2.7 and 2.8). If either of these arteries is compromised, a large portion of the brain can be affected. Luckily, the terminal branches of the internal carotid artery have important anastomotic connections with their twin from the other side, as well as from branches from a completely different arterial supply: the vertebral arterial system. Notice on the illustrations that there are areas where the anterior cerebral supply meets the middle cerebral supply; these areas are called the "watershed" regions – those regions where the two blood supplies meet and can partially overlap.

The vertebral arterial system

The **vertebral artery** begins from the subclavian artery in the neck and ascends up the neck by passing through the transverse foramina of the upper six vertebrae. The vertebral

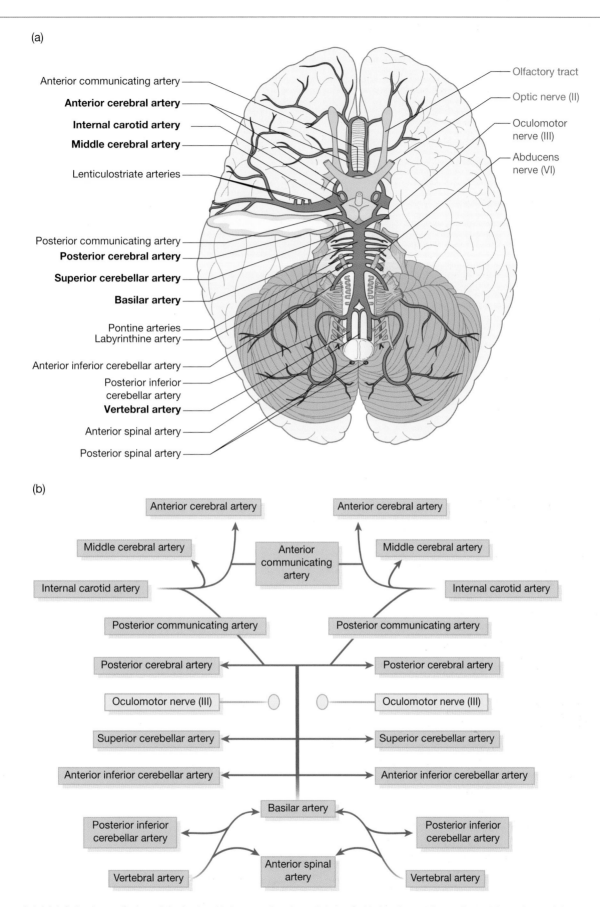

Figure 2.6 (a) Inferior (ventral) view of the brain with its associated arterial supply. Notice the two internal carotid arteries and the two vertebral arteries providing the blood supply to the brain through the cerebral arterial circle (of Willis). (b) A schematic diagram of the arterial supply of the brain. Notice the two internal carotid arteries and the two vertebral arteries providing the blood supply to the brain through the cerebral arterial circle (of Willis).

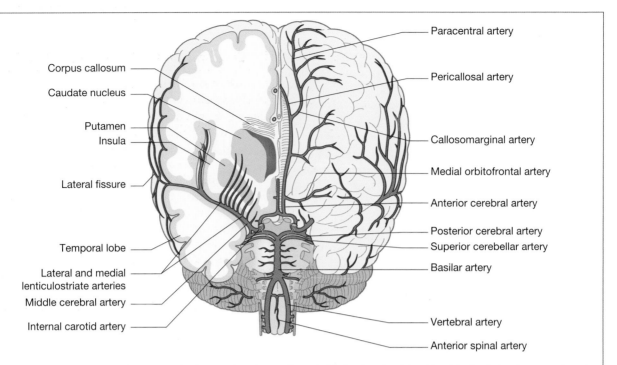

Figure 2.7 Anterior (frontal) view of the brain with its associated arterial supply. Notice that the right side of the brain has been sectioned to provide a more detailed view of the distribution of the middle cerebral artery.

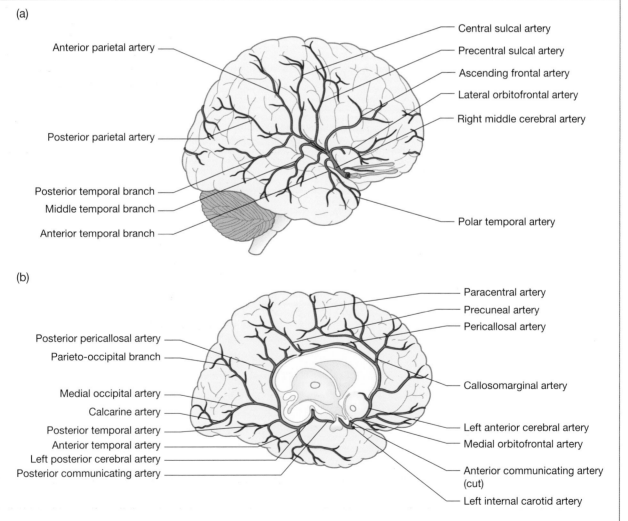

Figure 2.8 Lateral (a) and sagittal (b) views of the brain with its associated blood supply. Notice the distribution of the three cerebral arteries (anterior, middle, and posterior) and the regions of the brain where the vessels meet ("watershed" areas).

artery crosses medially over the arch of the atlas and then ascends into the cranial cavity through the **foramen magnum**, along with the spinal cord (Figure 2.5). Soon after it enters the cranial cavity, the vertebral artery gives off a **posterior inferior cerebellar artery** that supplies the region named, the posterior inferior aspect of the cerebellum. It also provides a small branch to the anterior surface of the spinal cord, the anterior spinal artery, which, interestingly, joins with the anterior spinal artery from the other vertebral artery to form a singular **anterior spinal artery**. The vertebral artery then joins the vertebral artery from the opposite side of the body to form a singular **basilar artery** that ascends the anterior (ventral) surface of the brain stem. The basilar artery supplies right and left **anterior inferior cerebellar arteries**, **labyrinthine arteries**, and **pontine arteries**. Just prior to its termination, it gives off right and left **superior cerebellar arteries** and then terminates as right and left **posterior cerebral arteries**. A well-known landmark is the third cranial nerve (**oculomotor, III**) passing between the superior cerebellar and posterior cerebral arteries. This can also be clinically relevant since a small aneurysm (berry aneurysm) on one of these arteries can impinge on this nerve and alter its ability to function (a change in extraocular muscle function; see Chapter 7 for details on oculomotor nerve lesions). The posterior cerebral arteries supply the occipital region of the ipsilateral cerebral hemisphere and have an important anastomotic connection with the carotid system through the **posterior communicating artery** (Figures 2.6, 2.7, and 2.8).

The cerebral arterial circle (of Willis)

The **cerebral arterial circle** (of Willis) is a continuous circle of arterial connections found on the base of the midbrain encircling the **pituitary gland**, the **mammillary bodies**, and the **optic nerves (II)**. It is supplied by branches of both internal carotid arteries (anterior and middle cerebral arteries) as well as by branches of the vertebral/basilar arteries (posterior cerebral arteries). In clockwise order (from an inferior view), the arteries that make up the cerebral arterial circle include the anterior communicating artery, the left anterior cerebral artery, the left internal carotid artery, the left posterior communicating artery, the left posterior cerebral artery, the basilar artery, the right posterior cerebral artery, the right posterior communicating artery, the right internal carotid artery, the right anterior cerebral artery, and its connection to the anterior communicating artery. This circle is extremely important as an anastomotic connection between the carotid and vertebral systems, as well as a right to left anastomotic connection. If any one vessel becomes compromised, then the other vessels can maintain blood flow to the brain (Figure 2.9).

While this anastomotic circle is an excellent device for balancing arterial blood flow to all regions of the brain, it is, sadly, not always complete or functional. Some individuals have variable sizes of these vessels and other individuals may be lacking one or more of the communicating arteries. This can be clinically problematic. For example, a patient without an anterior communicating artery who loses his anterior cerebral artery due to a thrombus, would lose blood supply to a large

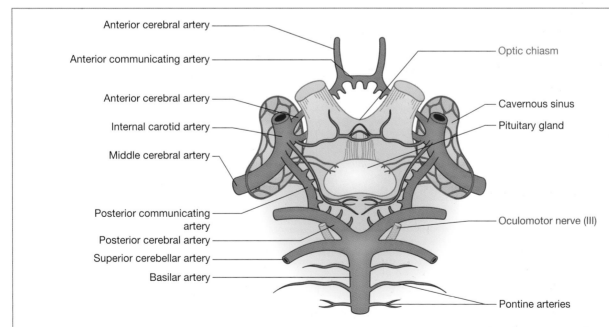

Figure 2.9 The cerebral arterial circle (of Willis) from an inferior (ventral) view. Notice the contributions of the internal carotid arteries and the basilar artery (from the fused vertebral arteries).

Clinical box 2.4

It is now quite easy to visualize the course and extent of the cerebral arterial supply with the use of non-invasive, magnetic resonance angiography (MRA). Using specialized settings on a magnetic resonance imager, the complete arterial blood supply to the brain can be viewed. This allows clinicians to observe aneurysms, obstructions, and anomalies in vessels. Once an MRA is produced, it can be rotated in all three planes, to visualize the entire blood supply to the brain. Try to identify the major vessels of the brain from this magnetic resonance angiogram.

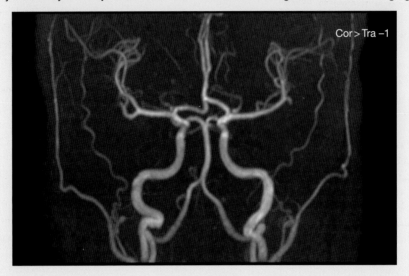

A more invasive procedure, angiography with contrast dye, can also be used to visualize the arterial supply or venous drainage of the brain. This technique has been available for a longer period of time and does not require a magnetic resonance imager. Chapter 18 provides more details on these imaging modalities.

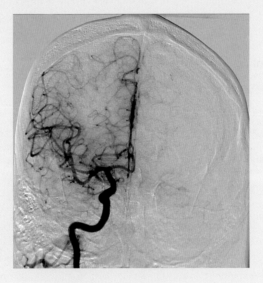

portion of the frontal portion of his ipsilateral cerebral hemisphere – a major neurologic loss.

Venous drainage

Removing blood from the cranial cavity is just as important as supplying blood to the brain. Not only does the venous drainage remove waste products and deoxygenated blood; it also makes sure that the volume of blood in the brain is not excessive, placing undue pressure on the brain and the brain stem (since they are housed in a non-expandable bony structure).

Small veins begin in the brain tissue, but instead of following the arterial system in reverse fashion (as is common in the rest of the body), these veins drain to peripherally located venous sinuses that are found encased in the **dura mater** of the **meninges**. The dura mater houses endothelium-lined venous structures (**dural**

Clinical box 2.5

Any disruption in blood supply to the brain for more than a few minutes can be quite serious since the brain requires a continuous oxygen supply. Loss of arterial supply to the brain is a **stroke** and can be due to a blockage of the supplying vessel (**ischemia**) or a rupture in the supplying vessel (**hemorrhage**). Knowing which type of loss has occurred is essential for proper treatment. For example, providing "clot busting" compounds to patients with ischemia can help remove the blockage and prevent irreparable damage. However, if "clot busting" compounds are given to a patient with a hemorrhage, this can produce even more devastating losses. Therefore, the type of stroke needs to be known before treatment is begun and this needs to be assessed quickly before the brain tissue dies from lack of oxygen supply. Current imaging techniques (CT and MRI) can be used to help differentiate between an ischemic stroke and a hemorrhagic stroke, providing vital information to the clinician prior to treatment.

Determining the severity of the stroke is dependent on knowing the detailed blood supply to the brain and knowing where the stroke occurred. By carefully examining Figures 2.6, 2.7 and 2.8, the specific areas of the brain supplied by the cerebral and cerebellar arteries can be determined. Note that the deep portions of the brain (basal ganglia and thalamus) are supplied by branches of the middle cerebral and posterior cerebral arteries (Pare and Kahn, 2012; Schmahmann, 2003).

Clinical box 2.6

Because so many structures are associated with the cavernous sinuses, any disruption of blood flow can lead to serious complications. For example, a blood clot in the cavernous sinus (**cavernous sinus thrombosis**) can place pressure on the cranial nerves that pass through the sinus, leading to extraocular muscle dysfunction (III, IV, and VI), as well as facial sensory deficits (V_1 and V_2).

An important aspect of the dural venous sinuses is that they do not have valves like typical veins, so that blood can flow in either direction (based on pressure gradients and gravity). This is also true of the ophthalmic veins, so that venous blood from the cavernous sinus can drain through the ophthalmic veins of the orbit and into an anastomosis with the facial veins (perhaps as a secondary drainage route to prevent increased intracranial venous pressure). Conversely, venous blood from facial veins can drain through the ophthalmic veins of the orbit and into the cavernous sinuses. If this facial blood contains bacteria from facial acne or other sources, then the contaminated blood can enter the cavernous sinus and produce a serious thrombosis. This is why the region of the face around the eyes and nose is referred to as the "**danger space**" of the face. Infections in this region should be monitored carefully to prevent progression into the cavernous sinuses.

venous sinuses). These sinuses primarily drain posteriorly and inferiorly to the **jugular foramen** in the skull, where the **internal jugular vein** begins, but there is an alternate, smaller drainage anteriorly through a venous connection that includes the **ophthalmic veins** and the **facial veins** (Figures 2.2 and 2.10).

The most superior dural venous sinuses are found in a fold of dura mater that separates the two cerebral hemispheres: the **falx cerebri**. In the inferior border of the falx cerebri is the **inferior sagittal sinus** that runs posteriorly and ends where it joins the **great cerebral vein** (of Galen) to form the **straight sinus**. In the superior border of the falx cerebri is the **superior sagittal sinus**, which also runs posteriorly and ends at the **confluence of the sinuses** (Figures 2.2). The confluence of the sinuses is located where four major venous sinuses join together and where two dura mater folds meet (the falx cerebri and the **tentorium cerebelli**). The four dural sinuses that join together are the superior sagittal sinus, the straight sinus, and the right and left **transverse sinuses**. The superior sagittal sinus enters the confluence superiorly, the straight sinus enters anteriorly along the plane where the falx cerebri meets the tentorium cerebella, while the transverse sinuses extend laterally from the

confluence of the sinuses where the tentorium cerebelli is attached to the cranial wall. (A smaller occipital sinus also joins the confluence inferiorly.) Normally, the venous drainage begins at the sagittal sinuses and the straight sinus, and continues into the confluence of sinuses and then drains out of the transverse sinuses laterally to enter the **sigmoid sinuses** that drain along the wall of the posterior cranial fossa to end at the jugular foramen – the beginning of the internal jugular vein. The sigmoid sinus gets its name from the "S" shaped course it takes along the posterior-lateral cranial wall.

Anteriorly, the major collection sites for venous blood are the **cavernous sinuses** located in the middle cranial fossa on either side of the **pituitary gland** (Figures 2.10 and 2.11). These sinuses communicate with each other by small **intercavernous sinuses** that encircle the pituitary. The sinuses also receive blood supply from the orbit by way of the **ophthalmic veins**, as well as by direct venous drainage from the brain and brain stem. The cavernous sinuses communicate with the posterior venous system by the petrosal sinuses. The **superior petrosal sinus** runs from the cavernous sinus to the junction of the transverse and sigmoid sinuses along the petrous (rock-like) portion of the

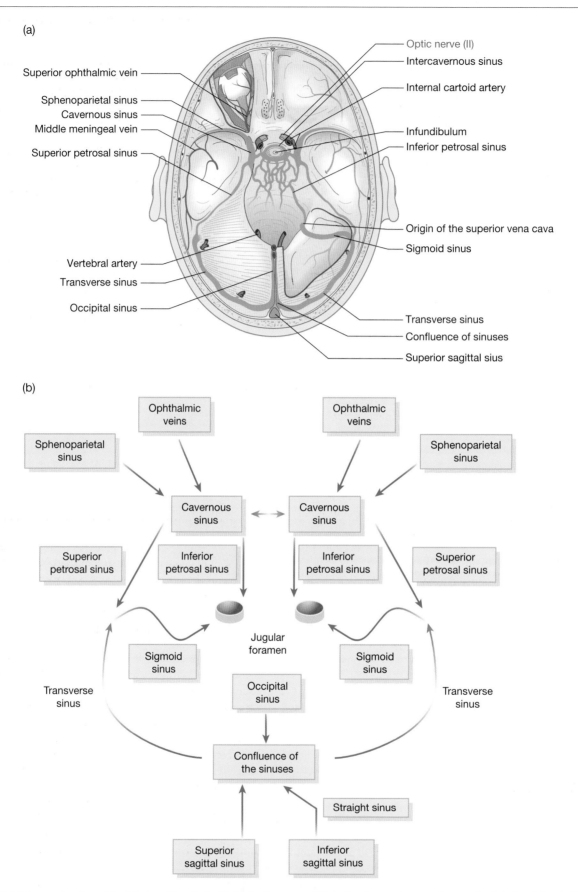

(a)

Optic nerve (II)
Intercavernous sinus
Internal cartoid artery

Superior ophthalmic vein
Sphenoparietal sinus
Cavernous sinus
Middle meningeal vein
Superior petrosal sinus

Infundibulum
Inferior petrosal sinus

Origin of the superior vena cava
Sigmoid sinus

Vertebral artery
Transverse sinus
Occipital sinus

Transverse sinus
Confluence of sinuses
Superior sagittal sius

(b)

Ophthalmic veins

Ophthalmic veins

Sphenoparietal sinus

Sphenoparietal sinus

Cavernous sinus ↔ Cavernous sinus

Superior petrosal sinus

Inferior petrosal sinus

Inferior petrosal sinus

Superior petrosal sinus

Jugular foramen

Sigmoid sinus

Sigmoid sinus

Transverse sinus

Occipital sinus

Transverse sinus

Confluence of the sinuses

Straight sinus

Superior sagittal sinus

Inferior sagittal sinus

Figure 2.10 (a) A superior view of the interior of the skull with the brain removed. Note the dura mater coverings on the interior of the skull that form the transverse sinuses, the petrosal sinuses, and the cavernous sinuses. In addition, note the primary drainage of the venous sinuses through the jugular foramen and the secondary drainage through the ophthalmic veins. (b) A diagrammatic view of the cerebral venous drainage. Note the primary drainage of the venous sinuses through the jugular foramen, as well as the multiple routes for anterior venous flow to reach the foramen. The secondary drainage of cerebral venous blood can occur as backflow through the ophthalmic veins to the veins of the face.

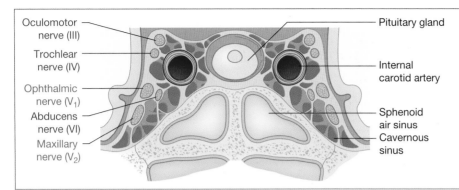

Figure 2.11 A frontal view of the cavernous sinuses surrounding the pituitary gland. Note the internal carotid artery in the each sinus, along with the cranial nerves that control eye movement (oculomotor, III; trochlear, IV; and abducens, VI) and sensation on the upper face (ophthalmic (V$_1$) and maxillary (V$_2$) divisions of the trigeminal nerve).

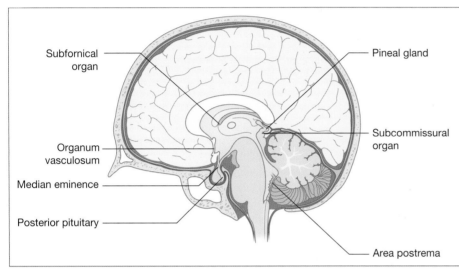

Figure 2.12 A midsagittal view of the brain with the areas that lack a blood-brain barrier indicated. These areas are located around the ventricles and are referred to as circumventricular organs.

temporal bone. The **inferior petrosal sinus** runs from the cavernous sinus to the junction of the sigmoid sinus and the jugular foramen – a more direct communication between the cavernous sinus and the internal jugular vein. These sinuses allow anterior venous blood to flow through the cavernous sinuses and eventually reach the internal jugular vein.

The cavernous sinuses have a number of important structures that course through them: the **oculomotor nerve (III)**, the **trochlear nerve (IV)**, the **abducens nerve (VI)** and two branches of the **trigeminal nerve (V)**, the **ophthalmic division (V$_1$)** and the **maxillary division (V$_2$)**, as well as the **internal carotid artery** which takes its characteristic "S" bend in the sinus (Figure 2.11).

The blood-brain barrier

Now that the arterial supply and the venous drainage of the brain are understood, it should be pointed out that the capillaries within the brain have a unique histology. The capillaries are typical type 1, continuous capillaries that normally restrict transport of products due to the presence of tight junctions between the cells. The capillaries in the central nervous system are further protected by a cell membrane lining on their outer surface from adjacent glial cells. These specific glial astrocytes create a thicker, more impermeable barrier than normal capillaries. This is the **blood-brain barrier** and it provides added protection to the neural tissues by preventing viruses, bacteria, and other harmful

agents from gaining access to the brain. Small molecules (CO$_2$, O$_2$) and lipid soluble compounds (thyroid hormones, steroids, melatonin) can diffuse across the blood-brain barrier, while all other substances are actively transported (glucose, peptides).

While the blood-brain barrier is an immunologically important barrier, it is not complete throughout the central nervous system. The regions where the barrier is faulty or does not exist are primarily found around the brain's ventricular system and are referred to as **circumventricular organs**. These include the **pineal gland**, the **subcommissural organ**, the **area postrema**, the **subfornical organ**, the **organum vasculosum**, the **median eminence**, and the **posterior pituitary** (Figure 2.12). It is not known why these areas lack a blood-brain barrier, but one hypothesis is that these structures have a secretory role or a blood sampling role and, therefore, need to be able to secrete into the blood (or sample from the blood) more readily than would be permitted with the barrier.

The blood-brain barrier can be compromised during clinical conditions such as inflammation, traumatic brain injury, or stroke. This can lead to an influx of immunological and anti-inflammatory products for repair and protection, as well as the influx of negative agents, such as viruses and bacteria. The disruption of the barrier has been implicated in a number of clinical conditions (meningitis, epilepsy, and multiple sclerosis, for example). Advances in magnetic resonance imaging have allowed visualization of blood-brain barrier permeability defects.

Clinical considerations

One take home message from this chapter should be that the cranial cavity is an enclosed space that provides protection to the brain as it floats in a fluid of cerebrospinal fluid. If anything abnormal occupies this enclosed space (excess blood, excess cerebrospinal fluid, a tumor), then increased pressure is produced that can damage the nervous tissue. Specific examples of this type of injury are provided below.

Case 1

While playing softball, the center fielder, Phil Johnson, and the left fielder, Mike Collins, run after a fly ball. They both arrive at the ball at the same time and Phil receives a hard blow to the left, lateral side of his head from a collision with Mike. He is knocked unconscious for a few moments, but, upon regaining consciousness, he states he feels OK and wants to continue playing. After the game, Phil arrives home and tells his wife that he feels slightly nauseous and wants to take a nap. He lies down to sleep and does not wake up.

During the collision, Phil fractured his skull and ruptured his left **middle meningeal artery** that runs between the skull and the outer layer of dura mater, producing an **epidural hematoma**. The artery bleeds into the epidural space putting pressure onto the dura and eventually onto the underlying brain. When only a small amount of bleeding has occurred, he feels OK. This is termed the **lucid interval**. As the bleeding continues, he may feel disoriented and nauseous. Once he falls asleep, the bleeding continues and places enough pressure onto the brain and the brain stem to compress the respiratory centers, which prevent him from breathing.

A rule of thumb is that anyone that suffers a blow to the head and is knocked unconscious should have their head visualized with computed tomography or magnetic resonance imaging. The physician would be looking for a smooth oval shaped structure that appears to be on the lateral surface of the brain between the brain tissue and the skull. The pool of blood collecting would be smooth sided because it is between the skull and the dura mater (Figure 2.13).

This is a relatively easy problem to treat, since the main goal is to reduce the pressure caused by the bleeding vessel. A surgeon can produce a small burr hole in the skull over the hematoma and allow the blood to drain, thereby reducing the pressure. If the bleeding does not stop on its own, then steps can be taken to prevent further bleeding, including ligating the artery.

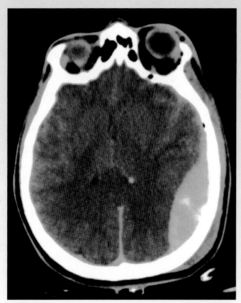
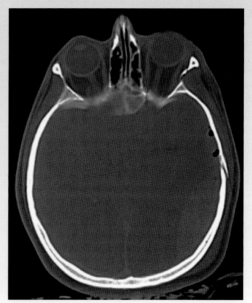

Brain window   Bone window

Figure 2.13 Two horizontal computed tomography examples from the same individual with an epidural hematoma. One example presents the blood clot (brain window) and the second example presents the skull fracture (bone window). Note the large blood-filled region on the left side of the skull, which has a smooth internal edge since the blood is pushing the dura mater against the brain.

Case 2

While driving home after a late night movie, Maxine Jones' car is hit in the side by a drunk driver who runs a red light. Maxine experiences a large lateral force through her head and neck from the collision. She is knocked unconscious by the blow and wakes up a few moments later disoriented with a broken left arm and many small lacerations. An ambulance arrives and takes her to the hospital, where she has her lacerations attended to and her arm set in a cast. Maxine mentions some disorientation to the attending physician who prescribes some pain reliever and tells her to follow up with her general physician. A few days later, Maxine begins feeling disoriented and has a small but constant headache, so she takes some aspirin to relieve the headache. The headaches get worse over the next 24–48 hours and she begins having nausea, difficulty speaking, and dizziness. She goes back to the emergency room and, when seen, is in obvious distress. She has immediate imaging of her head and a relatively large crescent shaped mass is seen over her right cerebral cortex. The mass is smooth on the side facing the skull, but has a roughened, indented surface facing the brain (Figure 2.14). This is a **subdural hematoma** and has occurred from a rupture of small bridging veins that cross from the dura mater to the arachnoid mater. The bleeding that occurs is slower than an epidural hematoma (venous versus arterial bleeding) and can actually be so slow that symptoms may not appear for months after an injury.

Maxine has emergency surgery to relieve the intracranial pressure and to stop the bleeding. A few weeks later, she has recovered fully, but she is discouraged from taking anything that might prevent her blood from clotting (aspirin) so that she does not have a recurrence.

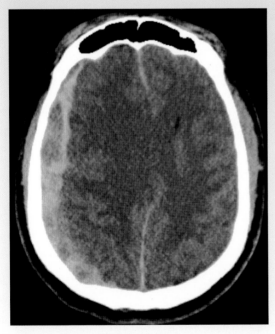

Horizontal view

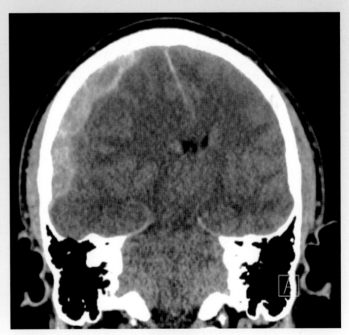

Frontal view

Figure 2.14 A horizontal and frontal computed tomography example from an individual with a subdural hematoma. Note the large blood-filled region on the right side of the skull, which has rough, irregular internal edges since the blood can infiltrate within the sulci of the brain.

Case 3

Jack Davidson has just enjoyed his retirement dinner from the accounting firm where he worked for 40 years. Upon arriving home, he has "the worst headache of his life" that radiates towards the back of his head and neck. He complains of nausea, blurry vision, and dizziness, and then collapses. His wife calls an ambulance and Jack arrives at the hospital unconscious with his breathing being artificially maintained. He has an emergency magnetic resonance image of his head and a large pool of blood is observed at the base of the brain in the area around the arterial cerebral circle (of Willis) (Figure 2.15). This is diagnosed as a **subarachnoid hemorrhage** and is caused by a rupture in one of the cerebral blood vessels in that area. This can be caused by acute head trauma, but, in Jack's case, it was most likely due to a cerebral aneurysm that ruptured. The bleeding would increase intracranial pressure rapidly, producing the headache and other symptoms.

Jack has emergency surgery to relieve the intracranial pressure and to try to repair the blood vessel (an aneurysm on the anterior communicating artery). Unhappily, the surgeon was not able to control the bleeding and Jack died postoperatively.

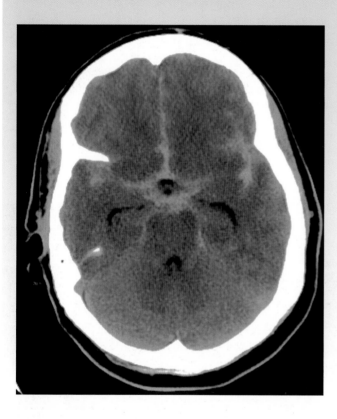

Figure 2.15 A horizontal computed tomography example from an individual with a subarachnoid hematoma. Note the large diffuse blood filled region at the base of the skull, and diffusing around the brain and the cerebrospinal fluid cisterns.

Case 4

Mrs Phyllis Armstrong, a 46-year-old mother of two teenagers, begins experiencing walking disturbances and feels clumsy. She mentions this to her physician during her yearly physical. The physician recommends that Phyllis have a brain magnetic resonance imaging scan to determine if anything is wrong. During the scan, it is noticed that Phyllis' ventricles are enlarged and that the posterior portion of her cerebellum has descended into the foramen magnum (**Chiari malformation**), obstructing the flow of **cerebrospinal fluid** out of the ventricles (Figure 2.16). This produces an **internal, non-communicating (obstructive) hydrocephalus**. After consulting with a neurosurgeon, Phyllis decides to have surgery to correct the placement of the cerebellum and, during the surgery, to have a cerebral shunt placed in the lateral ventricle that would allow drainage of the cerebrospinal fluid. The shunt would be run to the peritoneum where the fluid would be deposited for reabsorption.

The surgery is successful and Phyllis recovers fully, although she has yearly follow up to make sure that the hydrocephalus does not reoccur.

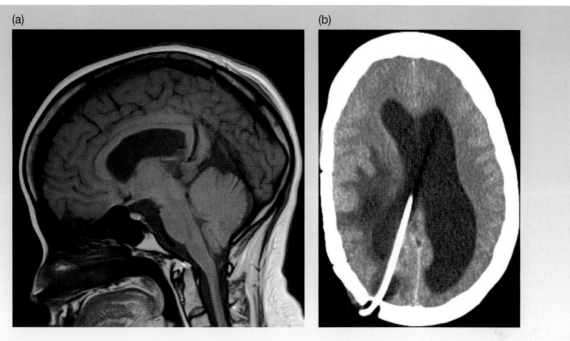

(a)   (b)

Figure 2.16 (a) A magnetic resonance image (MRI) of a patient with a Chiari malformation leading to hydrocephalus. Note the lower portion of the cerebellum in the spinal canal blocking the flow of cerebrospinal fluid and producing enlarged lateral ventricles indicating hydrocephalus. (b) A computer tomograph (CT) image of a patient with hydrocephalus who has an implanted shunt to divert excess cerebrospinal fluid to the peritoneum for reabsorption.

Case 5

Nancy Bates, a college student, returns to college after a spring break mission trip to Sub-Saharan Africa. A few days after she returns, she has flu-like symptoms with a headache and a high fever. She also develops a stiff neck. Nancy visits her local health clinic on campus and the astute physician, Dr Kathleen Foote, recognizes that the symptoms could indicate **meningitis** (an inflammation of the meninges). Dr Foote tries a few tests to help determine if meningitis is present. She asks Nancy to bend her neck forward (like bobbing her head "yes") and sees that Nancy's knee and hip flex at the same time. She also asks Nancy to rapidly rotate her head (as if she was indicating "no") and, as she does so, Nancy complains of the headache worsening. Dr Foote receives permission and performs a **lumbar puncture** to obtain **cerebrospinal fluid** for testing.

To perform the lumbar puncture, Nancy is asked to lie down on her side in the fetal position with her knees towards her chest. Dr Foote palpates the spinous processes of the fourth and fifth lumbar vertebrae (Figure 2.17). She disinfects and applies a local anesthetic to this region. She then inserts a needle through the skin and underlying tissue until the needle passes through the **ligamentum flavum** (first barrier) and then the **dura mater** (second barrier). At this point, the tip of the needle should be in the **subarachnoid space**, so Dr Foote can

measure the fluid pressure to determine if it is within normal range. She also collects a small quantity of the fluid and examines it for clarity and color. The fluid will be sent to the lab for testing to determine the presence of bacteria.

Immediately after the **spinal tap**, and prior to receiving the results, Dr Foote places Nancy on antibiotics to prevent any further complications of the meningitis. She also collects information from her about who she has had close contact with since her trip. These individuals will need to be notified about a potential exposure to meningitis. Happily, after a long course of antibiotics, Nancy recovered and went on to become a medical student and successful physician.

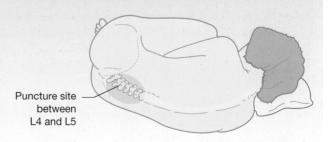

Puncture site
between
L4 and L5

Figure 2.17 The placement of a patient and the vertebral level location for the performance of a lumbar puncture (spinal tap).

Study questions

1. Hydrocephalus can be produced by which of the following:
a) blockade of cerebrospinal fluid production by the choroid plexus
b) inadequate drainage of cerebrospinal fluid through arachnoid granulations
c) overproduction of cerebrospinal fluid at arachnoid granulations
d) inadequate drainage of cerebrospinal fluid at the choroid plexus
e) blockade of cerebrospinal fluid production by the arachnoid granulations

2. When performing a spinal tap on a patient, the physician inserts the needle into the _____ to collect cerebrospinal fluid. The needle should be inserted inferior to the _____ vertebra to avoid damaging the spinal cord.
a) epidural space, 12th thoracic
b) subdural space, 12th thoracic
c) subarachnoid space, 12th thoracic
d) epidural space, 3rd lumbar
e) subdural space, 3rd lumbar
f) subarachnoid space, 3rd lumbar

3. The cerebral arterial circle (of Willis) is made of paired arteries from the right and left side as well as single, unpaired arteries. Which of the following is a single, unpaired artery in the cerebral arterial circle?
a) anterior communicating artery
b) posterior communicating artery
c) posterior cerebral artery
d) anterior cerebral artery
e) lateral communicating artery

4. A patient with a cavernous sinus thrombosis can have multiple cranial nerves involved, due to their course through the cavernous sinus. Which of the following is a major symptom of a cavernous sinus thrombosis?
a) paralysis of the facial muscles
b) tinnitus (ringing in the ear)
c) loss of vision
d) paralysis of the ocular muscles
e) paralysis of the muscles of mastication

5. In an epidural hematoma, which of the following vessels usually ruptures?
a) great cerebral vein (of Galen)
b) inferior sagittal sinus
c) posterior cerebral artery
d) anterior communicating artery
e) middle meningeal artery

6. An elderly male patient suffers a stroke that prevents blood flow in the left anterior cerebral artery just after the anterior communicating branch. On an illustration of the brain, mark off the area that would be affected by this condition. Explain the differences that would be found between a stroke that occurs in an arterial branch prior to the cerebral arterial circle compared to a stroke in a vessel that branches after the cerebral arterial circle.

For more self-assessment questions, visit the companion website at
www.wileyessential.com/neuroanatomy

FURTHER READING

For additional information on the blood vessels, meninges, and ventricles in neuroanatomy, the following textbooks and review articles may be helpful:

Blumenfeld H. 2002. *Neuroanatomy Through Clinical Cases*. Sinauer Associates, Sunderland, Massachusetts.

Felten DL, Shetty A. 2009. *Netter's Atlas of Neuroscience*, 2nd edition. Saunders Elsevier, Philadelphia, Pennsylvania.

Haines DE. 2012. *Neuroanatomy: An Atlas of Structures, Sections and Systems*, 8th edition. Lippincott Williams & Wilkin, Baltimore, Maryland.

Moore KL, Dalley AF, Agur AMR. 2014. *Moore Clinically Oriented Anatomy*, 7th edition. Lippincott, Williams & Wilkins, Philadelphia, Pennsylvania.

Obermeier B, Daneman R, Ransohoff RM. 2013. Development, maintenance and disruption of the blood-brain barrier. *Nat Med*, 19(12): 1584–1596.

Pare JR, Kahn JH. 2012. Basic neuroanatomy and stroke syndromes. *Emerg Med Clin North Am*, 30(3): 601–615.

Patestas MA, Gartner LP. 2006. *A Textbook of Neuroanatomy*. Blackwell Publishing, Malden, Massachusetts.

Prince EA, Ahn, SH. 2013. Basic vascular neuroanatomy of the brain and spine: What the general interventional radiologist needs to know. *Semin Intervent Radiol*, 30(3): 234–239.

Schmahmann JD. 2003. Vascular syndromes of the thalamus. *Stroke*, 34: 2264–2278.

Toulgoat F, Lasjaunias P. 2013. Vascular malformations of the brain. *Handb Clin Neurol*, 112: 1043–1051.

Wolburg H, Paulus W. 2010. Choroid plexus: biology and pathology. *Acta Neuropathol*, 119(1): 75–88.

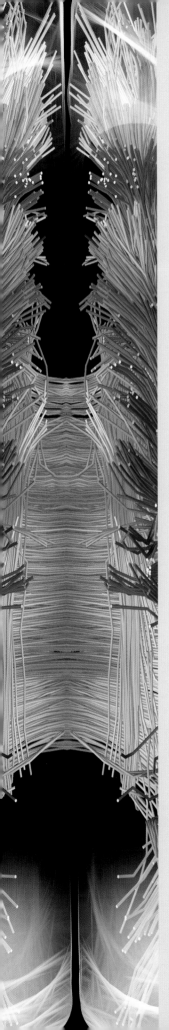

CHAPTER 3
Neurodevelopment

Learning objectives

1. Describe the stages of neural development.
2. Describe the development of the neural tube and its further growth and division into the adult brain structures.
3. Identify the cell types found in neural development.
4. Describe the time course of cellular development in the nervous system.
5. Discuss the different types of neurodevelopmental disorders.

Essential Clinical Neuroanatomy, First Edition. Thomas H. Champney.
© 2016 John Wiley & Sons, Ltd. Published 2016 by John Wiley & Sons, Ltd.
Companion website: www.wileyessential.com/neuroanatomy

Introduction

The development of the nervous system requires a complex orchestration of molecular signals that guide the growth and development of neural cells. This development begins with the formation of a simple tube out of ectoderm. The tube then grows and develops to form the primitive nervous system.

The nervous system begins development at three weeks of age and continues throughout the gestational period. Therefore, exposure to drugs, toxins, or trauma throughout a woman's pregnancy can have adverse effects on the neural development of her child.

Early neural development

As the bilaminar embryonic plate develops into a trilaminar embryo, one of the first structures formed is the **notochord** (an outgrowth of the endoderm that resides in the space between the endoderm and ectoderm). The notochord (which will develop into the vertebral column) induces the ectoderm below it to grow rapidly, forming a **neural plate**. The neural plate continues to grow more than the surrounding tissue and this produces a groove in the plate. As the groove continues to grow, its margins grow together, converting the neural groove into a **neural tube**. The neural tube first develops in the middle of the embryo and the tube then continues to grow towards the anterior and posterior ends of the embryo; much like a zipper fuses two pieces of cloth together (Figure 3.1).

The portion of the neural tube nearest the notochord develops into the **floor plate**, while the portion closest to the surface of the ectoderm develops into the **roof plate**. The area of tissue adjacent to the roof plate develops into specialized **neural crest cells**, which will migrate throughout the embryo, providing a multitude of different cells (Figure 3.2).

By the fourth week of development, the neural tube has grown the entire length of the embryo and the anterior end has expanded into three primary brain vesicles, the **forebrain** (prosencephalon), the **midbrain** (mesencephalon), and the **hindbrain** (rhombencephalon). In addition, the growth of the embryo has produced two primary curves in the neural tube. These curves (or flexures) are called the **cervical flexure** (in the

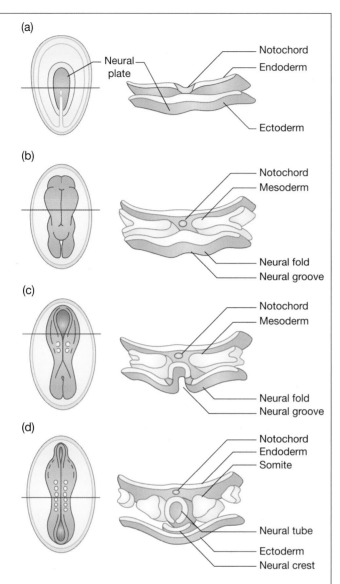

Figure 3.1 Cross-sectional and inferior view of neural development in a three-week-old embryo. Notice the early formation of the notochord (primitive vertebral column), which induces the adjacent ectoderm to develop into the neural plate. The rapid growth of the neural plate produces a neural groove which fuses together to form a neural tube. The neural tube will develop into the brain and spinal cord.

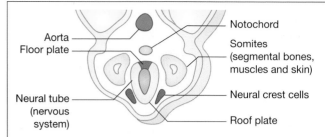

Figure 3.2 Cross-sectional view of neural development in a four-week-old embryo. Notice the formation of the floor plate and roof plate within the neural tube. Adjacent to the roof plate, neural cells will develop into neural crest cells that will distribute throughout the embryo. The neural crest cells will form the posterior (dorsal) root ganglia, the peripheral sensory nerves, the adrenal medulla, and non-neural tissues such as the flat bones of the skull, the melanocytes in the skin, and the odontoblasts in the teeth.

Clinical box 3.1

The neural crest cells produce numerous different cells in the developing embryo. Therefore, any problem with the growth or development of these cells can lead to both neural and non-neural consequences. For example, neural crest cells undergo an epithelial to mesenchymal transition that allows these cells to develop into non-neural cells such as melanocytes in the skin, odontoblasts in the teeth, enteroendocrine cells in the respiratory and gastrointestinal systems, as well as the flat bones in the skull. Disorder in this transition can lead to poor cellular development in these tissues.

Recent research into cancer metastasis has shown that the cells undergo a similar epithelial to mesenchymal transition to initiate metastasis, so this process can have additional clinical relevance.

hindbrain) and the **cephalic flexure** (in the midbrain). The cephalic flexure remains throughout development and is found in adults at the **midbrain flexure** that was mentioned in Chapter 1 (Figure 3.3a).

The cells surrounding the neural tube in the region that will become the spinal cord continue to grow outwards, creating two layers – a **mantle layer** near the center of the tube and a **marginal layer** on the periphery of the tube. The marginal layer is the primitive white matter (spinal tracts) and the mantle layer is the primitive gray matter of the spinal cord. The mantle layer near the floor plate is called the **basal plate**, while that portion near the roof plate is called the **alar plate**. The basal plate will develop into the anterior (ventral) horn of the spinal cord and contain motor neurons. The alar plate will develop into the posterior (dorsal) horn of the spinal cord and will contain sensory neurons (Figure 3.4).

At five weeks of age, the cells in the basal plate send out motor axons into the surrounding tissue. Some of the neural crest cells that remained near the alar plate have developed into sensory neurons which send processes out to the periphery and centrally into the alar plate. These cells will become the posterior (dorsal) root ganglia. This is a recurring theme throughout neural development – basal plate derivatives will become motor neurons, while alar plate derivatives will become sensory neurons. In the brain, further development has occurred by five weeks of age, such that the forebrain is divided into two

Figure 3.3 Lateral and sagittal view of neural development in a four (a) and five (b) week-old embryo. In the four-week-old embryo (a), notice the expansion of the anterior end of the neural tube forming the forebrain, midbrain, and hindbrain. Also, notice the bends in the neural tube: the cephalic flexure and the cervical flexure. In the five-week-old embryo (b), notice the differentiation of the forebrain into the telencephalon and diencephalon, and the differentiation of the hindbrain into the metencephalon and myelencephalon.

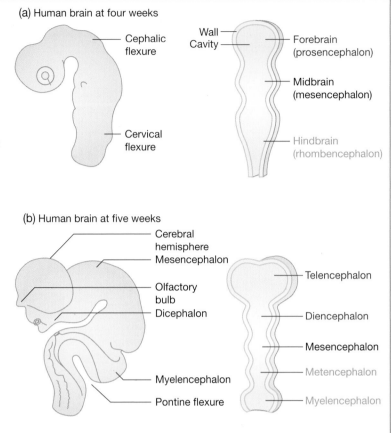

Figure 3.4 Cross-sectional view of spinal cord development in a five-week-old embryo. Notice the formation of the basal plates anteriorly for motor neuronal development and the formation of the alar plates posteriorly for sensory neuronal development.

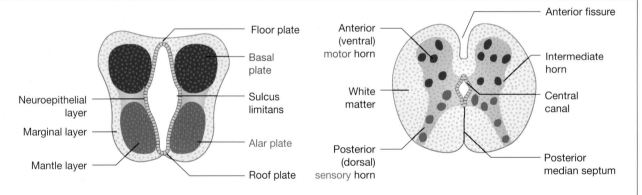

components: the **telencephalon** (cortex/limbic system/basal ganglia) and the **diencephalon** (hypothalamus/thalamus/epithalamus). The midbrain (**mesencephalon**) remains the midbrain, while the hindbrain further develops into the **metencephalon** (pons and cerebellum) and the **myelencephalon** (medulla oblongata) (Figure 3.3b).

As the region of the neural tube that becomes the spinal cord transitions into the myelencephalon, the alar plate moves laterally, while the basal plate moves medially. Therefore, neurons with motor activity will be medially placed and neurons

with sensory activity will be laterally placed. This is a good "rule of thumb" to keep in mind when learning the neuroanatomy of the brain stem: motor nuclei and their nerves tend to be medial (oculomotor (III), trochlear (IV), abducens (VI), hypoglossal (XII)), while sensory nuclei and their nerves tend to be lateral (trigeminal (V), vestibulocochlear (VIII)).

In the midbrain (mesencephalon), the sensory and motor components keep the typical arrangement, with the motor components placed anterior and medial, while the sensory components are posterior and lateral (Figure 3.5).

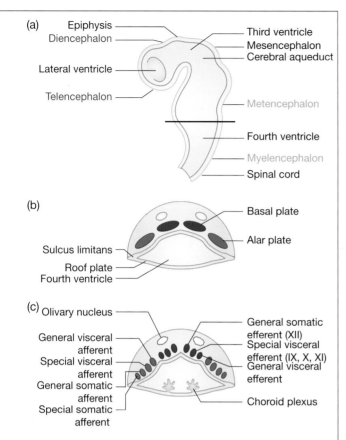

Figure 3.5 Cross-sectional view of hindbrain (myelencephalon) development in a five-week-old embryo. Notice the movement of the alar (sensory) plate laterally, while the basal (motor) plate moves medially. Therefore, sensory cranial nerve nuclei tend to be placed laterally, while motor cranial nerve nuclei are placed medially.

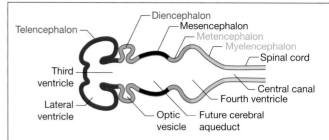

Figure 3.6 Coronal sectional through the developing central nervous system, indicating the expansion of the neural tube into the lateral ventricles (telencephalon), the third ventricle (diencephalon), the cerebral aqueduct (midbrain/mesencephalon), fourth ventricle (hindbrain/metencephalon and myelencephalon), and the central canal (spinal cord).

Neurodevelopment histology

The development of cells in the nervous system is tightly regulated by specific growth factors. The primitive neuroectodermal cells are induced from the ectoderm and then further differentiate into neural tube cells, roof plate, or floor plate cells. These precursor cells then differentiate into neuroblasts or gliablasts. The neuroblasts develop into neurons, while the gliablasts develop into glial cells: astrocytes or oligodendrocytes. The remaining undifferentiated cells line the central tube and develop into ependymal cells (Figure 3.7). Each of these steps in differentiation is controlled by stimulatory or inhibitory growth factors released by neighboring cells.

As the neural cells develop, they send out processes that will become dendrites and axons. These processes grow throughout the developing neural tissue, as well as into surrounding tissues. The growth of these processes is regulated by locally released factors that act as chemoattractants or chemorepulsants, guiding the direction of growth. In addition, target cells for the neuronal processes release compounds that act to support the growth and development of the neuronal cells. An excess amount of these processes grow into the periphery to contact target cells and then, as development continues, many of these processes are "pruned" to provide specific innervation to specific target cells. This is a unique way of ensuring that all target cells are innervated and that only the correct innervation remains after pruning.

In addition, nearby mesenchymal cells migrate into the developing neural tube and become **microglia** (macrophage-like cells). Other cells migrate out of the developing neural tube and migrate to distant tissues. These **neural crest cells** leave the posterior aspect of the neural tube and undergo an epithelial to mesenchymal transition (losing epithelial characteristics and acquiring characteristics of mesenchymal cells). Some of the neural crest cells retain neural-like properties and develop into the: 1) sensory ganglia associated with cranial and spinal nerves; 2) the sympathetic and parasympathetic ganglia; and 3) the adrenal medullary cells. Other neural crest cells undergo further differentiation and develop into the melanocytes

The development of the forebrain does not, however, follow this convention. It has a remarkable amount of growth in multiple directions that is task specific. For example, the posterior growth of the telencephalon (occipital lobe) contains visual sensation and processing, while the lateral growth of the telencephalon (temporal lobe) contains auditory sensation and processing.

While the cellular components of the nervous system are rapidly growing during weeks 4–6 of development, the central portion of the neural tube also grows in relation to the surrounding neural tissues. In the spinal cord, the central tube remains small and undeveloped and becomes the central canal. In the hindbrain, the growth of this region produces an enlargement of the central tube, leading to the formation of the fourth ventricle. The relatively small growth of the midbrain is reflected in the small remnant of the central tube – the cerebral aqueduct (of Sylvius). The explosive growth of the forebrain produces a concurrent expansion in the primitive central tube, leading to the development of the third ventricle and the large paired lateral ventricles. Recall that ependymal cells line the tube and in certain areas they expand to become the choroid plexus that produces cerebrospinal fluid (Figure 3.6).

Figure 3.7 Cellular development in the central nervous system begins with undifferentiated neuroectoderm (neuroepithelium) in the neural tube. Exposure to specific growth factors leads to the differentiation of neuroblasts or glioblasts. The neuroblasts become the neurons, while the glioblasts further differentiate into astrocytes or oligodendrocytes.

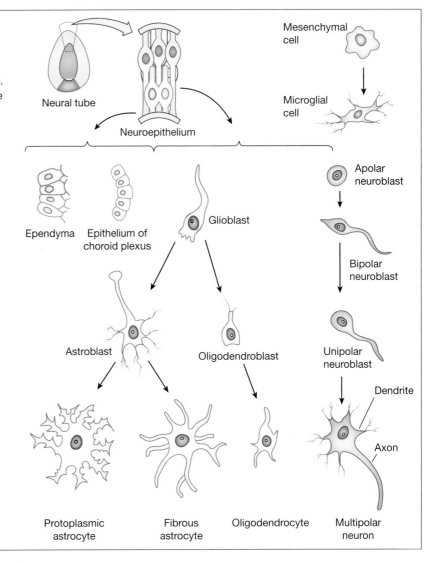

Clinical considerations

One take home message from this chapter is that the development of the nervous system occurs throughout a woman's pregnancy and that exposure to drugs or trauma at any time can have a major impact on the developing nervous system. Nutrition is also important for normal neural system development, with many women taking prenatal vitamins that include folic acid (folate) for this reason.

Women who drink alcohol during their pregnancy (even before they know they are pregnant) can negatively impact the neural development of their child. The facial structure of these children with **fetal alcohol syndrome** is markedly different than normal. They also have diminished intellectual development. While the molecular and biochemical effects of alcohol on the development of the nervous system are not fully understood, a simple preventative treatment is available: to strongly encourage women considering pregnancy to avoid alcohol consumption (Figure 3.8).

A common neural developmental defect is **spina bifida**. This occurs when the neural tube does not close appropriately

found in the skin, the odontoblasts found in teeth, the enteroendocrine cells found in the respiratory and digestive systems, and into the cells responsible for the formation of the flat bones in the skull.

during the fourth week of development. This can lead to a wide range of neural deficits. A minor variant of the disorder, **spina bifida occulta**, occurs when the lamina of the vertebrae do not form a "roof" over the spinal cord. This generally occurs in the lumbar region of the vertebrae and exposes the spinal cord to injury and trauma. Some children born with spina bifida occulta will present with dark hair on their lower back where the lumbar vertebral lamina would normally be found. It has been estimated that 10% of the population has some minor form of spina bifida which may go undetected throughout life.

More severe forms of spina bifida involve developmental disorders of the meninges or of the spinal cord itself. A **meningocele** is a cyst-like protrusion of the meninges through the lower back. A **meningomyelocele** has spinal cord material in the meningocele that is usually dysfunctional (Zerah and Kulkarni, 2013). These forms of spina bifida can be treated surgically (both *in utero* and after birth), but even with proper surgical correction there are quite often complications or neural deficits. It has been found that

women who have sufficient folic acid in their diet are much less likely to have children with spina bifida. This is why many food items are fortified with folic acid (since women may not know they are pregnant by the time neural tube closure begins) (Figure 3.9).

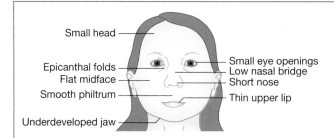

Figure 3.8 Typical facial characteristics of a child with fetal alcohol syndrome. These children will usually have delayed or reduced mental development as well.

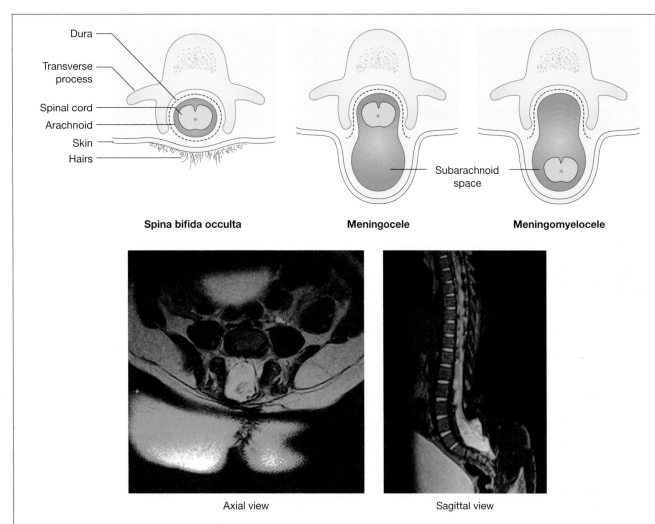

Figure 3.9 Characteristics of children born with neural tube defects (spina bifida) with meningocele or meningomyelocele. Children with spina bifida occulta typically present with dark hair over their lower back and will develop normally, although trauma to the lower back should be avoided. Magnetic resonance images (axial and sagittal) from a patient with meningocele. Note the hyperintense signal from the meningocele in the lower lumbar region.

Figure 3.10 Hydrocephalus in a child leads to enlarged ventricles that can place undue pressure on the brain. One mechanism to reduce the hydrocephalus is to place a one-way shunt from the ventricles to the peritoneum, where the excess fluid can drain and be resorbed (see Figure 2.16).

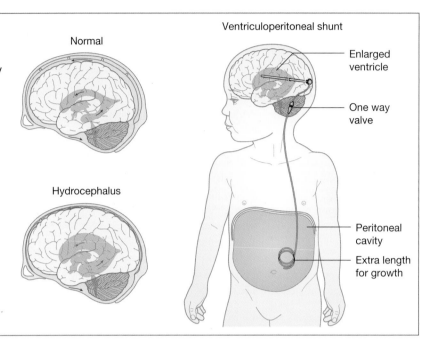

Normal

Hydrocephalus

Ventriculoperitoneal shunt

Enlarged ventricle

One way valve

Peritoneal cavity

Extra length for growth

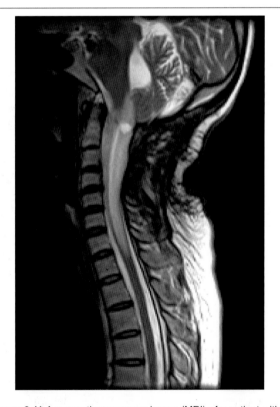

Figure 3.11 A magnetic resonance image (MRI) of a patient with a Chiari malformation and syringomyelia. Note the extension of the inferior aspect of the cerebellum into the spinal canal (Chiari malformation) and the formation of a hyperintense cyst in the center of the cervical spinal cord (syringomyelia).

A very severe form of spina bifida is termed **rachischisis** (myeloschisis) that involves a sheet of neural tissue that is incorporated into the skin with no protective membranes. Individuals with this disorder have dysfunctional spinal cords at the level of the lesion and below. This is a very debilitating disorder. Similar defects can be found in the anterior aspect of the neural tube and this can lead to **anencephaly** (the lack of cortical (telencephalon) development) or **microcephaly** (the reduced growth of the brain). While anencephaly is incompatible with life, children can be born and can live with microcephaly, although they usually have delayed or reduced mental capacities.

Another common developmental disorder is **hydrocephalus** – where cerebrospinal fluid is unable to drain properly and swelling of the lateral and third ventricles occurs. If this is determined at an early age, treatments can be used to drain the excess fluid to the abdomen via a shunt, preventing the expansion of the ventricles (Figure 3.10). Hydrocephalus can also be caused by the abnormal development of the inferior aspect of the cerebellum, which protrudes into the foramen magnum with the spinal cord. This can disrupt cerebrospinal fluid flow as well as place undue pressure on the brain stem. This defect (a **Chiari malformation**) can produce life-threatening events if the increased pressure on the brain stem alters neuronal firing from the cardiac and respiratory centers. A Chiari malformation can also disrupt cerebrospinal fluid flow through the central canal of the spinal cord, causing a cyst-like formation in the center of the spinal cord (**syringomyelia**) (Figure 3.11). This can lead to sensory or motor disturbances in that region of the spinal cord.

Case 1

Natalia Masters is a 14-year-old student who becomes pregnant. Afraid to discuss this with her parents, she doesn't tell anyone and begins wearing larger, baggy clothes. When she is six months pregnant, her mother finally notices the changes in her daughter and they discuss the pregnancy. Up to this point, Natalia has not been taking any extra nutritional supplements or visiting a doctor. She visits an obstetrician, Dr Janice Ward, for the first time and the health of the baby is assessed. The baby appears to be undersized for its developmental stage with a larger than normal head, but otherwise appears to be normal.

Natalia delivers a baby girl two weeks before her due date and Dr Ward notices a dark hair patch on the baby's lower back, as well as an enlarged head with slightly bulging fontanelles. Dr Ward suggests that the baby be watched carefully during her postnatal growth, since she may have **hydrocephalus** and **spina bifida**. She also convinces Natalia and her parents to allow an ultrasound and MRI of the infant (since exposure to radiation would not be recommended). Upon examination, a slight enlargement of the cerebral ventricles, along with the bulging fontanelles, suggests a developing hydrocephalus. In the lower back, it appears that the posterior aspects of the vertebrae in the lumbar region have not fully developed, but this is difficult to assess since the bones have not fully formed in an infant. With this information, Natalia and her parents take the infant, Joyce, home.

For the next two years, Joyce is taken care of by Natalia and her parents. She develops more slowly than other children her age and, at age two, suffers a convulsion. She is rushed to the hospital where she is treated. The consulting pediatrician, Dr Jeff Broscone, suggests that Joyce has a shunt surgically placed between her fourth ventricle and her abdomen to relieve the pressure that is developing in her brain due to the hydrocephalus (Figure 3.10). Natalia and her parents agree and the surgery is successful in shunting excess cerebrospinal fluid to her abdomen. Dr Broscone also suggests that Joyce's lower back is monitored carefully for any problems with her vertebral growth, as well as monitoring for any neural disturbances in her lower extremities that could be due to compression or compromise of the lumbar spinal nerves.

After her shunt surgery, Joyce continues to develop at a normal pace and, while restricted from participating in contact sports, she maintains a relatively normal lifestyle.

Case 2

Ken and Karen Godfrey are anticipating the birth of their first child. Karen became pregnant at 28 years of age and saw her obstetrician, Dr Pamela Gordon, throughout her pregnancy. She took prenatal vitamins including folic acid, avoided alcohol, and ate a healthy diet. During her prenatal checkups, Dr Gordon examined Karen's child with ultrasound and noted that the child's head appeared smaller than normal. Karen had a normal delivery of a baby boy within one week of the due date. However, on examining the infant, Charles, Dr Gordon noticed that his head was smaller than normal. Upon measurement, it was found that Charles' head was one and a half standard deviations below normal size for an infant of that age and weight. This is not considered **microcephaly** (below two standard deviations), but Dr Gordon suggested that the Godfreys watch the development of Charles closely, especially looking for neurodevelopmental milestones (Figure 3.12).

Over the next five years, Charles develops more slowly than his peers and, when tested, has a lower than normal IQ. His head remains smaller than normal, although not less than two standard deviations below normal. The Godfreys are cautioned that Charles may not achieve normal intellectual development, but otherwise can live a full and healthy life.

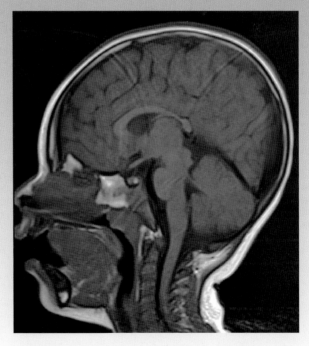

Figure 3.12 A magnetic resonance image of a child with microcephaly. Note that all of the anatomy is correctly positioned, although the overall dimensions of the skull and brain are decreased.

Study questions

1. The neural plate and neural tube develop from the:
a) endoderm
b) mesoderm
c) ectoderm
d) amnion
e) yolk sac

2. The mantle layer of the developing spinal cord is subdivided into two components: the alar plate and the basal plate. The alar plate is for _____, while the basal plate is for _____.
a) Sensation, motor activity
b) motor activity, sensation
c) sympathetic activity, parasympathetic activity
d) parasympathetic activity, sympathetic activity
e) autonomic motor, skeletal motor
f) skeletal motor, autonomic motor

3. All of the following develop from neural crest cells and undergo an epithelial to mesenchymal transition except for:
a) sensory ganglia cells
b) adrenal medullary cells
c) melanocytes
d) odontoblasts
e) ependymal cells

4. Pregnant women should have sufficient _____ in their diet to prevent neural tube defects.
a) fiber
b) folic acid
c) vitamin C
d) vitamin D
e) vitamin A

5. During pregnancy, a woman can consume _____ glasses of beer or wine per day.
a) 0
b) 2
c) 4
d) 6
e) 10

For more self-assessment questions, visit the companion website at
www.wileyessential.com/neuroanatomy

FURTHER READING

For additional information on neuroembryology, the following textbooks and review articles may be helpful:

Blumenfeld H. 2002. *Neuroanatomy Through Clinical Cases*. Sunderland, Massachusetts: Sinauer Associates.

Copp AJ, Greene ND. 2013. Neural tube defects – disorders of neurulation and related embryonic processes. *Wiley Interdiscip Rev Dev Biol*, 2(2): 213–227.

Haines DE. 2012. *Neuroanatomy An Atlas of Structures, Sections, and Systems*. 8th edition. Baltimore, Maryland: Lippincott Williams & Wilkins.

Moore KL, Dalley AF, Agur AMR. 2014. *Moore Clinically Oriented Anatomy*, 7th edition. Lippincott, Williams & Wilkins, Philadelphia.

Netter FH. 2011. *Atlas of Human Anatomy*, 5th edition. Saunders Elsevier, Philadelphia.

Raybaud C, Ahmad T, Rastegar N, Shroff M, Al Nassar M. 2013. The premature brain: developmental and lesional anatomy. *Neuroradiology*, 55 (Suppl 2): 23–40.

Sadler TW. 2010. *Langman's Medical Embryology*, 11th edition. Lippincott, Williams & Wilkins, Philadelphia.

Zerah M, Kulkarni AV. 2013. Spinal cord malformations. *Handb Clin Neurol*, 112: 975–991.

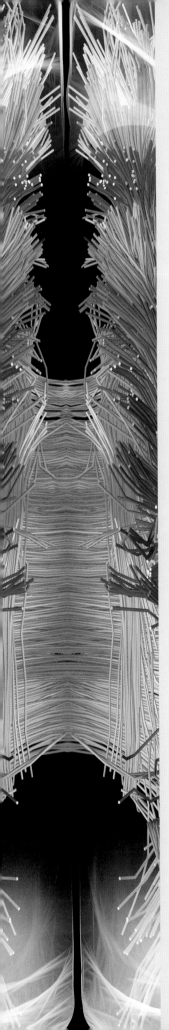

CHAPTER 4
Spinal cord

Learning objectives

1. Describe the relationship between the spinal nerves and the vertebrae.
2. Describe the length and distribution of the spinal cord in the vertebral canal.
3. Identify the meningeal coverings of the spinal cord.
4. Identify the somatotopic organization of the spinal cord gray matter.
5. Identify the major components and pathways of a spinal cord cross section.

Spinal cord structure   50

Relationship of spinal cord with vertebrae
1. Extends to L1/L2 level
2. Thirty-one pairs of spinal nerves
   a) Eight cervical nerves
   b) Twelve thoracic nerves
   c) Five lumbar nerves
   d) Five sacral nerves
   e) One coccygeal nerve
3. First seven cervical nerves exit **above** their respective vertebra
4. C8 exits between C7 and T1 vertebrae
5. All other spinal nerves exit **below** their respective vertebra
6. Conus medullaris
7. Cauda equine
8. Filum terminale (externum and internum)

Spinal cord meninges
1. Epidural space
2. Dura mater
3. Subdural space
4. Arachnoid mater
5. Subarachnoid space – cerebrospinal fluid
6. Pia mater – denticulate ligaments

Spinal cord cross section
1. Gray matter
   a) Anterior (ventral) horn
      i. Somatic motor – skeletal muscle
      ii. Cervical enlargement (C5–T1)
      iii. Lumbosacral enlargement (L1–S3)
      iv. Anterior (ventral) rootlets – ventral root

Essential Clinical Neuroanatomy, First Edition. Thomas H. Champney.
© 2016 John Wiley & Sons, Ltd. Published 2016 by John Wiley & Sons, Ltd.
Companion website: www.wileyessential.com/neuroanatomy

Introduction

In the next six chapters, the regional anatomy of the central nervous system will be covered. This will begin at the spinal cord and then proceed rostrally through the medulla oblongata, pons, midbrain, cerebrum, and cerebellum. The major focus of these chapters will be the anatomical arrangement of the nuclei and tracts, with the function of these structures provided secondarily. The chapters following this anatomical introduction will attempt to consolidate these individual regions into a coherent whole. This will take place by discussing the entire extent of individual pathways, focusing on their function and their deficits when lesioned.

Spinal cord relationships

Remember that the spinal cord is made of five distinct regions: the cervical region with eight cervical nerves, the thoracic region with 12 thoracic nerves, the lumbar region with five lumbar nerves, the sacral region with five sacral nerves, and the coccygeal region with one coccygeal nerve. This produces a total of 31 pairs of spinal nerves.

While there are eight cervical nerves, there are only seven cervical vertebrae. Therefore, the first seven cervical nerves exit above their respective vertebrae while the eighth cervical nerves exit between the seventh cervical and first thoracic vertebrae. All other spinal nerves exit below their respective vertebrae (Figure 4.1).

Recall that the spinal cord is housed in the vertebral canal. The extent of the spinal cord within the canal is not equal. The spinal cord begins at the foramen magnum and descends through the vertebral canal to the first or second lumbar vertebrae (L1 or L2). Therefore the spinal cord is shorter than the vertebral canal. Those nerves that exit the spinal cord in the cervical region, exit horizontally through their associated intervertebral foramina. Those nerves that exit the spinal cord more distally, such as the lower thoracic and lumbar spinal nerves, must descend in the vertebral canal to reach their associated intervertebral foramina. Therefore, below the level of the second lumbar vertebrae, only descending spinal nerve roots are observed, with no intervening spinal cord. This collection of descending spinal nerve roots is termed the **cauda equina**.

The distal end of the spinal cord narrows as it ends and is termed the **conus medullaris**. At the end of the conus medullaris, the pia mater continues as a small thread distally within the vertebral canal, to attach at the coccygeal region (the filum terminale internum). The extension of the dura mater at the distal end of the vertebral canal is the filum terminale externum.

The spinal meninges, the connective tissue layer coverings of the spinal cord, extend throughout the vertebral canal. The outermost layer, the **dura mater**, has a small space between it and the vertebral canal. This is the **epidural space** and contains small amounts of fat and venous blood vessels. Clinically, anesthetic can be injected into this region, which then diffuses through the dura mater to anesthetize the local spinal nerves. Deep to the dura mater, is a small potential space (the subdural

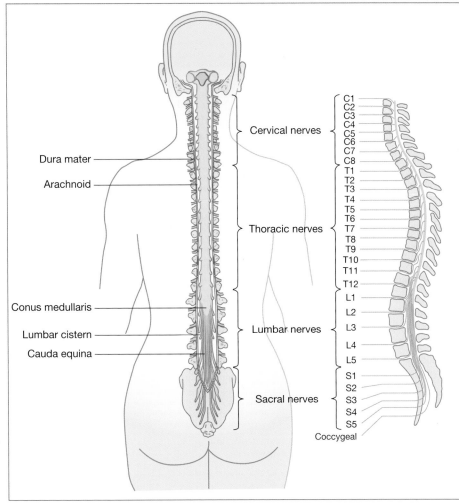

Figure 4.1 The five regions of the spinal cord with their associated spinal nerves. Note that the spinal cord ends at the upper lumbar vertebral levels (L1 or L2) and that the spinal nerves descend through the vertebral canal to exit below their respective vertebra.

space). The **arachnoid mater** extends from the surface of the spinal cord (pia mater) to the dura mater. The arachnoid mater is made of filamentous connective tissue and therefore creates a space amongst these filaments, the **subarachnoid space**. The subarachnoid space contains the cerebrospinal fluid, which circulates around the spinal cord, acting as a liquid buffer and shock absorber. The **pia mater** is a thin layer of connective tissue that tightly adheres to the spinal cord. From the lateral edges of the spinal cord portions of pia mater extend laterally to attach to the dura mater and provide additional support for the spinal cord. These lateral extensions of pia mater are denticulate (dentate) ligaments.

Spinal cord anatomy

The spinal cord is made of two major regions: the **gray matter** that contains neuronal cell bodies, as well as axons, and the **white matter** that contains only axons. Recall that they received their names because, when viewed with the naked eye, the gray matter (with less myelin) appeared darker in color than the white matter (which has a greater ratio of myelin wrapped axons) (Figure 4.2).

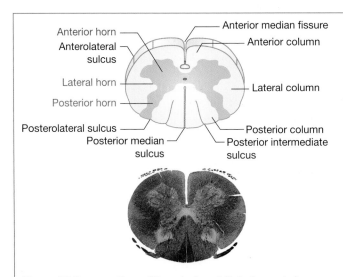

Figure 4.2 Cross sections of the spinal cord. Note the central gray matter divided into three regions (anterior, lateral, and posterior horns). Also the peripheral white matter is divided into three regions (anterior, lateral, and posterior columns). The anterior horn and columns are associated with motor (efferent) functions, while the posterior horn and columns are associated with sensory (afferent) functions.

Gray matter

The gray matter of the spinal cord is subdivided into various regions, with the largest being the **anterior (ventral) horn**. The anterior horn contains the neuronal cell bodies that innervate skeletal muscle. This is referred to as somatic (voluntary) motor innervation as opposed to visceral (involuntary) motor innervation that innervates cardiac and smooth muscle. Since the upper and lower extremities contain large quantities of skeletal muscle, there are corresponding enlargements within the spinal cord to accommodate the increased numbers of motor neurons necessary to drive these muscles. The cervical enlargement (C5–T1) is responsible for the upper extremity, while the lumbosacral enlargement (L1–S3) is responsible for the lower extremity. The motor axons which leave the spinal cord do so through an **anterior (ventral) root**. Therefore, the anterior root is a motor root containing efferent motor fibers.

Another region of gray matter in the spinal cord is the **lateral horn** (intermediolateral cell column), which is adjacent to the anterior horn. The lateral horn is enlarged in the thoracic and upper lumbar regions, as well as the upper sacral region of the spinal cord. The neuronal cell bodies within this column are responsible for visceral (involuntary) motor innervation to smooth muscles. This is the location of preganglionic autonomic nerve cell bodies. **Preganglionic sympathetic** nerve cell bodies are located between the first thoracic and second lumbar spinal segments (T1–L2) and provide all of the preganglionic sympathetic fibers for the body. **Preganglionic parasympathetic** nerve cell bodies are located between the second sacral and fourth sacral spinal segments (S2–S4). These preganglionic parasympathetic cell bodies provide innervation to the smooth muscles of the lower gastrointestinal tract, the bladder, and the reproductive organs.

The third region of gray matter in the spinal cord is the **posterior (dorsal) horn**, which is where sensory neuronal cell bodies reside. Peripheral receptors activate sensory nerves, which course with the major nerves throughout the body and enter the spinal cord through the **posterior (dorsal) roots**. Just prior to entering the spinal cord, the posterior (dorsal) roots have an enlargement where their cell bodies are found, the **posterior (dorsal) root ganglia**. Recall that these cell bodies are part of a **pseudounipolar neuron**, with a short projection into the central nervous system and a longer projection from the periphery to the ganglion. Once the sensory nerve enters the spinal cord through the posterior horn, it has a number of options available. It can synapse on an interneuron and this interneuron can project to a corresponding motor neuron, producing a fast-acting reflex response (Figure 4.3). The sensory nerve can also ascend in the spinal cord to the medulla oblongata, where it will synapse.

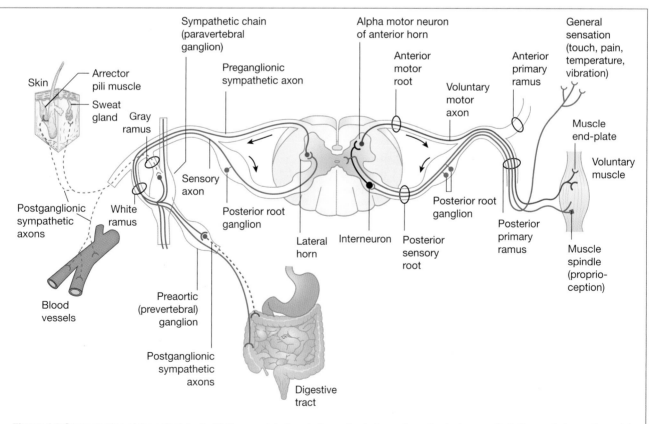

Figure 4.3 Cross section of the spinal cord with its associated posterior and anterior roots and spinal nerve. Note the posterior roots contain sensory (afferent) fibers (along with their cell bodies in the posterior root ganglion), while the ventral root contains motor (efferent) axons.

Clinical box 4.1

The sensory distribution of each spinal nerve displayed on the body is a dermatome. The specific dermatomal distribution is clinically relevant, because it indicates at which level of the spinal cord an injury has occurred. By testing for regional loss of sensation, a clinician can determine whether the neural loss is due to a peripheral nerve lesion or to a central spinal cord injury. If the sensory loss is displayed in a dermatomal pattern, then the clinician is able to pinpoint the damage to a specific spinal cord level. Note the characteristic banding of the dermatomes over the body. Notably important dermatome spinal cord levels are C6 for the thumb, C7 for the middle finger and C8 for the fifth digit; T4 for the nipple, T10 for the umbilicus, L5 for the first (big) toe, S1 for the last (small) toe and S5 for the anal region.

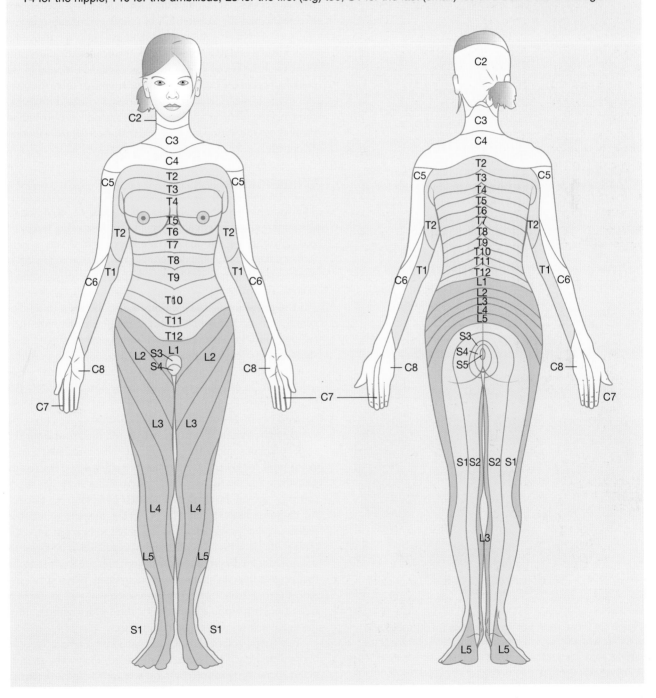

Clinical box 4.2

The gray matter of the spinal cord has been subdivided into ten Rexed regions based on the types of neurons present and the specific functional attributes of the regions. Six of these Rexed laminae (indicated by Roman numerals) are found in the posterior (dorsal) horn and contain neuronal relay nuclei for afferent (sensory) nerve fibers. One of the layers (the nucleus dorsalis (of Clarke)) is only found in the lower spinal cord and is a large proprioceptive relay nucleus sending information to the cerebellum.

The lateral horn contains the autonomic efferent (motor) cell bodies: the preganglionic sympathetic cell bodies (T1–L2) and the preganglionic parasympathetic cell bodies (S2–S4). This region is Rexed lamina VII.

The anterior (ventral) horn contains the cell bodies for the skeletal motor efferent fibers and is the ninth Rexed lamina (IX). This lamina has a medial, central, and lateral component that contains cell bodies that are specific for medial musculature (neck and trunk) and lateral musculature (extremities) respectively.

While these neuroanatomical distinctions are histologically and physiologically definable, trauma to the spinal cord will generally affect large portions of the gray matter, with little regard to the distribution of neurons in the Rexed laminae.

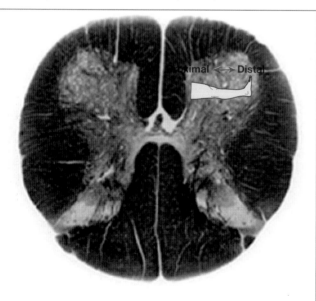

Figure 4.4 Cross section of the spinal cord with its associated posterior and anterior horns and columns. Note that within the anterior horn, the distribution of motor neurons is precisely arranged, with neurons providing distal muscles in the lateral aspect of the horn, while neurons providing proximal muscles are located in the medial portion of the horn. This organized arrangement of neurons is described as a somatotopic distribution.

Recall that the spinal nerves are mixed nerves with both sensory and motor axons. Compare this to the posterior and anterior roots that contain only sensory or motor axons respectively. Therefore, a loss of a spinal nerve will produce a loss of motor and sensory function, while the loss of one of the roots of a spinal nerve will only produce a loss of one modality, either sensory or motor (Figure 4.3).

An important concept that will be developed throughout this text is the highly specific distribution of axons within a neuronal region. In the anterior horn of the spinal cord, this is exemplified by the distribution of motor neurons throughout the horn. This distribution is not random, but is specific and is anatomically oriented. For example, the neurons that drive the muscles of the lateral side of the hand would be located in the lateral aspect of the horn, while the neurons that drive the muscles of the medial side of the hand would be located medial to those neurons. This produces a specific anatomical distribution throughout the ventral horn termed a somatotopic distribution (Figure 4.4).

White matter

The white matter of the spinal cord is made of ascending or descending axons, referred to as tracts. The **ascending tracts** are generally bringing information into the central nervous system (sensory axons), while the **descending tracts** are bringing information to the spinal cord from upper portions of the central nervous system.

The **posterior (dorsal) columns** are ascending tracts that contain the sensory axons from the periphery that have their cell bodies in the posterior (dorsal) root ganglia and send their central projection into the spinal cord through the posterior root and posterior horn. These axons continue into the white matter that is posterior and medial to the posterior horn – the posterior (dorsal) columns. The axons ascend through the spinal cord in a highly organized fashion, with the axons from the lower extremity more medially placed and the axons from the upper extremity more laterally placed. These medially placed axons from the lower extremity are referred to as the **fasciculus gracilis**, while the more laterally placed axons from the upper extremity are the **fasciculus cuneatus**. Therefore, the fasciculus cuneatus is not found in the lower thoracic or lumbar regions of the spinal cord. It is presumed to begin at approximately the sixth thoracic (T6) spinal cord level. The axons in the columns are **first order axons**, since they are the first axons that project into the central nervous system. When they synapse, the next axon in the communication pathway would be a second order neuron, followed by a third order neuron, until the signal reaches the cortex (Figure 4.5).

The lateral columns of white matter contain both ascending (sensory) tracts and descending (motor) tracts. The ascending tracts are the **spinocerebellar tracts** and the **spinothalamic tracts**. The spinocerebellar tracts are subdivided into anterior (ventral) and posterior (dorsal) tracts – both sets of tracts projecting to the cerebellum, but each taking a different route.

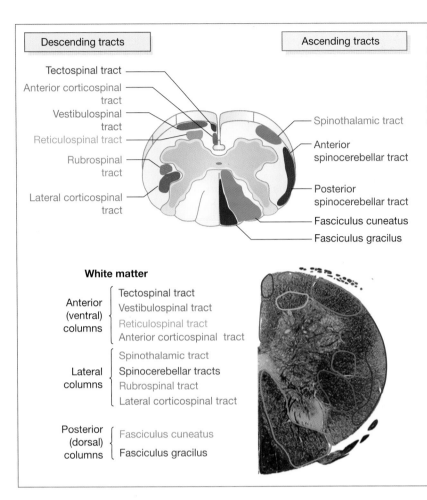

Descending tracts		Ascending tracts

Tectospinal tract

Anterior corticospinal tract

Vestibulospinal tract

Reticulospinal tract

Rubrospinal tract

Lateral corticospinal tract

Spinothalamic tract

Anterior spinocerebellar tract

Posterior spinocerebellar tract

Fasciculus cuneatus

Fasciculus gracilus

White matter

Anterior (ventral) columns
- Tectospinal tract
- Vestibulospinal tract
- Reticulospinal tract
- Anterior corticospinal tract

Lateral columns
- Spinothalamic tract
- Spinocerebellar tracts
- Rubrospinal tract
- Lateral corticospinal tract

Posterior (dorsal) columns
- Fasciculus cuneatus
- Fasciculus gracilus

Figure 4.5 The white matter tracts in the spinal cord contain ascending (sensory) fibers (in green) and descending fibers (in reds or browns). The descending fibers can provide motor (efferent) information to the spinal cord (red) or descending sensory information from the brain to the spinal cord (brown).

Details of the spinocerebellar tracts will be discussed in the chapter on the cerebellum, but, at this point, it is relevant to know that these tracts provide information to the cerebellum about the positioning of the limbs and trunk in space (proprioception). The **spinothalamic tracts** (also referred to as the anterolateral system) are composed of second order sensory neurons whose cell bodies are in the posterior (dorsal) horn on the opposite (contralateral) side of the tract. These axons carry pain and temperature information to the thalamus and the cortex. Therefore, pain and temperature sensory information from the right upper extremity synapses in the right posterior horn and the second order neurons project to the left side of the spinal cord (contralateral side) through the **anterior white commissure** and ascend in the spinothalamic tract. This is typical of many second order sensory neurons; they decussate (cross over) and ascend on the contralateral side. A collection of second order axons can also be referred to as a **lemniscus** and, therefore, the spinothalamic tract can be called the **spinothalamic lemniscus**. This is important clinically because the pathway for pain and temperature is physically separated from the general sensation pathway at the level of the spinal cord. This means that patients with spinal cord lesions may present with a loss of pain and temperature on one side of the body and a loss of general sensation on the opposite side of the body. This is an important concept to keep in mind when assessing patients with spinal cord lesions (Figure 4.5).

The lateral columns of white matter also contain descending (motor) tracts. These tracts include the **lateral corticospinal tract** and the **rubrospinal tract**. The lateral corticospinal tract is the primary descending tract in the spinal cord. It carries upper motor neurons from the cortex to the anterior (ventral) horn of the spinal cord to drive peripheral skeletal muscle. This is a clinically important tract, since it is responsible for the major innervation of skeletal muscles below the neck. The **rubrospinal tract** descends through the spinal cord from the red nucleus of the midbrain (an area to be discussed in future chapters) to the anterior horn of the spinal cord in the cervical and upper thoracic levels. The relevance of the rubrospinal tract is still being debated (Figure 4.5).

The third and final group of tracts in the white matter of the spinal cord are the descending tracts in the anterior (ventral) column. There are four primary descending tracts in the anterior column: the **anterior corticospinal tract**, the **tectospinal tract**, the **reticulospinal tract**, and the **vestibulospinal tract**. The names of these tracts designate the origin and the endpoint for each of these tracts. The **anterior corticospinal**

tract carries fibers from the cortex to the anterior horn and is thought to direct skeletal muscle action for trunk musculature. This is a smaller tract with less clinical significance then the lateral corticospinal tract. However, when the lateral corticospinal tract is lesioned, some muscular function may remain due to the presence of the anterior corticospinal tract. The other three descending tracts carry information from higher levels of the central nervous system to the spinal cord. Therefore, although they are descending tracts, they are not driving skeletal muscle action directly. For example, the **tectospinal tract** arises in the tectum of the midbrain and carries visual and auditory information to the upper spinal cord for head and neck reflex action. The **reticulospinal tract** arises from the reticular system within the pons and medulla of the brain stem and is responsible for modifying motor activity and muscle tone in the spinal cord,

mediating autonomic (sympathetic and parasympathetic) action in the spinal cord and other reflex functions. The **vestibulospinal tract** arises from the vestibular nuclei and provides balance information to the spinal cord. All of these tracts provide a variety of sensory information to the spinal cord for integration of spinal cord function, primarily reflex adjustments for posture and balance (Figure 4.5) (Table 4.1).

Central canal

Within the central portion of the gray matter is a small tubular structure, the **central canal**. The central canal is lined by ependymal cells and contains cerebrospinal fluid. Recall from the second chapter that the central canal is part of the central cerebrospinal fluid system (Figure 4.6).

Table 4.1 White matter tracts found in the spinal cord. Note that the posterior columns contain ascending tracts, while the anterior columns contain descending tracts. The lateral columns contain both ascending and descending tracts.

Spinal Cord Tracts

Posterior (dorsal) columns – ascending tracts (sensory: fine touch, proprioception)
    Fasciculus gracilis – lower extremity
    Fasciculus cuneatus – upper extremity

Lateral columns – ascending and descending tracts
    Lateral corticospinal tract – descending (motor: skeletal muscle)
    Rubrospinal tract – descending (motor: cerebellum to skeletal muscle)
    Spinothalamic (anterolateral) tract – ascending (sensory: pain and temperature)
    Posterior (dorsal) spinocerebellar – ascending (sensory: proprioception to cerebellum)
    Anterior (ventral) spinocerebellar – ascending (sensory: proprioception to cerebellum)

Anterior (ventral) columns – descending tracts
    Anterior corticospinal tract – descending (motor: skeletal muscle)
    Vestibulospinal tract – descending (sensory: vestibular, balance to motor neurons)
    Reticulospinal tract – descending (sensory: pain gating, autonomic to motor neurons)
    Tectospinal tract – descending (sensory: visual to cervical motor neurons)

Figure 4.6 The central canal of the spinal cord (indicated by the arrows) is lined with ependymal cells and contains cerebrospinal fluid.

Central canal

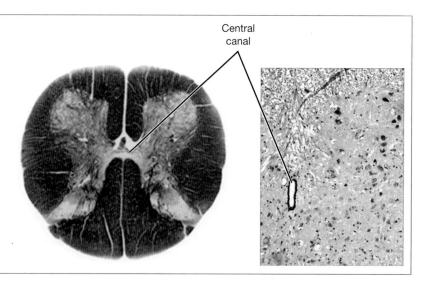

Intervertebral foramen

When the anterior root and the posterior root join together to form a **spinal nerve**, the nerve exits the vertebral canal through an **intervertebral foramen** (a space formed by the two vertebrae). Any compression in the intervertebral foramen can damage the spinal nerve passing through the space. This would produce both motor and sensory losses from the same (**ipsilateral**) side as the side of compression. Sensory deficits usually precede motor deficits, since the sensory axons are more sensitive.

Intervertebral discs

Between the individual vertebral bodies are connective tissue structures that act as shock absorbers and "spacers" for the vertebrae. These **intervertebral discs** have an inner gelatinous substance, the **nucleus pulposus**, and an outer fibrous ring, the **annulus fibrosus**. (Figure 4.7) Clinically, these discs can degenerate with age and, when under pressure, can herniate (or bulge) into the vertebral canal or the intervertebral foramen. This herniated disc compresses the anterior portion of the spinal cord or the spinal nerve within the intervertebral foramen. Consider how these two points of compression could produce different symptoms in patients.

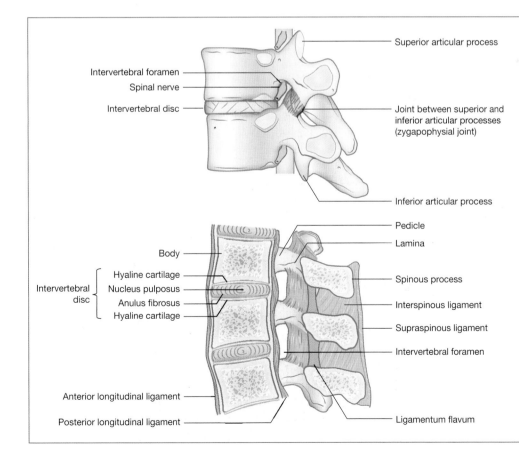

Figure 4.7 The vertebral column with the vertebrae, intervertebral discs, and the intervertebral foramena. Note how each spinal nerve passes through an intervertebral foramen and how a herniated intervertebral disc could place pressure on the anterior spinal cord or the spinal nerve.

Clinical box 4.4

The vascular supply to the spinal cord consists of spinal arteries that run the length of the spinal cord. There are two posterior spinal arteries found near the posterior (dorsal) horns and one anterior spinal artery found near the anterior median fissure. Each posterior spinal artery supplies a posterior (dorsal) horn (gray matter) and its associated posterior (dorsal) columns (white matter). The anterior spinal artery supplies anterior (ventral) horns and lateral horns (gray matter) as well as the anterior (ventral) columns and lateral columns (white matter). Notice that the anterior spinal artery supplies both the left and right sides of the anterior spinal cord. Therefore, the loss of the anterior spinal artery can produce large neural deficits – generally efferent (motor) deficits.

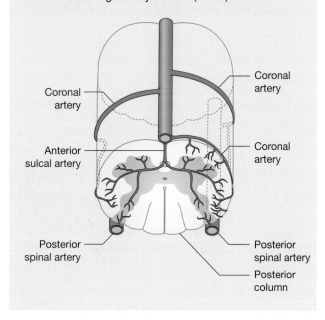

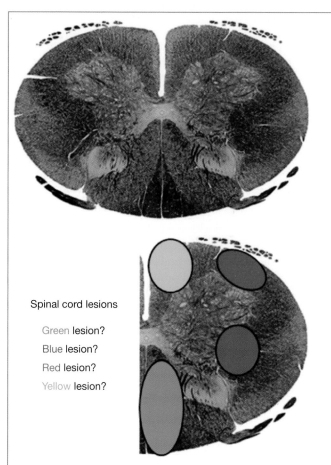

Spinal cord lesions

Green lesion?

Blue lesion?

Red lesion?

Yellow lesion?

Figure 4.8 For each of the colored lesions, identify the clinical loss that would occur (sensory or motor deficit on the same (ipsilateral) or opposite (contralateral) side of the body), as well as the actual white matter tracts damaged by the lesion.

Clinical considerations

One take home message from this chapter should be that the spinal cord has a central region (**gray matter**) that contains neural cell bodies for incoming sensory information and for outgoing motor control, as well as an outer region (**white matter**) that contains axons either ascending to the upper portions of the central nervous system or descending axons from the brain stem and cortex. Realize that a **complete transection of the spinal cord** will damage both regions, but that the damage to the white matter is more detrimental since all connections with the spinal cord distal to the lesion are lost. Therefore, a lesion at the T4 level produces a gray matter loss of T4 neuronal cell bodies and, more importantly, a loss of all the axons in the white matter distal to T4. No sensory innervation will ascend past T4 and no motor control will be able to descend below T4. Consider the ramifications of a lesion of this type on both the sensory and motor symptoms. Would pain and temperature be affected to the same degree as general sensation? (See Figure 4.8.)

Case 1

Jack Robinson, a 46-year-old roofer, falls from the ladder while trying to climb down from the roof. He falls on his back, hitting a rock at his T2 vertebra, shattering the vertebra and damaging the underlying spinal cord. He is rushed immediately to a nearby emergency room where he is treated for the vertebral fracture and other small injuries. During Mr Robinson's initial assessment in the emergency room, Dr Kimberly Hastings tests his upper and lower extremities for motor and sensory function. All of Mr Robinson's motor and sensory functions are normal in his upper extremities, head, and neck, but he has deficits in his trunk and lower extremities. During careful testing, it is found that he can't feel general sensation over most of his abdomen and both of his lower extremities as well as having a loss of most motor control in his lower extremities. By consulting a **dermatome map**, Dr Hastings concludes that Mr Robinson has damaged his spinal cord at the T4 or T5 level (Figure 4.9). Recall that the vertebral level and the spinal cord level are not the same, so that a fracture of a vertebra will generally affect a lower portion of the spinal cord.

Since Mr Robinson has damaged his entire cord at that level, he loses all sensation (pain, temperature, and general sensation) because both sides of the cord are damaged. If he had only hemi-sected his spinal cord, Mr Robinson would have lost general sensation from the ipsilateral side of the lesion, while losing pain and temperature from the contralateral side of the lesion. Why would this difference in loss of sensation occur?

After being stabilized, Dr Hastings arranged for Mr Robinson to be transferred to a regional spinal cord injury center where he was able to receive extended treatment for his spinal cord injury. With excellent treatment and persistence by Mr Robinson, he was able to regain some function of his lower extremities, although he was unable to make a full recovery.

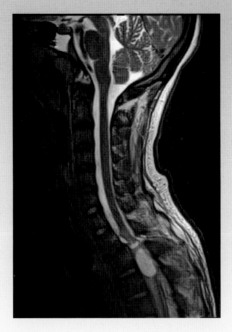

Figure 4.9 Sagittal margnetic resonance image (MRI) of a patient with a complete spinal cord transection. Note the transection occurred at the T2 vertebral level, producing a lower thoracic spinal cord injury.

Case 2

Mrs Carolyn Kennedy, an overweight 82-year-old widow, experiences tingling sensations on her left leg and onto her foot. This is especially apparent after she has been standing for a long period of time. This can be slightly relieved by lying down. It begins to interfere with her daily activities, so she mentions it to her general internist, Dr Scott Chambers, at her next visit. Dr Chambers suspects that she has a herniated disc that is causing compression on her fifth lumbar spinal nerve where it exits the intervertebral foramen. He recommends that Mrs Kennedy have an MRI of her lower spine to determine if there is a herniated disc (Figure 4.10).

After undergoing the procedure, Mrs Kennedy met with Dr Chambers, who showed her a protrusion of the intervertebral disc between her fourth and fifth lumbar vertebrae, which was causing compression of the fifth lumbar spinal nerve exiting just below that point. Because of her age and condition, Dr Chambers recommended a non-invasive course of action, since surgical repair of the herniation could be problematic for Mrs Kennedy. He suggested that she receive corticosteroid injections in the local area to reduce inflammation, that she attempt to lose some weight (putting less strain on the lumbar vertebrae), and that she limit placing her full weight on the vertebrae. He also suggested that physical therapy might be beneficial.

While these treatments all provided some relief to Mrs Kennedy, they did not alleviate the condition and she continued to have symptoms related to the nerve compression until she died peacefully in her sleep at age 86.

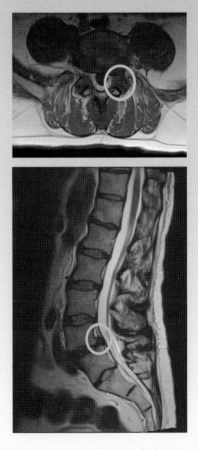

Figure 4.10 Magnetic resonance images (axial and sagittal) of a herniated intervertebral disc between L4 and L5. Note the bulging disc on the patient's left side (axial view).

Study questions

1. The seventh cervical nerve exits _____ its respective vertebra and the fifth thoracic nerve exists _____ its respective vertebra.
a) above, above
b) below, below
c) above, below
d) below, above

2. A lesion of the posterior (dorsal) columns of the spinal cord damages:
a) ipsilateral, first order sensory axons
b) contralateral, first order sensory axons
c) ipsilateral, second order sensory axons
d) contralateral, second order sensory axons
e) ipsilateral, upper motor corticospinal axons
f) contralateral, upper motor corticopinal axons

3. A lesion produces damage to both ascending and descending tracts in the spinal cord. The only place this lesion could be found is in the:
a) posterior (dorsal) columns
b) lateral columns
c) anterior (ventral) columns
d) central columns
e) rostral columns

4. The anterior (ventral) horns of gray matter in the spinal cord are largest in the
a) cervical and thoracic sections
b) cervical and lumbar sections
c) thoracic and lumbar sections
d) thoracic and sacral sections
e) cervical and sacral sections

5. Preganglionic autonomic cell bodies are found in the lateral gray matter of the spinal cord in the:
a) cervical and thoracic sections
b) cervical and lumbar sections
c) thoracic and lumbar sections
d) thoracic and coccygeal sections
e) cervical and sacral sections

For more self-assessment questions, visit the companion website at
www.wileyessential.com/neuroanatomy

FURTHER READING

For additional information on the spinal cord, the following textbooks and review articles may be helpful:

Bican O, Minagar A, Pruitt AA. 2013. The spinal cord: a review of functional neuroanatomy. *Neurol Clin*, 31(1): 1–18.

Blumenfeld H. 2002. *Neuroanatomy Through Clinical Cases*. Sinauer Associates, Sunderland, Massachusetts.

Felten DL, Shetty A. 2009. *Netter's Atlas of Neuroscience*, 2nd edition. Saunders Elsevier, Philadelphia, Pennsylvania.

Haines DE. 2012. *Neuroanatomy: An Atlas of Structures, Sections and Systems*, 8th edition. Lippincott Williams & Wilkin, Baltimore, Maryland.

Moore KL, Dalley AF, Agur AMR. 2014. *Moore Clinically Oriented Anatomy*, 7th edition. Lippincott, Williams & Wilkins, Philadelphia, Pennsylvania.

Patestas MA, Gartner LP. 2006. *A Textbook of Neuroanatomy*. Blackwell Publishing, Malden, Massachusetts.

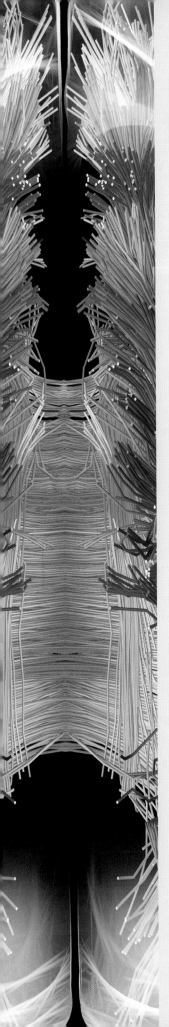

CHAPTER 5
Medulla oblongata

Learning objectives

1. Identify the major structures seen on cross sections of the medulla oblongata.
2. Describe and identify the major components of cranial nerves IX–XII.
3. Describe the major functions of cranial nerves IX–XII.
4. Localize lesions in the medulla oblongata based on provided symptoms.

Essential Clinical Neuroanatomy, First Edition. Thomas H. Champney.
© 2016 John Wiley & Sons, Ltd. Published 2016 by John Wiley & Sons, Ltd.
Companion website: www.wileyessential.com/neuroanatomy

Introduction

In this chapter, the ascending white matter tracts presented in the spinal cord will be followed into the **medulla oblongata** of the **brain stem** as they pass to higher levels of the central nervous system. Likewise, the descending white matter tracts will be followed as they pass through the medulla. Finally, the cranial nerve nuclei and other associated nuclei found in the medulla oblongata will be discussed. One take home message for the medulla oblongata is that this is a major site for **decussation** – where axons from one side cross over to the opposite (contralateral) side.

Brain stem anatomy

The brain stem is the structure that connects the spinal cord, the cerebrum, and the cerebellum, and is where the majority of the cranial nerve nuclei and tracts originate. The brain stem is made of three components; the **medulla oblongata**, the **pons**, and the **midbrain**. The medulla connects the spinal cord with the pons and is the site of the lower four cranial nerves and their nuclei (cranial nerves IX–XII). The pons contains the majority of axons that pass into and out of the cerebellum (the pontocerebellar tracts) along with the fifth through eighth cranial nerves (V–VIII) and their associated nuclei. The midbrain is the most superior portion of the brain stem and contains axons of passage along with the third and fourth cranial nerves (III and IV) and their associated nuclei (Figures 5.1, 5.2, 5.3, 5.4). Each of these components will be covered in a separate chapter.

Anatomy of the medulla oblongata

The medulla appears as the superior dilated portion of the spinal cord. The medulla's inferior border is at the **foramen magnum**, just superior to the first cervical nerves, and its superior border is at the **pontomedullary junction**. From an anterior view, there are two long parallel ridges medially that are called the **pyramids** and contain the axons of the **corticospinal tracts**. Just lateral to these ridges are two bulges referred to as the **inferior olives**. Between the pyramid and the inferior olive on each side is a groove, the **preolivary sulcus**. Likewise, on the opposite (more lateral) side of the inferior olive is another

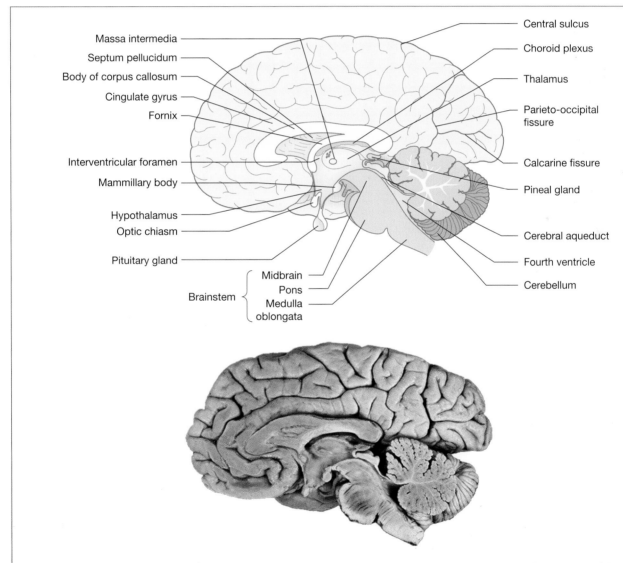

Figure 5.1 The three major regions of the brain stem (the midbrain, the pons, and the medulla oblongata) on a sagittal section of the brain.

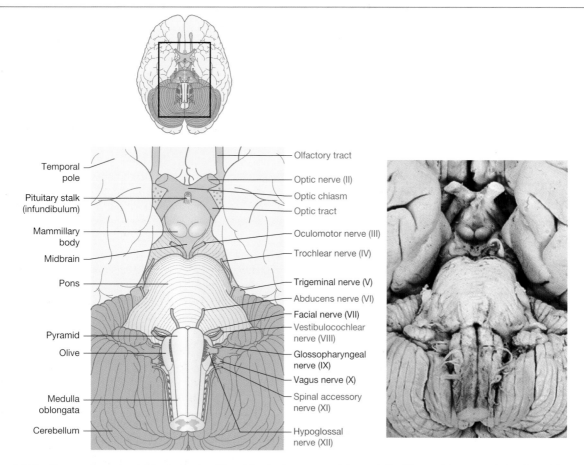

Figure 5.2 The three major regions of the brain stem (the midbrain, the pons, and the medulla oblongata) on a sagittal section of the brain. Identify as many of the structures on this photograph using the labels from Figure 5.1.

groove, the **postolivary sulcus**. Specific cranial nerves exit from each of these sulci and can be used as anatomic landmarks (cranial nerve XII (hypoglossal) from the preolivary sulcus and cranial nerves IX (glossopharyngeal) and X (vagus) from the postolivary sulcus) (Figure 5.3). From a posterior view, two small parallel ridges are seen on both sides and these represent the **nucleus gracilis** and **nucleus cuneatus**: the sensory nuclei for the axons in the posterior (dorsal) columns of the spinal cord (Figure 5.4).

Cross section of the caudal medulla oblongata

When examining a cross section of the medulla, it is important to recognize the nuclei and tracts present at that level. Recall that the clinical cross-section views are an inferior view, with posterior at the lower part of the field and anterior at the upper part of the field (as if you are looking at the patient from the foot of their bed while they are supine – on their back). If a portion of the medulla were damaged (lesioned) then knowing the nuclei present, the tracts that pass through, and their relationships can lead to an accurate diagnosis of the problem. The

Temporal pole
Pituitary stalk (infundibulum)
Mammillary body
Midbrain
Pons
Pyramid
Olive
Medulla oblongata
Cerebellum

Olfactory tract
Optic nerve (II)
Optic chiasm
Optic tract
Oculomotor nerve (III)
Trochlear nerve (IV)
Trigeminal nerve (V)
Abducens nerve (VI)
Facial nerve (VII)
Vestibulocochlear nerve (VIII)
Glossopharyngeal nerve (IX)
Vagus nerve (X)
Spinal accessory nerve (XI)
Hypoglossal nerve (XII)

Figure 5.3 The three major regions of the brain stem (the midbrain, the pons, and the medulla oblongata) from an inferior view of the brain. Note the cranial nerves associated with each region.

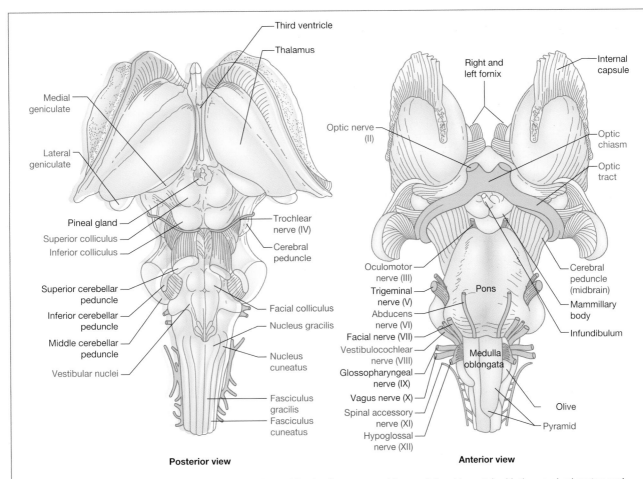

Figure 5.4 The three major regions of the brain stem (the midbrain, the pons, and the medulla oblongata) with the cerebral cortex and cerebellum removed. Note the cranial nerves associated with each region.

caudal medulla can be particularly problematic since both sensory and motor fibers **decussate** (cross over) at this point. Therefore, lesions at this level of the medulla can produce major functional losses.

There are two types of sensory nuclei present in the caudal medulla. The **nucleus gracilis** and **nucleus cuneatus** contain second order sensory cell bodies that have synapsed with axons that travel through the fasciculus gracilis and cuneatus in the spinal cord. The axons from these nuclei **decussate** (cross over) from one side to the other and then ascend in the **medial lemniscus** to synapse in the **thalamus**. As a general rule, as soon as first order sensory neurons synapse on second order cell bodies, the second order axons decussate to the other side (recall this happened in the spinal cord with the spinothalamic tract). Likewise, when the term lemniscus is used, it refers to decussated second order sensory axons – in this case, second order sensory axons for fine touch and proprioception from one side of the body below the head. The other type of sensory nucleus present in the caudal medulla is the **spinal nucleus of the trigeminal nerve (V)**

(Figures 5.5, 5.6). It contains second order cell bodies for general sensation, pain, and temperature from the face, nasal cavity, oral cavity, pharynx, and larynx. It will be described in greater detail in subsequent sections.

The tracts found in the caudal medulla include the continuation of ascending and descending tracts that were found in the spinal cord. The ascending tracts include the terminal ends of the **fasciculus gracilis and cuneatus**, where they synapse on the cell bodies in the **nucleus gracilis and cuneatus**, respectively. The ascending **spinocerebellar tracts** pass through the lateral medulla on their way to the cerebellum, while the ascending, second order **spinothalamic tracts** travel through the lateral medulla on their way to the **thalamus**, carrying pain and temperature information from the contralateral side of the body. Recall that the descending **corticospinal tracts** travel through the spinal cord bringing cortical motor information to the spinal cord. These same axons are found in the **pyramids** in the medulla, where they **decussate** to form the **lateral corticopinal tracts**. The other descending tracts in the spinal cord (**rubrospinal,**

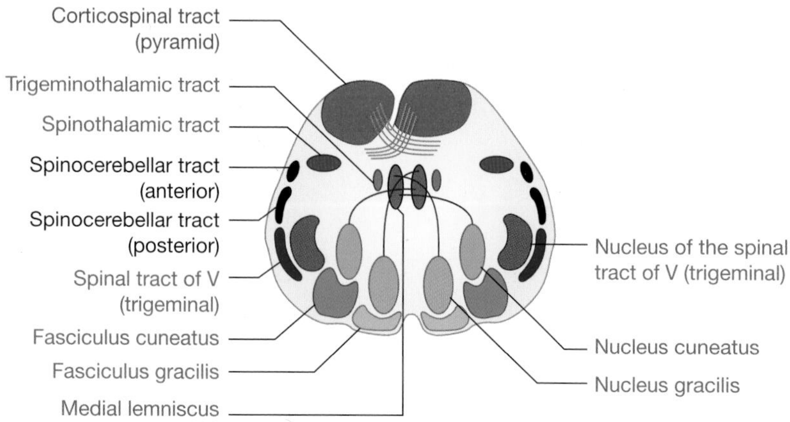

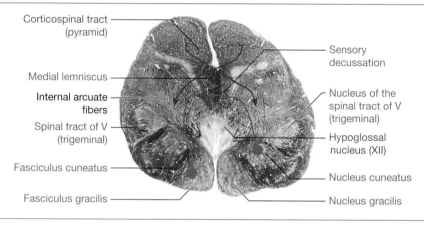

Corticospinal tract (pyramid)
Trigeminothalamic tract
Spinothalamic tract
Spinocerebellar tract (anterior)
Spinocerebellar tract (posterior)
Spinal tract of V (trigeminal)
Fasciculus cuneatus
Fasciculus gracilis
Medial lemniscus

Nucleus of the spinal tract of V (trigeminal)
Nucleus cuneatus
Nucleus gracilis

Figure 5.5 A drawing of a clinically oriented cross section through the caudal medulla oblongata. Note the three sensory nuclei present (the nucleus gracilis, the nucleus cuneatus, and the nucleus of the spinal tract of the trigeminal). Also, note the decussation of the second order sensory axons into the medial lemniscus, along with the decussation of the motor axons in the corticospinal tract.

Corticospinal tract (pyramid)
Medial lemniscus
Internal arcuate fibers
Spinal tract of V (trigeminal)
Fasciculus cuneatus
Fasciculus gracilis

Sensory decussation
Nucleus of the spinal tract of V (trigeminal)
Hypoglossal nucleus (XII)
Nucleus cuneatus
Nucleus gracilis

Figure 5.6 A myelin-stained clinically oriented cross section through the caudal medulla oblongata. Note the lighter staining sensory nuclei present (the nucleus gracilis, the nucleus cuneatus, and the nucleus of the spinal tract of the trigeminal). Also, note the decussation of the second order sensory axons into the medial lemniscus, along with the decussation of the motor axons in the corticospinal tract.

vestibulospinal, tectospinal, and anterior corticospinal tracts) also pass through the medulla on their way to the spinal cord. Two new tracts found in the medulla are the **trigeminothalamic tract** and the **medial lemniscus**. Both of these tracts are composed of second order decussated sensory axons – one set from the contralateral head and another set from the contralateral body (Figures 5.5, 5.6).

A good way to consolidate this information is to describe the type of fibers and course they take whenever a neural tract is encountered.

Cross section of the rostral medulla oblongata

In the rostral medulla, there are seven type of nuclei present. Beginning posteriorly at the midline is the **hypoglossal nucleus**. Just posterior and lateral to this nucleus is the **dorsal motor nucleus** of the vagus nerve (X). More posteriorly and slightly lateral are the four **vestibular nuclei** associated with cranial nerve number VIII (**vestibulocochlear**). Just anterior to the vestibular nuclei is the **nucleus solitarius** (a sensory

nucleus for taste). Lateral to the nucleus solitarius is the continuation of the **spinal nucleus of the trigeminal nerve (V)**. Just anterior to the nucleus solitarius is the **nucleus ambiguous**, a large centrally placed nucleus that is responsible for skeletal muscle motor control of the pharynx and larynx. Finally, on the lateral side of the ventral rostral medulla, is the **inferior olive**, a relay nucleus involved in cerebellar function. Notice the large number of nuclei in the rostral medulla compared to the caudal medulla. The hypoglossal nuclei, the dorsal motor nucleus of the vagus, and the nucleus ambiguous are motor nuclei, while the vestibular nuclei, nucleus solitaries, and spinal nucleus of the trigeminal nerve are sensory nuclei (Figure 5.7a).

The tracts that pass through the rostral medulla are a continuation of the tracts seen in the caudal medulla. These include the anteriorly placed **corticospinal tract**, the laterally placed **spinothalamic tract**, the **rubrospinal tract**, and the more medially placed **trigeminothalamic tract** and **medial lemniscus**. The **nucleus solitarius** with its solitary fasciculus and the **spinal nucleus and tract of the trigeminal nerve (V)** are also present. Notice that these tracts are in the same

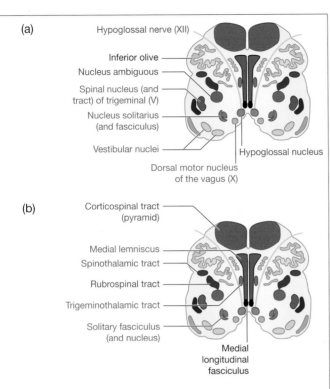

(a)
- Hypoglossal nerve (XII)
- Inferior olive
- Nucleus ambiguous
- Spinal nucleus (and tract) of trigeminal (V)
- Nucleus solitarius (and fasciculus)
- Vestibular nuclei
- Hypoglossal nucleus
- Dorsal motor nucleus of the vagus (X)

(b)
- Corticospinal tract (pyramid)
- Medial lemniscus
- Spinothalamic tract
- Rubrospinal tract
- Trigeminothalamic tract
- Solitary fasciculus (and nucleus)
- Medial longitudinal fasciculus

Figure 5.7 A drawing of a clinically oriented cross section through the rostral medulla oblongata with the nuclei (a) or tracts (b) highlighted. Note the three motor nuclei (hypoglossal (XII), dorsal motor nucleus of the vagus (X), and the nucleus ambiguous), along with the three sensory nuclei (vestibular nuclei, nucleus solitarius, and spinal nucleus of the trigeminal (V)).

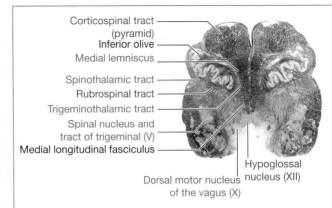

- Corticospinal tract (pyramid)
- Inferior olive
- Medial lemniscus
- Spinothalamic tract
- Rubrospinal tract
- Trigeminothalamic tract
- Spinal nucleus and tract of trigeminal (V)
- Medial longitudinal fasciculus
- Hypoglossal nucleus (XII)
- Dorsal motor nucleus of the vagus (X)

Figure 5.8 A myelin-stained clinically oriented cross section through the rostral medulla oblongata. Note the nuclei and tracts present. Consider the ramifications of lesions in various parts of the cross section.

approximate position as they were in the caudal medulla. A new tract that first appears in the rostral medulla is the **medial longitudinal fasciculus** (MLF). This tract is a relay tract between the three nuclei that control the ocular muscles, the vestibular system, and the motor control of neck musculature. This tract coordinates eye motion and neck motion, so that individuals can have a clear and continuous visual experience. Finally, the axons arising in the **hypoglossal nucleus** pass anteriorly and slightly laterally through the rostral medulla to exit the brain stem as the hypoglossal nerve (XII) in the **preolivary sulcus** (Figures 5.7b, 5.8).

It is important to be able to recognize the location of the nuclei and tracts within the rostral medulla. Knowing this location allows clinicians to pinpoint lesions based on specific symptoms. As an example, if a patient presents with a sensory and motor loss on the same side of the body below the neck along with a motor loss to the opposite side of the tongue, a clinician could surmise that a lesion occurred within the anterior and medial portions of the rostral medulla contralateral to the side of the sensory and motor loss. To confirm this location, a magnetic resonance image of the brain and brain stem could be obtained with an emphasis on the medulla oblongata.

Cranial nerves

There are three cranial nerves associated with the medulla oblongata. These are the glossopharyngeal nerve (IX), the vagus nerve (X), and the hypoglossal nerve (XII). The spinal accessory nerve (XI) is not associated with any portion of the brain stem, but will be discussed in this section for completeness (Table 5.1). When discussing cranial nerve lesions, it is important to be able to distinguish if a lesion has occurred in the axons of the nerve or if a lesion occurred at one of the nuclei supplying that nerve. For example, a nerve lesion may produce multiple symptoms, while a lesion of a nucleus may have only specific symptoms associated with the function of that nucleus.

Glosspharyngeal nerve (IX)

The **glossopharyngeal nerve (IX)** is primarily a sensory nerve bringing to the central nervous system general sensation from the middle ear, pharynx, and posterior tongue, as well as taste sensation from the posterior one-third of the tongue. The **pseudounipolar axons** travel in the glossopharyngeal nerve and have their cell bodies in ganglia associated with the nerve. They synapse on second order cell bodies in the **nucleus solitarius** (solitary nucleus) for taste or in the **spinal nucleus of the trigeminal (V)** for general sensation, pain, and temperature. As an aside, this is another case where a nucleus in the brain is poorly named. The spinal nucleus of the trigeminal (V) actually receives general sensation, pain, and temperature input from the face, nasal cavity, oral cavity, pharynx, and larynx. The majority of these fibers are conveyed by the trigeminal nerve (V), although some sensation is carried by the facial (VII), glossopharyngeal (IX), and vagus (X) nerves. This means that the second order

Clinical box 5.1

Three additional areas in the medulla oblongata include the **reticular formation**, the **raphe nuclei**, and the **area postrema**. The reticular formation is a column of poorly defined, diffusely arranged neurons found throughout the brain stem. In the medulla, it is located centrally between the nucleus ambiguous and the medial lemniscus (blue circle below). The reticular formation has numerous functions, including mediation of cardiovascular and respiratory functions, involvement in awareness (sleep, consciousness, alertness, habituation), pain modulation and maintenance of muscle tone, balance, and motor coordination. The reticulospinal tracts originate from this region. The raphe nuclei are located medially within the reticular formation (purple ovals below). These nuclei have numerous functions, including pain modulation through descending pathways that mediate incoming pain sensations in the spinal cord. These nuclei have projections throughout the central nervous system, with serotonin as the primary neurotransmitter. Therefore, pharmacologic compounds that alter serotonin activity (many antidepressants, for example) have a major impact on the raphe and its projections. Because of the numerous functions associated with the reticular formation and the raphe nuclei, lesions in these areas can have a major impact on basic homeostatic neural function.

The area postrema (orange circles below) is located adjacent to the dorsal motor nucleus of the vagus in the medulla. It is one of the circumventricular organs found outside of the blood-brain barrier. This allows the area postrema to respond to toxins in the blood and can induce vomiting. It is referred to as the emetic center.

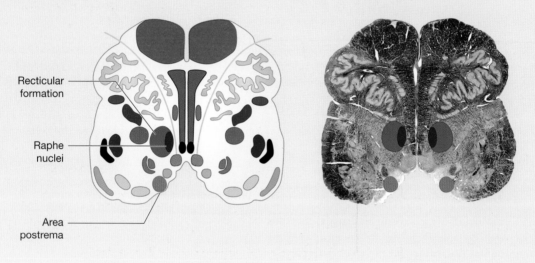

Recticular formation

Raphe nuclei

Area postrema

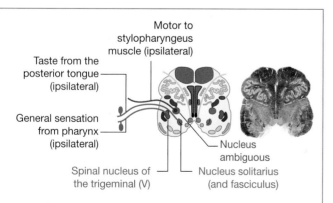

Motor to stylopharyngeus muscle (ipsilateral)

Taste from the posterior tongue (ipsilateral)

General sensation from pharynx (ipsilateral)

Spinal nucleus of the trigeminal (V)

Nucleus ambiguous

Nucleus solitarius (and fasciculus)

Figure 5.9 A drawing and a myelin-stained clinically oriented cross section through the rostral medulla oblongata indicating the location of the nuclei and fibers associated with the glossopharyngeal nerve (IX).

sensory cell bodies for general sensation from the glossopharyngeal nerve are found in the spinal nucleus of the trigeminal (V). These second order axons, like most second order sensory axons, decussate and then ascend in the contralateral **trigeminothalamic tract** to synapse in the thalamus (Figures 5.9, 5.10).

The glossopharyngeal nerve also provides motor innervation to a single muscle, the stylopharyngeus muscle. The cell bodies for this motor nerve are found in the **nucleus ambiguous**. The final function of the glossopharyngeal nerve is providing preganglionic parasympathetic autonomic motor innervation to the parotid gland. The preganglionic parasympathetic cell bodies are found in the **inferior salivatory nucleus** and pass through the glossopharyngeal nerve to synapse in the **otic ganglion**. The inferior salivatory nucleus is found in the same relative position as the

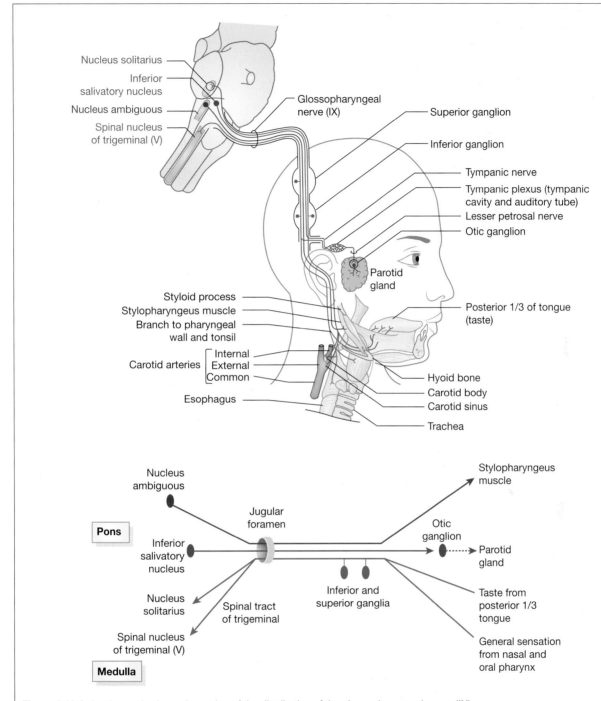

Figure 5.10 A drawing and schematic version of the distribution of the glossopharyngeal nerve (IX).

dorsal motor nucleus in the medulla, just at a more rostral level (Figures 5.10, 5.16).

The glossopharyngeal nerve exits the medulla in the **post-olivary sulcus** and exits the skull through the **jugular foramen**. A lesion of the glossopharyngeal nerve will produce a decrease in ipsilateral salivary production, as well as a loss of sensory sensation from the ipsilateral middle ear and pharynx. This sensory deficit is best revealed by a loss of the gag reflex.

Vagus nerve (X)

The **vagus nerve (X)** is a highly complex and multi-functional nerve. The vagus carries general sensory innervation from the larynx as well as some small portions from the pharynx and middle ear. It also carries taste sensations from the base of the tongue and the epiglottis. Additionally, it brings visceral sensation from the heart, the lungs, and the gastrointestinal tract (proximal to the left colic flexure). All

Heart, lung, GI,
cardiac/smooth muscle
(ipsilateral)

Soft palate, pharynx,
larynx, skeletal muscles
(ipsilateral)

Taste and visceral
sensation from
larynx, heart, lungs,
GI (ipsilateral)

General sensation
from larynx
(ipsilateral)

Nucleus
ambiguous

Spinal nucleus of
the trigeminal (V)

Dorsal
motor nucleus
of the vagus (X)

Nucleus solitarius
(and fasciculus)

Figure 5.11 A drawing and a myelin-stained clinical cross section through the rostral medulla oblongata indicating the location of the nuclei and fibers associated with the vagus nerve (X).

of these **pseudounipolar** sensory fibers have cell bodies in ganglia associated with the vagus nerve. The sensory fibers for taste and visceral sensation synapse on second order neurons in the **nucleus solitarius**. The general sensory fibers synapse on second order neurons in the **spinal nucleus of the trigeminal (V)**.

The vagus nerve provides motor innervation to the ipsilateral skeletal muscles of the soft palate, pharynx, and larynx. The cell bodies for this innervation are found in the **nucleus ambiguous**. The vagus nerve also provides autonomic motor innervation to the cardiac muscle of the heart and the smooth muscle of the lungs and gastrointestinal system (to the left colic flexure). The preganglionic parasympathetic cell bodies for this autonomic innervation are found in the **dorsal motor nucleus**, while the postganglionic parasympathetic cell bodies are found in the wall of the organ that is innervated (Figures 5.11, 5.12, 5.16).

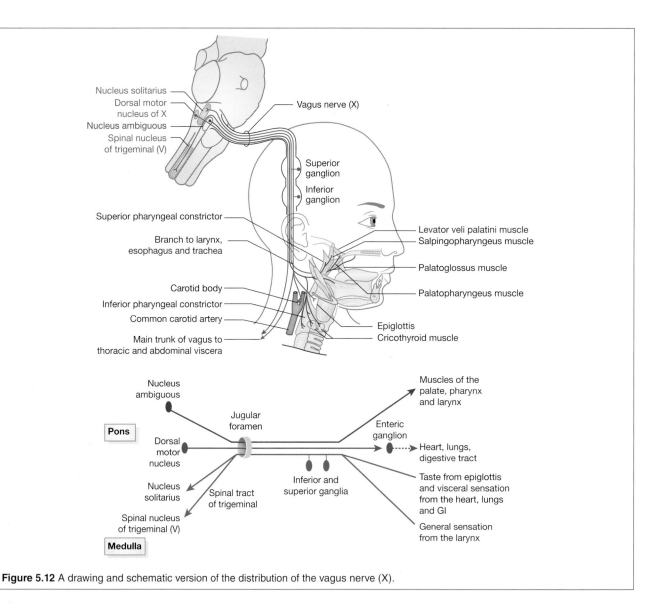

Figure 5.12 A drawing and schematic version of the distribution of the vagus nerve (X).

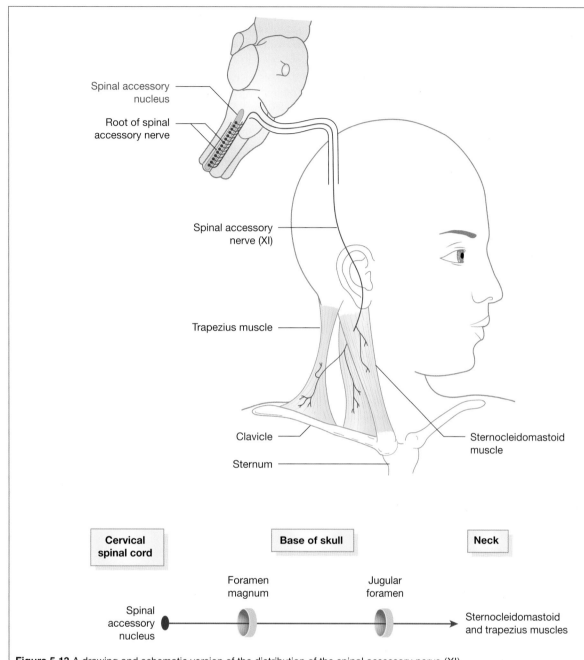

Figure 5.13 A drawing and schematic version of the distribution of the spinal accessory nerve (XI).

The vagus nerve exits the medulla in the postolivary sulcus and exits the skull through the jugular foramen. A lesion of the vagus nerve in this region produces multiple symptoms, with the sensory and motor functions of the larynx being heavily involved (superior and recurrent laryngeal nerves). Patients with unilateral vagus nerve lesions have difficulty speaking (usually a hoarse whisper), while patients with bilateral lesions can present with respiratory emergencies. Vagus nerve lesions can also have marked effects on respiration, heart rate, and gastrointestinal function.

Spinal accessory nerve (XI)

The **spinal accessory nerve (XI)** is a cranial nerve that is not associated with any brain stem nuclei. It is a motor nerve that supplies the ipsilateral sternocleidomastoid and trapezius muscles. It has its motor cell bodies in the upper cervical spinal cord and these axons ascend through the vertebral canal and **foramen magnum** to exit the skull through the **jugular foramen**, along with the glossopharyngeal nerve (IX) and the vagus nerve (X) (Figures 5.13, 5.16). A lesion of the spinal accessory nerve produces an ipsilateral loss of motor control to the sternocleidomastoid and trapezius muscles, preventing patients from shrugging their shoulder or moving their chin to their opposite shoulder.

Hypoglossal nerve (XII)

The **hypoglossal nerve (XII)** arises from the hypoglossal nucleus in the rostral medulla and exits the brain stem in the preolivary sulcus. The nerve exits the skull through the **hypoglossal canal** to innervate the ipsilateral tongue musculature (Figures 5.14, 5.15, 5.16). A lesion of the hypoglossal nucleus or nerve produces an inability to protrude the tongue. This is demonstrated by asking patients to stick out their tongue, with the tongue pointing towards the side of the lesion.

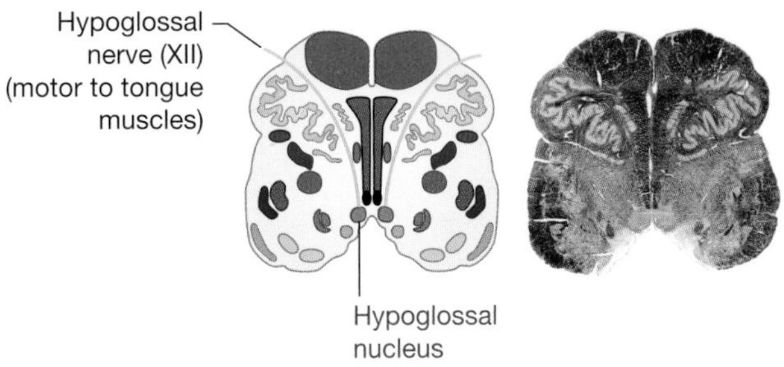

Figure 5.14 A drawing and a myelin-stained clinical cross section through the rostral medulla oblongata indicating the location of the nuclei and fibers associated with the hypoglossal nerve (XII).

Clinical considerations

At this point, it is important to be able to describe the symptoms that would be present if any of these cranial nerves were lesioned. In addition, lesions to specific portions of the medulla will produce specific symptoms and these should be correlated (Figure 5.17). One method for testing this knowledge is to close your eyes and point to a cross section of the medulla. Where your finger lies, describe the type of lesion that occurs and the symptoms that would be present. This is called "pin the tail on the lesion" and can be used throughout the study of the nervous system.

Table 5.1 The composition and course of the four cranial nerves associated with the medulla oblongata.

Glossopharyngeal nerve (IX):
Sensory: General sensation from the posterior one-third of tongue, nasal and oral pharynx and middle ear, taste sensation from the posterior one-third of the tongue and chemoreception from the carotid body, first order cell bodies in the inferior (petrosal) and superior (jugular) ganglia, first order axons enter the skull through the jugular foramen, enter the medullary brain stem in the postolivary sulcus, the general sensation fibers project to the spinal trigeminal nucleus, the taste, and chemoreception fibers project to the nucleus solitarius.
Motor: Nucleus ambiguous, axons exit postolivary sulcus in medulla, exit the skull through the jugular foramen, innervate the stylopharyngeus muscle.
Autonomic: Inferior salivatory nucleus (preganglionic parasympathetic), axons exit postolivary sulcus in medulla, become tympanic plexus in middle ear, form lesser petrosal nerve, exit the skull through the foramen ovale, synapse in the otic ganglion; postganglionic parasympathetic fibers innervate the parotid salivary gland.

Vagus nerve (X):
Sensory: General sensation from the larynx, epiglottis and small portion of external auditory meatus, taste from the epiglottis, chemoreception from the carotid sinus and aortic arch, and diffuse visceral sensation from the thoracic and abdominal viscera, first order cell bodies in the inferior (nodose) and superior (jugular) ganglia, first order axons enter the skull through the jugular foramen, enter the medullary brain stem in the postolivary sulcus, the general and visceral sensation fibers project to the spinal trigeminal nucleus, the taste, and chemoreception fibers project to the nucleus solitarius.
Motor: Nucleus ambiguous, axons exit postolivary sulcus in medulla, exit the skull through the jugular foramen, innervate the muscles of the palate, pharynx, and larynx.
Autonomic: Dorsal motor nucleus of the vagus (X) (preganglionic parasympathetic), axons exit postolivary sulcus in medulla, exit the skull through the jugular foramen; postganglionic parasympathetic cell bodies and axons are found in the walls of the organs and innervate the cardiac muscle of the heart and the smooth muscle of the respiratory system and digestive system (to the left colic flexure).

Spinal accessory nerve (XI):
Motor: Anterior horn cells of upper cervical nerves, axons ascend through the foramen magnum, exit the skull through the jugular foramen, innervate the trapezius and sternocleidomastoid muscles.

Hypoglossal nerve (XII):
Motor: Hypoglossal nucleus, axons exit preolivary sulcus in medulla, exit the skull through the hypoglossal canal, innervate intrinsic and extrinsic muscles of the tongue.

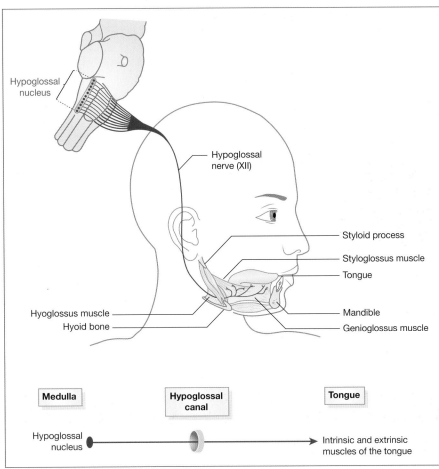

Figure 5.15 A drawing and schematic version of the distribution of the hypoglossal nerve (XII).

Hypoglossal nucleus

Hypoglossal nerve (XII)

Styloid process

Styloglossus muscle

Tongue

Hyoglossus muscle

Hyoid bone

Mandible

Genioglossus muscle

Medulla	Hypoglossal canal	Tongue

Hypoglossal nucleus

Intrinsic and extrinsic muscles of the tongue

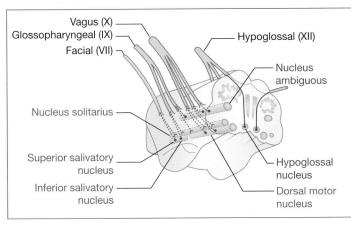

Vagus (X)

Glossopharyngeal (IX)

Facial (VII)

Hypoglossal (XII)

Nucleus ambiguous

Nucleus solitarius

Superior salivatory nucleus

Inferior salivatory nucleus

Hypoglossal nucleus

Dorsal motor nucleus

Figure 5.16 A three-dimensional drawing of the rostral medulla oblongata and the pons, indicating the location of the nuclei and fibers of the cranial nerves.

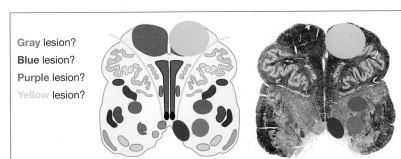

Gray lesion?

Blue lesion?

Purple lesion?

Yellow lesion?

Figure 5.17 Identify the functional loss, including on which side of the patient's body the loss would be found as well as the nuclei or tracts involved in each of the colored lesions indicated.

Case 1

Jonathan Jones, a 35-year-old banker, is involved in a major car accident. He is unconscious when paramedics arrive and he is transported to the hospital for observation and treatment. He regains consciousness and he has a head CT and MRI. A fracture of the base of the skull near the jugular foramen is observed (Figure 5.18). The resident in charge, Dr Christine Logan, begins a neurologic exam to determine if any losses have occurred. Which of the cranial nerves could be affected by a fracture at the jugular foramen? What specific tests would be used to determine which nerves are functional?

After determining that Mr Jones' right glossopharyngeal nerve (IX) has been severed as it passes through the jugular foramen, but that the vagus nerve (X) and spinal accessory nerve (XI) are intact, Dr Logan realizes that Mr Jones will have an ipsilateral loss of sensation from the middle ear and the pharynx as well as a loss of taste sensation from the posterior one third of the tongue on the affected side. In addition, he will have an inability to produce saliva from his ipsilateral parotid gland. After recovery from the accident, it is hoped that some neural regrowth may occur in the severed nerve, as well as compensation from other nerves in the area to reduce the amount of lost sensation. Two years after the

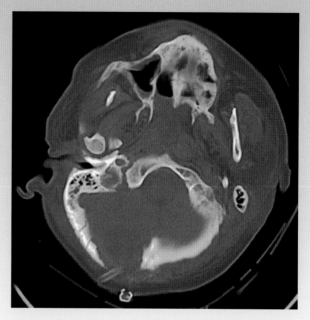

Figure 5.18 A computer tomograph (CT) of a patient with a right basal skull fracture involving the jugular foramen. Note the discontinuity of bone in the right middle portion of the field.

accident, during a routine follow up, Mr Jones has regained the majority of his lost sensation.

Case 2

Paul Wilson, a 62-year-old stock broker, suffers a small ischemic stroke while jogging on his treadmill at home. His wife calls an ambulance and he is rushed to the emergency room with assisted ventilation. The emergency room physician, Dr Charles Allen, performs a detailed physical examination and observes a bilateral loss of both general sensation and motor control below Mr Wilson's neck, although his motor reflexes are intact and actually slightly increased. Based on these symptoms, where would a stroke likely have occurred?

Why would a stroke at this location produce bilateral losses?

Dr Allen informs Mr and Mrs Wilson that the stroke occurred in the caudal medulla of the brain stem (Figure 5.19) (Pongmoragot, *et al.*, 2013) at an area where both descending and ascending tracts cross over, thus producing bilateral losses of both sensation and motor control. Sadly, he has to discuss with them the poor prognosis for Mr Wilson's recovery.

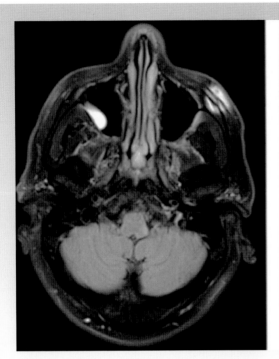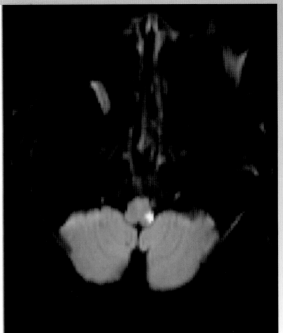

Figure 5.19 Magnetic resonance images of a stroke (infarct) in the medulla oblongata. Note the hyperintense signal from the left posterior medulla.

Study questions

1. A lesion in the nucleus gracilis would produce a loss of:
a) pain and temperature from the ipsilateral lower extremity
b) pain and temperature from the contralateral lower extremity
c) fine touch and proprioception from the ipsilateral lower extremity
d) fine touch and proprioception from the contralateral lower extremity
e) general sensation from the contralateral upper extremity

2. A lesion in the spinothalamic tract in the rostral medulla would produce a loss of:
a) pain and temperature from the ipsilateral side of the body
b) pain and temperature from the contralateral side of the body
c) fine touch and proprioception from the ipsilateral side of the body
d) fine touch and proprioception from the contralateral side of the body
e) general sensation from the contralateral side of the body

3. A patient presents with the inability to protrude (stick out) the tongue on the right side. This is due to a lesion in the:
a) postolivary sulcus on the right side
b) postolivary sulcus on the left side
c) preolivary sulcus on the right side
d) preolivary sulcus on the left side
e) pontomedullary junction on the right side
f) pontomedullary junction on the left side

4. A 22-year-old male patient presents with a loss of voluntary motor control on the right side of his body. This is due to a lesion in the:
a) pyramid of the rostral medulla on the right side
b) pyramid of the rostral medulla on the left side
c) lateral part of the rostral medulla posterior to the inferior olive on the right side
d) lateral part of the rostral medulla posterior to the inferior olive on the left side
e) posterior part of the medulla adjacent to the fourth ventricle on the right side
f) posterior part of the medulla adjacent to the fourth ventricle on the left side

5. A lesion in the nucleus ambiguous of the rostral medulla would produce a loss in:

a) general sensation from the contralateral face, oral cavity, pharynx, and larynx

b) general sensation from the ipsilateral face, oral cavity, pharynx, and larynx

c) pain sensation from the contralateral face, oral cavity, pharynx, and larynx

d) pain sensation from the ipsilateral face, oral cavity, pharynx, and larynx

e) voluntary motor control from the contralateral pharynx and larynx

f) voluntary motor control from the ipsilateral pharynx and larynx

For more self-assessment questions, visit the companion website at
www.wileyessential.com/neuroanatomy

FURTHER READING

For additional information on the medulla oblongata, the following textbooks and review articles may be helpful:

Angeles Fernández-Gil M, Palacios-Bote R, Leo-Barahona M, Mora-Encinas JP. 2010. Anatomy of the brainstem: a gaze into the stem of life. *Semin Ultrasound CT MR,* 31(3): 196–219.

Blumenfeld H. 2002. *Neuroanatomy Through Clinical Cases.* Sinauer Associates, Sunderland, Massachusetts.

Felten DL, Shetty A. 2009. *Netter's Atlas of Neuroscience,* 2nd edition. Saunders Elsevier, Philadelphia, Pennsylvania.

Haines DE. 2012. *Neuroanatomy: An Atlas of Structures, Sections and Systems,* 8th edition. Lippincott Williams & Wilkin, Baltimore, Maryland.

Moore KL, Dalley AF, Agur AMR. 2014. *Moore Clinically Oriented Anatomy,* 7th edition. Lippincott, Williams & Wilkins Philadelphia, Pennsylvania.

Patestas MA, Gartner LP. 2006. *A Textbook of Neuroanatomy.* Blackwell Publishing, Malden, Massachusetts.

Pongmoragot J, Parthasarathy S, Selchen D, Saposnik G. 2013. Bilateral medial medullary infarction: a systematic review. *J Stroke Cerebrovasc Dis,* 2(6): 775–780.

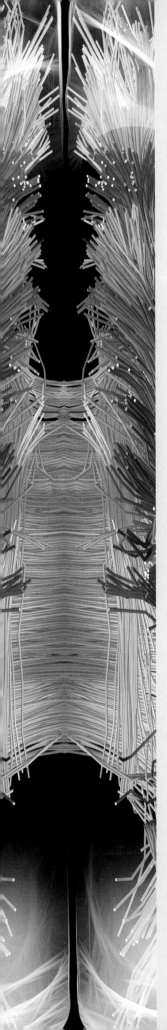

CHAPTER 6
Pons

Learning objectives

1. Identify the major components of the pons.
2. Describe the components of the trigeminal nerve (V).
3. Describe the components of the abducens nerve (VI).
4. Describe the components of the facial nerve (VII).
5. Describe the components of the vestibulocochlear nerve (VIII).
6. Describe the fourth ventricle from rostral to caudal.
7. Describe lesions of the trigeminal (V), abducens (VI), facial (VII), and vestibulocochlear (VIII) nerves.

Essential Clinical Neuroanatomy, First Edition. Thomas H. Champney.
© 2016 John Wiley & Sons, Ltd. Published 2016 by John Wiley & Sons, Ltd.
Companion website: www.wileyessential.com/neuroanatomy

Cross section of the caudal pons 80

Nuclei
1. Abducens nucleus
2. Facial nucleus
3. Spinal nucleus of trigeminal (V)

Tracts
1. Corticospinal tracts, corticobulbar tracts, and corticopontine tracts
2. Medial longitudinal fasciculus (MLF)
3. Medial lemniscus
4. Trigeminothalamic tract
5. Spinothalamic tract
6. Spinal tract of trigeminal (V)
7. Rubrospinal and tectospinal tracts
8. Middle cerebellar peduncle – pontocerebellar tract

Cross section of the middle pons 82

Nuclei
1. Main sensory nucleus of the trigeminal (V)
2. Motor nucleus of the trigeminal (V)
3. Mesencephalic nucleus of the trigeminal (V)
4. Locus coeruleus (noradrenergic)
5. Raphe nuclei (serotonergic)

Tracts
1. Corticospinal tracts, corticobulbar tracts, and corticopontine tracts
2. Medial longitudinal fasciculus (MLF)
3. Medial lemniscus
4. Trigeminothalamic tract
5. Spinothalamic tract
6. Middle cerebellar peduncle – pontocerebellar tract (transverse pontine)

Cross section of the rostral pons 82

Nuclei
1. Mesencephalic nucleus of the trigeminal (V)
2. Locus coeruleus (noradrenergic)
3. Raphe nuclei (serotonergic)

Tracts
1. Corticospinal tracts, corticobulbar tracts, and corticopontine tracts
2. Pontocerebellar tract (transverse pontine)
3. Medial longitudinal fasciculus (MLF)
4. Medial lemniscus
5. Trigeminothalamic tract
6. Spinothalamic tract
7. Lateral lemniscus
8. Superior cerebellar peduncle – efferent axons from cerebellum

Cranial nerves associated with the pons 83

Trigeminal nerve (V)
1. Main sensory nucleus – ipsilateral face (V_1, V_2, and V_3)
   a) Trigeminal nerve branches
   b) Trigeminal (semilunar) ganglion
   c) Spinal tract of V
   d) Spinal nucleus of V or sensory nucleus – synapse (second order)
   e) Ascend in trigeminothalamic tract
   f) Thalamus (VPM) – synapse (third order)
   g) Cortex (postcentral gyrus)
2. Mesencephalic nucleus – proprioception
3. Motor nucleus – ipsilateral muscles (motor root, V_3)
   a) Innervation of first branchial arch muscles
   b) Four muscles of mastication
   c) Four other muscles
4. Trigeminal lemniscus (trigeminothalamic tract)
5. Lesion of the trigeminal nerve (V)
   a) Ipsilateral effects – all sensation from face (V_1, V_2, and V_3)
   b) Eight muscles affected (muscles of mastication)
   c) Trigeminal neuralgia (tic douloureux)

Abducens nerve (VI)
1. Abducens nucleus
2. Exits at pontomedullary junction – medially
3. Innervates the ipsilateral lateral rectus
4. Lesion of the abducens nerve (VI)
   a) Ipsilateral effect – lateral rectus nonfunctional
   b) Eye deviates medially (strabismus), double vision (diplopia)

Facial nerve (VII)
1. Facial nucleus – motor
2. Superior salivatory nucleus – parasympathetic (nervus intermedius)
3. Exits at pontomedullary junction – laterally
4. Innervates all facial muscles, stapedius, stylohyoid, posterior belly digastric
5. Innervates lacrimal, sublingual, and submandibular glands
6. Taste from anterior twothirds tongue
   a) Lingual nerve
   b) Chorda tympani
   c) Facial nerve – cell body in geniculate ganglion
   d) Nucleus solitarius (gustatory nucleus) – synapse (second order)
   e) Thalamus (VPM) – synapse (third order)
   f) Cortex (postcentral gyrus)
7. Lesion of the facial nerve (VII)
   a) Ipsilateral effect – facial muscle paralysis
   b) Also loss of stapedius, stylohyoid, posterior belly digastricmuscles

c) Loss of parasympathetic to lacrimal, sublingual, and submandibular glands

d) Bell's palsy

Vestibulocochlear nerve (VIII)

1. Vestibular pathways
   a) Bipolar axons from the semicircular canals and utricle/saccule
   b) Vestibulocochlear nerve – cell bodies in vestibular ganglion
   c) Some axons project directly to cerebellum
   d) Majority synapse in four ipsilateral vestibular nuclei (second order)
   e) Vestibular nuclei project to:
      i. Spinal cord
         a) Medial vestibulospinal tract – cervical region
         b) Lateral vestibulospinal tract – entire spinal cord
      ii. Eye motor nuclei (III, IV, VI) – medial longitudinal fasiculus (MLF)
      iii. Cerebellum – inferior cerebellar peduncle
      iv. Thalamus (ventral posterior nucleus) to the cortex
2. Auditory pathways
   a) Bipolar axons from the cochlea (tonotopic)
   b) Vestibulocochlear nerve – cell bodies in spiral ganglion

c) Posterior and anterior cochlear nuclei – synapse (second order)

d) Bilateral projections – trapezoid body (decussation)

e) Synapse in superior olivary nuclei

f) Ascend in lateral lemniscus to inferior colliculus (synapse)

g) Brachium of inferior colliculus to medial geniculate nucleus

h) Auditory cortex (area 41)

3. Lesion of the vestibulocochlear nerve (VIII)
   a) Vestibular effects – balance, coordination, vertigo, nystagmus
   b) Auditory effects – tinnitus, unilateral loss (peripheral)
   c) Acoustic neuroma

Introduction

In this chapter, the tracts presented in the spinal cord and medulla will be followed into the **pons** of the **brain stem**. In addition, the cranial nerve nuclei and other associated nuclei found in the pons will be discussed. One take home message for the pons is that it is a major site for cerebellar input and output. The majority of fibers that enter or leave the cerebellum pass through the pons. The pons is also the site for the nuclei for the fifth through eighth cranial nerves (V–VIII).

Anatomy of the pons

The pons, when viewed inferiorly/anteriorly, is most noticeable as a large set of fibers extending into the cerebellum (the **middle cerebellar peduncle**). At the border between the pons and the medulla (the **pontomedullary junction**), three cranial nerves can be seen exiting on each side. The most medially placed nerve is the **abducens nerve (VI)**. The laterally placed nerves are the **facial nerve (VII)** and the **vestibulocochlear nerve (VIII)**. A more rostrally placed cranial nerve that pierces the middle cerebellar peduncle is the **trigeminal nerve (V)** (Figure 6.1). The distribution and function of these nerves will be discussed below.

To view the pons from a superior/posterior view, the cerebellum must be removed by sectioning through the cerebellar peduncles (superior, middle, and inferior). This opens up the diamond-shaped **fourth ventricle** with the floor of the fourth ventricle represented by the superior aspect of the pons. The lateral extensions of the fourth ventricle are the outlets for cerebrospinal fluid to circulate in the subarachnoid space (the **lateral foramina** (of Luschka)), along with a singular midline outlet: the midline foramen (of Magendie) (Figure 6.2).

Cross section of the pontomedullary junction

Many of the structures observed in the rostral medulla continue into the pontomedullary junction. For example, the **corticospinal tracts** are found in the anterior aspect of a cross-sectional view – much like the pyramids in the medulla. Intermixed with the corticospinal axons are motor axons from the cortex that project to cranial nerve nuclei (**corticobulbar axons**) and motor axons that project to pontine nuclei (**corticopontine axons**). The pontine nuclei then send decussating axons into the opposite lobe of the cerebellum via the middle cerebellar peduncle. Recall in the middle of the medulla, the relationship of the **medial longitudinal fasciculus**, the **medial lemniscus**,

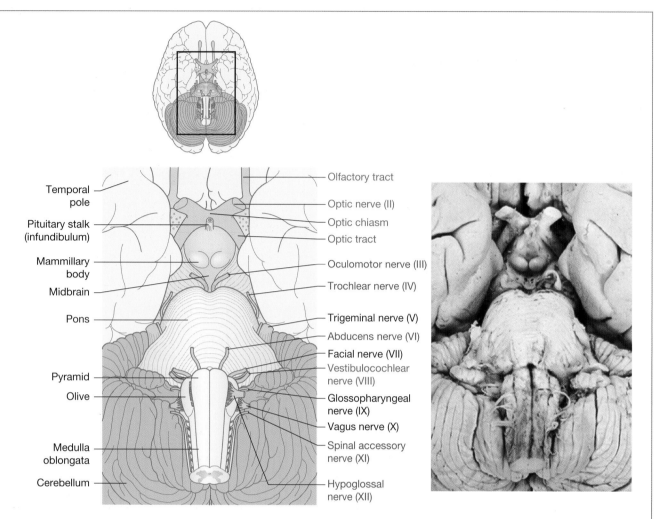

Figure 6.1 The three major regions of the brain stem (the midbrain, the pons, and the medulla oblongata) from an inferior view of the brain. Note the cranial nerves associated with the pons: the trigeminal (V), the abducens (VI), the facial (VII), and the vestibulocochlear (VIII).

the **trigeminothalamic tract**, and the **spinothalamic tract**. These tracts occupy similar positions in the section of the pontomedullary junction, with the most noticeable change being the compression and lateral motion of the medial lemniscus. While the medial lemniscus is "upright" in the medulla, here it is "rounded up" into a more circular structure that is closely related to the two other sensory tracts, the trigeminothalamic and spinothalamic tracts. The **spinal tract** and **nucleus of the trigeminal (V)** are also present in the pontomedullary junction in the same location as in the medulla. A new bilateral tract found at the pontomedullary junction is the **inferior cerebellar peduncle**, which primarily contains axons entering the cerebellum from the brain stem and spinal cord (Figure 6.3).

The nuclei found in the pontomedullary junction are the **cochlear** and **vestibular nuclei** associated with the **vestibulocochlear nerve (VIII)**. These nuclei contain the second order neuronal cell bodies from the cochlea (hearing) and the vestibular apparatus (balance).

Cross section of the caudal pons

There are three types of nuclei present in the caudal pons: two that are motor nuclei and one that is sensory. The **abducens nucleus** is the site of the motor neuronal cell bodies for the lateral rectus muscle in the eye. The axons from these cell bodies course directly through the substance of the pons and exit from the medial aspect of the pontomedullary junction. The **facial nucleus** is the site of the motor neuronal cell bodies for the facial musculature. The course of these axons is circuitous, with the axons progressing superiorly around the abducens nucleus before exiting the pons laterally at the pontomedullary junction. Clinically, it is important to point out that this unique course of the facial axons puts them in close proximity to the abducens nucleus, so that damage to the nucleus can also include damage to the nearby facial nerve fibers. The sensory nuclei present in the caudal pons are the continuation of the **spinal nucleus of the trigeminal (V)**. These contain second order cell bodies for sensation from the head (Figure 6.4).

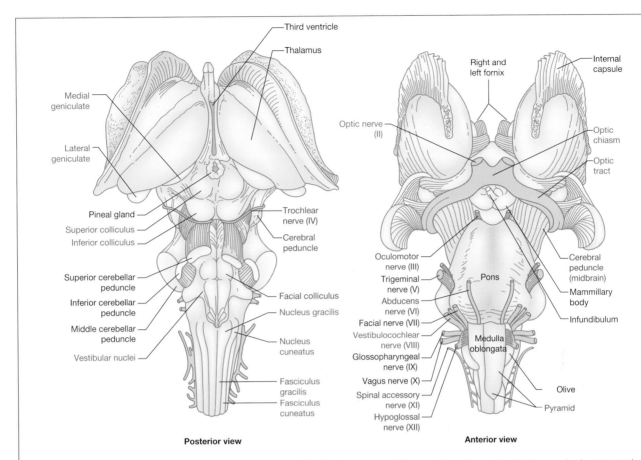

Posterior view

Anterior view

Figure 6.2 The three major regions of the brain stem (the midbrain, the pons, and the medulla oblongata) with the cerebral cortex and cerebellum removed. Note the cranial nerves associated with the pons.

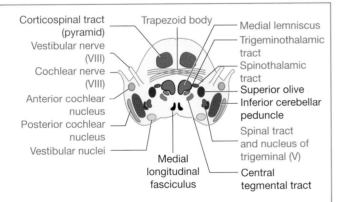

Figure 6.3 A drawing of a clinically oriented cross section through the pontomedullary junction. Note the numerous sensory and motor tracts including the medial lemniscus, trigeminothalamic tract, the spinothalamic tract, the spinal tract and nucleus of the trigeminal (V), the corticospinal tract, and the medial longitudinal fasciculus.

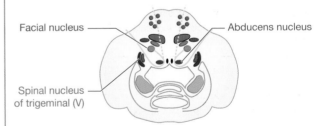

Figure 6.4 A drawing of a clinically oriented cross section through the caudal pons with the nuclei present highlighted. Note the abducens nerve (VI) and its nucleus, the unique course of the facial nerve (VII), along with the spinal tract and nucleus of the trigeminal (V).

The tracts found in the caudal pons include the continuation of ascending and descending tracts that were found in the medulla. For example, the **spinocerebellar tracts** pass

through the pons to enter the cerebellum via the inferior cerebellar peduncle. The second order **spinothalamic tracts**, **trigeminothlamic tracts**, and the **medial lemniscus** travel through the pons to reach the **thalamus**. Recall that the medial lemniscus is "rounded up" in the pontomedullary junction and, in the caudal pons, it is stretched out horizontally in a lateral to medial direction. Although these sensory tracts have changed their position as they course through the pons and medulla, the **medial longitudinal fasciculus** has remained in the same posterior position. The motor tracts also continue through the pons and include the **corticospinal tracts**, **corticobulbar tracts**, and the **corticopontine tracts**. The other descending tracts seen in the medulla (**rubrospinal**, **tectospinal**) also pass through the caudal pons on their way to the spinal cord. Notice that the **vestibulospinal tract** is no longer present since it arose from the vestibular nuclei, which are found in more caudal sections of the brain stem (Figures 6.5, 6.6).

Remember to keep in mind that the tracts are made of axons that are passing through these cross sections, so they will be seen in sections above and below the section of interest. If possible, describe the type of fibers and course they take whenever a neural tract is encountered.

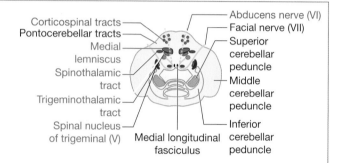

Corticospinal tracts — Pontocerebellar tracts — Medial lemniscus — Spinothalamic tract — Trigeminothalamic tract — Spinal nucleus of trigeminal (V) — Medial longitudinal fasciculus

Abducens nerve (VI) — Facial nerve (VII) — Superior cerebellar peduncle — Middle cerebellar peduncle — Inferior cerebellar peduncle

Figure 6.5 A drawing of a clinically oriented cross section through the caudal pons with the neural tracts highlighted. Note the location of the medial lemniscus, trigeminothalamic tract, the spinothalamic tract, the spinal tract and nucleus of the trigeminal (V), the corticospinal tract, the cerebellar peduncles, and the medial longitudinal fasciculus.

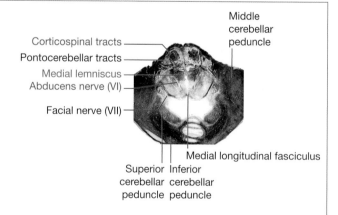

Corticospinal tracts — Pontocerebellar tracts — Medial lemniscus — Abducens nerve (VI) — Facial nerve (VII)

Middle cerebellar peduncle — Medial longitudinal fasciculus — Superior cerebellar peduncle — Inferior cerebellar peduncle

Figure 6.6 A myelin-stained clinically oriented cross section through the caudal pons. Note the location of the medial lemniscus, the corticospinal tract, the cerebellar peduncles, and the medial longitudinal fasciculus.

Cross section of the middle pons

When examining a cross section of the middle of the pons, the middle and superior cerebellar peduncles are quite prominent. The nuclei that are present in this portion of the pons include nuclei associated with the **trigeminal nerve (V)**: the **main sensory nucleus**, the **motor nucleus,** and the **mesencephalic nucleus**. These nuclei are found in the postero-lateral portion of the pons. Their functions will be described in the section on the trigeminal nerve (V). Other prominent nuclei in this section of the pons are the **locus coeruleus** and the **raphe nuclei**. The locus ceruleus has projections throughout the brain which are **noradrenergic** (utilizing norepinephrine as a neurotransmitter). It is found in the postero-lateral portion of the pons in a close relationship with the **mesencephalic nucleus of the trigeminal (V)**. The raphe nuclei axons are also widely distributed throughout the brain and are **serotonergic** (utilizing serotonin as a neurotransmitter). The raphe nuclei (and the associated reticular formation) are found medially in the pons, just inferior to the **medial longitudinal fasciculus**. Both of these nuclear groups have multiple functions, including awareness, attention, and arousal.

The tracts found in the middle pons include the same ascending and descending tracts that are found in other sections of the pons. The three sensory tracts (**spinothalamic, trigeminothalamic,** and the **medial lemniscus**) continue traveling through the pons to the **thalamus**. Recall that the medial lemniscus is "rounded up" in the pontomedullary junction and, in the caudal pons it is laid out horizontally in a lateral to medial direction. In the middle pons, it is still flattened, but is moving slightly lateral carrying the trigeminothalamic tract with it. The **medial longitudinal fasciculus** has not changed its postero-medially placed position. The motor tracts also continue through the pons and include the **corticospinal tracts**, **corticobulbar tracts**, and the **corticopontine tracts**. Transverse fibers can be observed in the region of the corticospinal tracts and these are the **pontocerebellar tract** (**transverse pontine fibers**). These fibers originate from the contralateral pontine nuclei and ascend into the cerebellum through the middle cerebellar peduncle (Figures 6.7, 6.8).

Cross section of the rostral pons

In the rostral pons, the majority of the nuclei and tracts present in the middle pons are in very similar locations. The **medial lemniscus** and the other two sensory tracts (spinothalamic and trigeminothalamic) have moved more laterally, the middle cerebellar peduncle is no longer seen, and a small second order sensory tract, the **lateral lemniscus**, is first observed. The lateral lemniscus is a set of second order axons associated with hearing that ascend to the inferior colliculi of the midbrain (with their cell bodies in the cochlear nuclei). At this point, all three cross sections of the pons and the two sections of the medulla should be reviewed, so that the tracts that course through them can be identified and followed (Figures 6.9, 6.10).

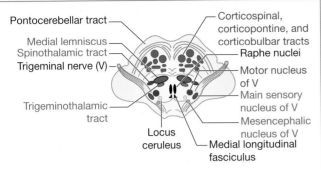

Figure 6.7 A drawing of a clinically oriented cross section through the middle pons. Note the three main nuclei associated with trigeminal nerve (motor nucleus, sensory nucleus, and mesencephalic nucleus) as well as the location of the medial lemniscus, trigeminothalamic tract, the spinothalamic tract, the corticospinal tract, and the medial longitudinal fasciculus.

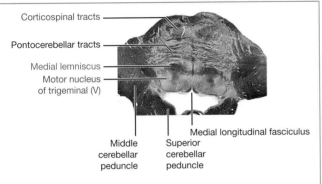

Figure 6.8 A myelin-stained clinically oriented cross section through the middle pons. Note the location of the medial lemniscus, the corticospinal tract, the cerebellar peduncles, and the medial longitudinal fasciculus.

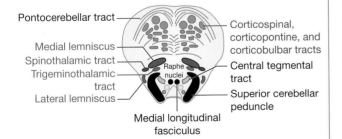

Figure 6.9 A drawing of a clinically oriented cross section through the rostral pons. Note the location of the medial lemniscus, trigeminothalamic tract, the spinothalamic tract, the corticospinal tract, the superior cerebellar peduncle, and the medial longitudinal fasciculus.

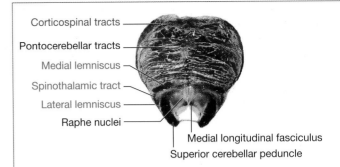

Figure 6.10 A myelin-stained clinically oriented cross section through the rostral pons. Note the location of the medial lemniscus, the corticospinal tract, the superior cerebellar peduncle, and the medial longitudinal fasciculus.

Clinical box 6.1

Three additional areas of clinical interest in the pons include the **reticular formation**, the **raphe nuclei**, and the **locus coeruleus**. The location and function of the reticular formation and raphe nuclei in the medulla were described in the previous chapter. They have a similar diffuse distribution in the middle of the pons. While the raphe nuclei have a large axonal network throughout the central nervous system, utilizing serotonin as the neurotransmitter (Hornung, 2003), the locus coeruleus also has a large distributed neural network, but uses norepinephrine as its neurotransmitter. This noradrenergic innervation is believed to be important in arousal, attentiveness, and stress responsiveness, as well as emotional modulation (Szabadi, 2013). Pharmacologic agents that disrupt norepinephrine activity have a major impact on the locus coeruleus and its projections.

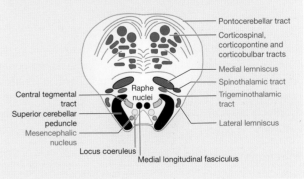

Cranial nerves

There are four cranial nerves associated with the pons. These are the **trigeminal nerve (V)**, **abducens nerve (VI)**, **facial nerve (VII)**, and **vestibulocochlear nerve (VIII)** (Table 6.1). When discussing cranial nerve lesions, it is important to be

Table 6.1 The composition and course of the four cranial nerves associated with the pons.

Trigeminal nerve (V):

Sensory: General sensation from the face (three main branches: ophthalmic (V_1), maxillary (V_2), and mandibular (V_3)), first order axons enter the skull through the superior orbital fissure (V_1), foramen rotundum (V_2) or foramen ovale (V_3), first order cell bodies in the trigeminal ganglion, axons enter the mid pons, the general sensation fibers project to the main sensory nucleus, the pain/temperature fibers project to the spinal trigeminal nucleus, and the proprioceptive fibers project to the mesencephaic nucleus.

Motor: Motor nucleus of trigeminal (V), axons exit mid pons, exit skull through the foramen ovale (V_3), innervate four muscles of mastication and four small accessory muscles.

Autonomic: No direct autonomic innervation, but the braches of the trigeminal nerve carry parasympathetic fibers that originate from the facial nerve (VII) and glossopharyngeal nerve (IX).

Abducens nerve (VI):

Motor: Abducens nucleus, axons exit medial pontomedullary junction, pass anteriorly through cavernous sinus, enter orbit through superior orbital fissure, innervate lateral rectus muscle.

Facial nerve (VII):

Sensory: General sensation from a small portion of the external auditory meatus and taste from the anterior two-thirds of the tongue, first order axons enter the skull through the stylomastoid foramen (general sensation) or via the chorda tympani nerve (taste), first order cell bodies in the geniculate ganglion, axons enter the lateral pontomedullary junction (as part of nervus intermedius), the general sensation fibers project to the spinal trigeminal nucleus and the taste fibers project to the nucleus solitarius.

Motor: Facial nucleus, axons loop posteriorly around abducens nucleus, exit lateral pontomedullary junction, enter skull through internal acoustic meatus, give off chorda tympani in middle ear, supply stapedius muscle, exit skull through stylomastoid foramen, supply muscles of facial expression as well as stylohyoid muscle and posterior belly of digastric muscle.

Autonomic: Superior salivatory nucleus (preganglionic parasympathetic), axons exit lateral pontomedullary junction (as part of nervus intermedius), enter skull through internal acoustic meatus, give off greater petrosal nerve, give off chorda tympani in middle ear. Greater petrosal nerve courses across petrous bone synapses in pterygopalatine ganglion; postganglionic parasympathetic fibers supply the nasal mucosa and the lacrimal gland. Chorda tympani courses through the middle ear, joins lingual nerve and synapses in the submandibular ganglion; postganglionic parasympathetic fibers supply the submandibular and sublingual salivary glands.

Vestibulocochlear nerve (VIII):

Sensory: First order vestibular axons arise in the ampullae of the semicircular canals or the maculae of the utricle and saccule within the temporal bone, first order cell bodies in vestibular ganglion, axons exit skull through internal acoustic meatus, enter the lateral pontomedullary junction, project to the four vestibular nuclei.

First order auditory axons arise in the organ of Corti of the cochlea within the temporal bone, first order cell bodies in spiral ganglia, axons exit skull through internal acoustic meatus, enter the lateral pontomedullary junction, project to the two cochlear nuclei.

able to distinguish if a lesion has occurred in the axons of the nerve or if a lesion occurred at one of the nuclei supplying that nerve. For example, a nerve lesion may produce multiple symptoms, while a nuclear lesion may have only specific symptoms associated with the function of that particular nucleus.

Trigeminal nerve (V)

The **trigeminal nerve (V)** is a mixed nerve with a large somatosensory component. Its peripheral axons carry tactile, pain, and temperature sensation from the face, orbit, nasal, and oral cavities into the pons, with their cell bodies found in the **trigeminal (semilunar) ganglion** (similar to a posterior (dorsal) root ganglion). The axons travel by way of three divisions of the nerve: the **ophthalmic division (V_1)**, the **maxillary division (V_2)**, and the **mandibular division (V_3)**. The axons

for fine touch synapse on the **main sensory nucleus**, while the axons for crude touch, pain, and temperature descend in the **spinal tract of the trigeminal (V)** to synapse on the **spinal nucleus of the trigeminal nerve (V)** in the pons and medulla. Note that the separation of sensory modalities (fine touch versus pain and temperature) is the same as observed in the spinal cord. The second order axons (like virtually all second order sensory axons) decussate across the pons or the medulla and ascend up the brain stem in the **trigeminothalamic tract** to synapse in the thalamus (Figure 6.11). Therefore, the spinal tract of the trigeminal (V) that is seen in the medulla and pons contains first order axons from peripheral sensory nerves that synapse in the spinal nucleus of the trigeminal (V). Recall that general sensory fibers found in the facial (VII), glossopharyngeal (IX), and vagus (X) nerves also contribute to the spinal tract of the trigeminal.

The proprioceptive (position sense) component from the muscles innervated by the trigeminal nerve (V) are carried in the mandibular division (V$_3$). These axons arise in the muscles and relay their state of contractility back to the brain. The first order axons have their cell bodies in the **mesencephalic nucleus** in the rostral pons and midbrain (Figure 6.11).

The motor component of the trigeminal nerve arises in the **motor nucleus of the trigeminal (V)** and passes out of the cranium on the third division of the nerve (**mandibular division (V$_3$)**) (Figure 6.11). It supplies eight muscles that embryologically arise from the first branchial arch and include the four muscles of mastication (temporalis, masseter, medial, and lateral pterygoid), the mylohyoid, the anterior belly of the digastric, the tensor tympani, and the tensor veli palatini muscles.

The three branches of the trigeminal nerve enter the skull through three different foramen (**ophthalmic (V$_1$) – superior orbital fissure**; **maxillary (V$_2$) – foramen rotundum**; **mandibular (V$_3$) – foramen ovale**). Two of the branches (V$_1$ and V$_2$) pass through the **cavernous sinus** before joining together at the trigeminal ganglion. The combined nerve exits the ganglion and enters the pons at the level of the middle cerebellar peduncle. Once inside the pons, the fine touch fibers enter the main sensory nucleus, the pain and temperature fibers descend in the spinal tract of the trigeminal (V) and the proprioceptive fibers ascend into the mesencephalic nucleus (Figure 6.12). The distribution of the fibers to these nuclei is highly organized and has a somatotopic arrangement (including the contributions from the facial (VII), glossopharyngeal (IX), and vagus (X) nerves).

A lesion of the trigeminal nerve will produce a large ipsilateral somatosensory loss from the face, oral, and nasal cavities, as well as an ipsilateral loss to the muscles of mastication. On the other hand, patients can also present with an increased sensitivity to sensation over the region of the face supplied by parts of the trigeminal nerve (notably the maxillary division (V$_2$)). This is referred to as **trigeminal neuralgia** or **tic douloureux**. This can be quite debilitating to patients, and treatments include the use of local anesthetics or, in severe cases, actual transection of the peripheral nerves.

Abducens nerve (VI)

The **abducens nerve (VI)** is a motor nerve that drives one extraocular muscle: the lateral rectus muscle. Since the lateral rectus produces abduction of the eye, the nerve was named the abducens nerve. The cell bodies for this innervation are found in the **abducens nucleus** (Figure 6.13). The ipsilateral axons from the nucleus descend directly through the pons and exit at the pontomedullary junction.

From the pontomedullary junction, the abducens nerve (VI) courses anteriorly across the base of the skull, passes through the **cavernous sinus**, and exits the skull through the **superior orbital fissure** into the orbit (Figure 6.14). A lesion of the abducens nerve produces diplopia (double vision), since the eyes will not move together in synchrony (especially when looking laterally on the side of the lesion).

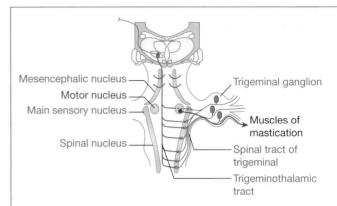

Figure 6.11 A drawing of a posterior view of the brain stem with the trigeminal nuclei and tracts highlighted. Note the location of the nuclei and tracts within the regions of the brain stem.

Facial nerve (VII)

The **facial nerve (VII)** is a mixed nerve with a large motor component (contrasted with the trigeminal nerve (V) that has a large sensory component). The motor cell bodies are found in the **facial nucleus** and supply all of the muscles from the embryological second branchial arch (the muscles of facial expression, the stapedius muscle, the stylohyoid muscle, and the posterior belly of the digastric muscle). The axons from the facial nucleus have a unique course through the pons, angling posteriorly around the abducens nucleus and then passing laterally to exit at the **pontomedullary junction** (Figure 6.15).

The second motor component of the **facial nerve (VII)** is the autonomic component – the parasympathetic innervation of the submandibular, sublingual, and lacrimal glands. The preganglionic parasympathetic cell bodies are found in the **superior salivatory nucleus** (located in the rostral medulla/caudal pons in the same positional space as the dorsal motor nucleus and the inferior salivatory nucleus) (Figures 5.16, 6.16, 6.18). The axons course through the pons to exit with the facial nerve (VII). The axons that control the lacrimal gland and the nasal cavity glands exit the facial nerve on the greater petrosal nerve, become part of the nerve of the pterygoid canal, and synapse in the **pterygopalatine ganglion**. The postganglionic parasympathetic axons from this ganglion travel on branches of the trigeminal nerve (V) to reach their target organs. The axons that control submandibular and sublingual gland function exit the facial nerve on the chorda tympani, join with the lingual nerve (of the trigeminal (V)) and synapse in the **submandibular ganglion**. Short postganglionic parasympathetic axons travel to their target organs – the submandibular and sublingual salivary glands.

The small sensory component of the **facial nerve (VII)** is taste from the anterior two-thirds of the tongue. These sensory axons begin in the tongue and are carried by the lingual nerve (of the trigeminal (V)), the chorda tympani nerve, and the facial nerve (VII) into the pons. The cell bodies of these pseudounipolar axons are in the **geniculate ganglion** and their central projections enter the pons to synapse

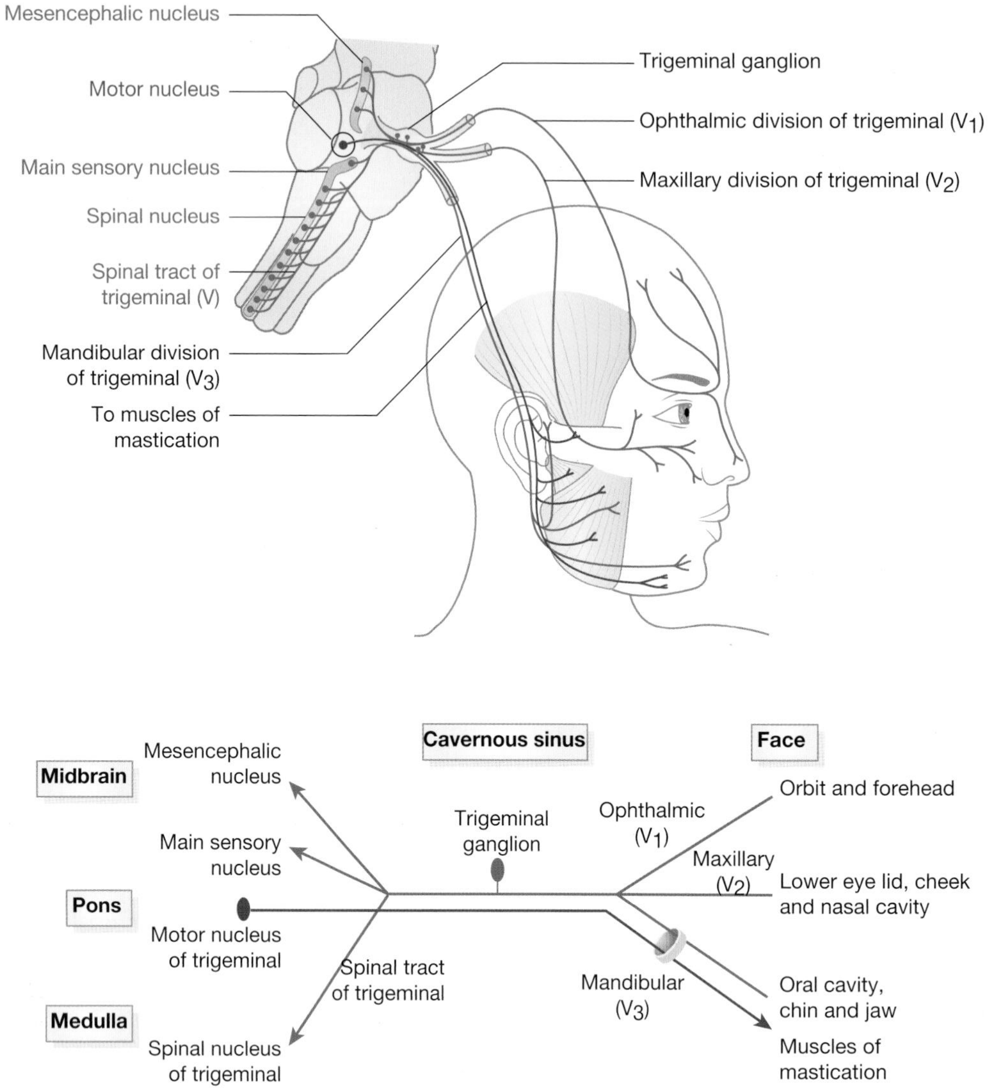

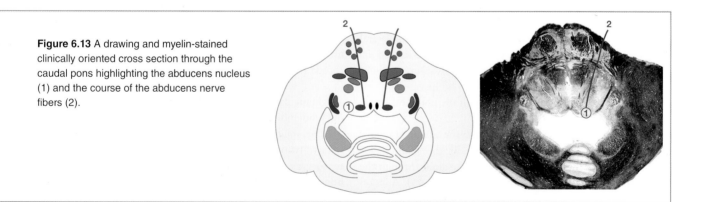

Mesencephalic nucleus

Motor nucleus

Main sensory nucleus

Spinal nucleus

Spinal tract of trigeminal (V)

Mandibular division of trigeminal (V₃)

To muscles of mastication

Trigeminal ganglion

Ophthalmic division of trigeminal (V₁)

Maxillary division of trigeminal (V₂)

Midbrain

Mesencephalic nucleus

Main sensory nucleus

Pons

Motor nucleus of trigeminal

Spinal tract of trigeminal

Medulla

Spinal nucleus of trigeminal

Cavernous sinus

Trigeminal ganglion

Face

Ophthalmic (V₁)

Orbit and forehead

Maxillary (V₂)

Lower eye lid, cheek and nasal cavity

Mandibular (V₃)

Oral cavity, chin and jaw

Muscles of mastication

Figure 6.12 A drawing and schematic version of the distribution of the trigeminal nerve (V).

Figure 6.13 A drawing and myelin-stained clinically oriented cross section through the caudal pons highlighting the abducens nucleus (1) and the course of the abducens nerve fibers (2).

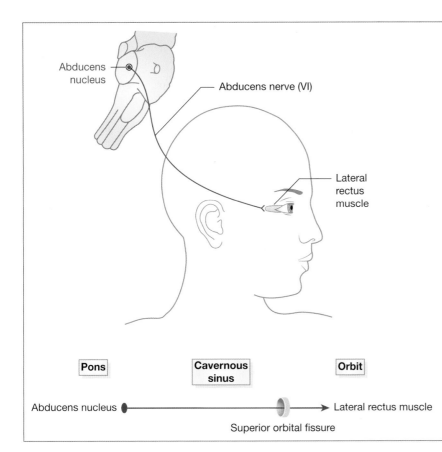

Figure 6.14 A drawing and schematic version of the distribution of the abducens nerve (VI).

in the **nucleus solitarius** (gustatory nucleus). The second order neurons from the solitary nucleus ascend ipsilaterally to the parabrachial nucleus and the thalamus, with third order neurons projecting to the cortex. There can also be a small general sensory component of the facial nerve from the external ear. The first order cell bodies are in the geniculate ganglion and synapse in the **spinal nucleus of the trigeminal (V)**. The second order cell bodies decussate and ascend on the contralateral side through the **trigeminothalamic tract**.

The parasympathetic and sensory components of the facial nerve (VII) are often combined into a separate nerve bundle referred to as the **nervus intermedius**, which can be distinguished from the lower motor neurons in the facial nerve. Since this is a separate nerve bundle, it can, on occasion, be lesioned independently.

The **facial nerve (VII)** exits the pons at the lateral pontomedullary junction, crosses the cranial cavity, and enters the skull in the **internal acoustic meatus**. Within the petrous portion of the temporal bone, the facial nerve gives off branches (greater petrosal nerve, chorda tympani nerve, nerve to stapedius) before exiting the skull through the **stylomastoid foramen** (Figure 6.16). The nerve can experience

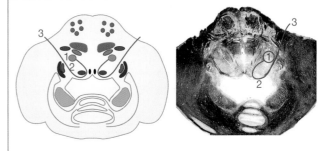

Figure 6.15 A drawing and myelin-stained clinically oriented cross section through the caudal pons highlighting the facial nucleus (1) and the course of the facial nerve fibers (2 and 3).

compression syndromes or lesions throughout its course in the temporal bone. For example, a glioblastoma (**acoustic neuroma**) at the internal acoustic meatus will produce deficits in the motor, autonomic, and sensory components of the facial nerve (VII), while a lesion of the nerve at the stylomastoid foramen will only produce a loss in motor function (muscles of facial expression).

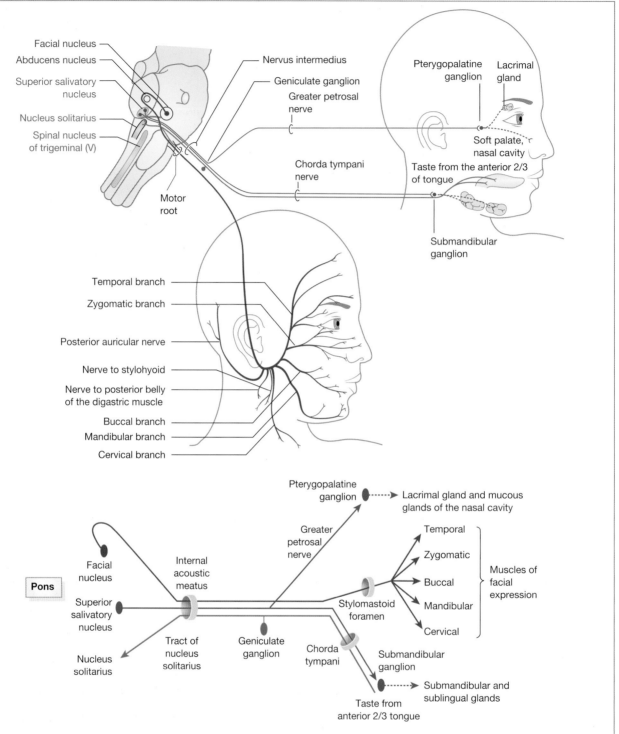

Figure 6.16 A drawing and schematic version of the distribution of the facial nerve (VII) with its motor, autonomic, and sensory components highlighted.

Vestibulocochlear nerve (VIII)

The **vestibulocochlear nerve (VIII)** is a purely sensory nerve that arises from the **vestibular apparatus** (semicircular canals/utricle) and the **cochlea** within the petrous portion of the temporal bone. The vestibular portion of the nerve has its bipolar cell bodies in the **vestibular ganglion,** with peripheral projections from the vestibular apparatus and central projections to the four **vestibular nuclei** in the medulla. Some of

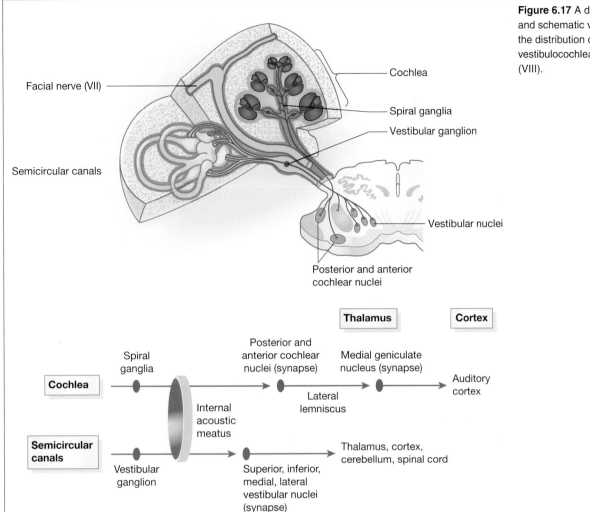

Figure 6.17 A drawing and schematic version of the distribution of the vestibulocochlear nerve (VIII).

Facial nerve (VII)

Semicircular canals

Cochlea

Spiral ganglia

Vestibular ganglion

Vestibular nuclei

Posterior and anterior cochlear nuclei

Thalamus

Cortex

Spiral ganglia

Posterior and anterior cochlear nuclei (synapse)

Medial geniculate nucleus (synapse)

Cochlea

Internal acoustic meatus

Lateral lemniscus

Auditory cortex

Semicircular canals

Vestibular ganglion

Superior, inferior, medial, lateral vestibular nuclei (synapse)

Thalamus, cortex, cerebellum, spinal cord

these projections go directly to the cerebellum, but the majority synapse in the four ipsilateral vestibular nuclei (Figure 6.17). The vestibular nuclei have a multitude of projections, including to the spinal cord (**vestibulospinal tracts**), to the control of eye muscle movement (via the **medial longitudinal fasciculus**), to the cerebellum (via the **inferior cerebellar peduncle**), and to the cortex (via the **thalamus**). Therefore, the vestibular input is directed throughout the central nervous system.

The cochlear portion of the nerve has its bipolar cell bodies in the **spiral ganglia** of the cochlea, with the peripheral projections arising from specific portions of the cochlea and the central projections synapsing in the two **cochlear nuclei** (Figure 6.17). The second order axons from the cochlear nuclei project bilaterally to ascend in the **lateral lemniscus**, with some of the axons synapsing in the **superior olive**, while others bypass the superior olive and ascend directly to the **inferior colliculus** in the midbrain. From the midbrain, these auditory

projections continue to the thalamus (**medial geniculate**) and then on to the cortex. Recall how sensation from the body is very specifically arranged in the central nervous system (somatotopic distribution). In a similar way, sound is carried to the central nervous system with specific tones (frequencies) distributed in an organized fashion (a **tonotopic** distribution).

The **vestibulocochlear nerve (VIII)** arises within the temporal bone of the skull and exits medially through the **internal acoustic meatus** (with the facial nerve (VII)). It crosses the cranial cavity and enters the brain stem at the lateral **pontomedullary junction**. The vestibular axons project to the vestibular nuclei, while the cochlear axons project to the cochlear nuclei. A lesion of the nerve at the internal acoustic meatus or at the pontomedullary junction would produce the same deficits: a loss of hearing from the ipsilateral side and disturbances in balance (vertigo). This nerve, along with its projections, is covered in more detail in Chapter 13 on the auditory and vestibular systems.

Clinical box 6.2

Utilizing Figure 6.18, notice the distribution of the sensory and motor nuclei in the medulla and pons especially concentrating on the arrangement of similar functional nuclei (e.g. the dorsal motor nucleus of the vagus, inferior salivatory nucleus, and superior salivatory nucleus). Also, identify how lesions of specific regions of the brain stem can have multiple effects depending on the nuclei and tracts involved.

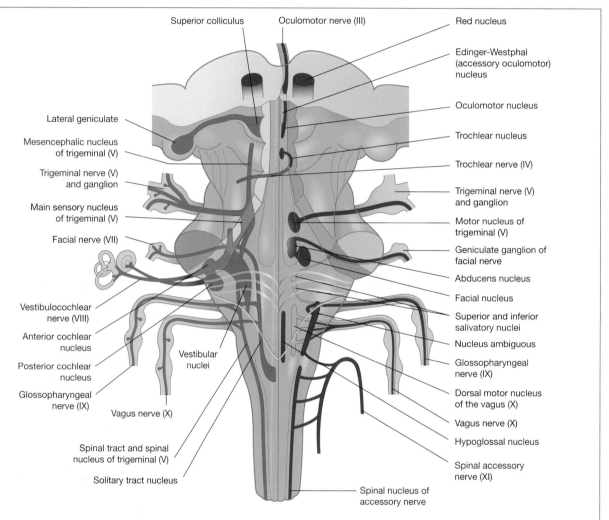

Figure 6.18 A three-dimensional drawing of the brain stem with the nuclei and tracts highlighted. Note the sensory nuclei and tracts on the left hand side and the motor nuclei and tracts on the right hand side.

Clinical considerations

At this point, it is important to be able to describe the symptoms found in patients who have had any of these cranial nerves or their branches lesioned. In addition, lesions to specific portions of the pons will produce specific symptoms (Figures 6.19 and 6.20). As mentioned previously, try to construct a visual, three-dimensional model of the spinal cord, medulla, and pons, so that the neural tracts can be followed throughout their course in the brain stem (Figure 6.18).

Pontine lesions

Red lesion?

Blue lesion?

Green lesion?

Yellow lesion?

Black lesion?

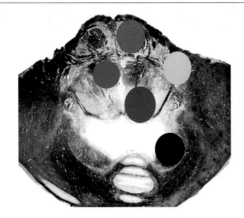

Figure 6.19 Identify the functional loss, including on which side of the patient's body the loss would be found, as well as the nuclei or tracts involved in each of the colored lesions. Remember to consider both the nuclei present and the tracts passing through the lesioned area.

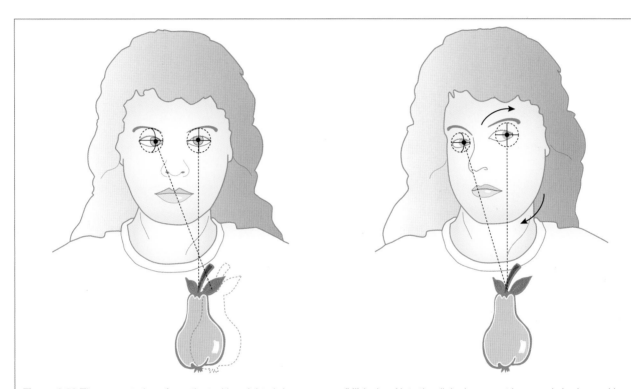

Figure 6.20 The presentation of a patient with a right abducens nerve (VI) lesion. Note the diplopia present in normal viewing and how the diplopia can be relieved by the patient rotating her head to accommodate for the loss of innervation to the right lateral rectus muscle.

Case 1

Catherine Williams, a 47-year-old school teacher, begins experiencing a "ringing" in her left ear and has some difficulty hearing. She thinks this is just an effect of age and deals with it by turning up the volume on audio equipment. A few months later, she begins to feel a "tingling" in the muscles of her face on the left side. She mentions this to her primary care physician at her annual checkup and is referred to a neurologist, Dr Peter Wondel. He takes a detailed history and performs a neurologic examination. After examining Ms Williams, he suggests that she have an MRI of the head – specifically in the region of the temporal bone. He thinks she may have an **acoustic neuroma**, which would be visible on the MRI. He describes the neuroma as slowly dividing cells that support and enwrap two cranial nerves: the facial nerve (VII) and the vestibulocochlear nerve (VIII). The increase in the number of cells has compressed the nerves as they pass through a narrow canal in the bones of the skull producing the symptoms.

Once the MRI is complete, Dr Wondel confirms the neuroma (Figure 6.21) and suggests that Ms Williams have brain surgery to remove the mass and reduce the pressure on the cranial nerves. He mentions the risks and side effects that can occur with the surgery, including the loss of hearing on the affected side, paralysis of the facial muscles on the affected side, and disturbances in balance. Ms Williams decides to wait on the surgery until the symptoms become more problematic, since she was assured by Dr Wondel that waiting will not cause problems in other parts of her nervous system. Six months later, after another MRI and visit with Dr Wondel, Ms Williams decides to have the surgery during her summer break from teaching. The surgery is successful in removing the mass and Ms Williams has no facial nerve deficits, but she does have a 50% loss of hearing from her left ear which she will have for the rest of her life.

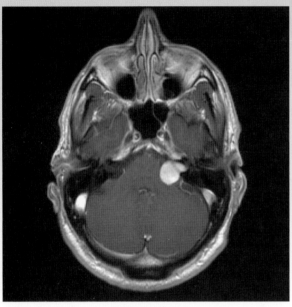

Horizontal MRI

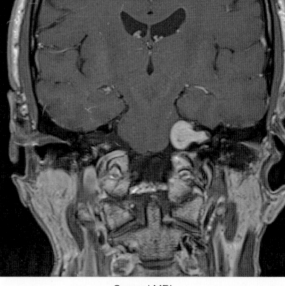

Coronal MRI

Figure 6.21 Acoustic neuroma (vestibular schwanoma) is apparent as a white circular or "lollipop" structure on the left side of the brain stem in both the horizontal and coronal views.

Case 2

A 53-year-old medical doctor, Dr Constance Armstrong, was attending a vigorous hot yoga class when she suddenly experienced a period of light headedness and tingling over her body and then she collapsed. Paramedics were called to the yoga studio. They noted a large contusion on Dr Armstrong's left occipital region, produced by the fall, and transported her to the hospital. After awakening in the hospital, Dr Armstrong noticed that she had no general sensation, pain or temperature sensation from the left side of her body or from the left side of her face. She did not notice any motor deficits.

At the hospital, she was evaluated by the emergency room physician, who immediately called for a neurological consultation. The neurologist on call, Dr Michael Christianson, evaluated Dr Armstrong and suspected that she had experienced a stroke somewhere in her brain stem, since there are only a few places were the general sensation, pain, and temperature for both the face and body are in the same area. Dr Christianson ordered an MRI of Dr Armstrong's brain and observed damage to an area on the right side of the pons just anterior to the superior cerebellar peduncle (Figure 6.22). Based on all of the available information, Dr Christianson believed that an ischemic stroke had occurred and he gave Dr Armstrong anticoagulants to prevent further blood clots and to help break up the clot that produced the stroke.

Luckily, the loss produced by the ischemia was small and localized to the rostral pons. The anticoagulants limited the amount of damage. Six months following the episode, Dr Armstrong had regained most of the sensation from her face and from portions of her thorax and abdomen, but she still had sensation losses from the upper and lower right extremities.

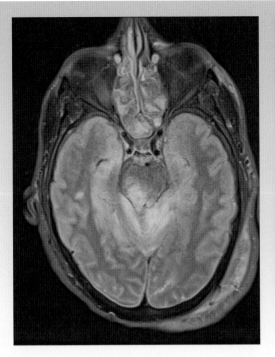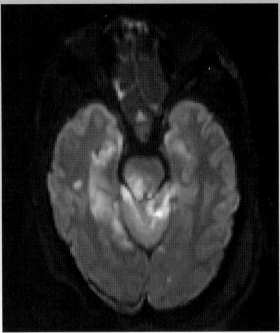

Figure 6.22 Axial magnetic resonance images of a patient with stroke (infarct) in the pons. Note the hyperintense area in the posterior pons as well as portions of the cerebellum.

Study questions

1. If a 34-year-old female patient has a lesion that produces a loss of sensation over her jaw with a loss of motor control to her muscles of mastication, then the lesion has affected the:
a) first (ophthalamic) portion of the trigeminal nerve (V)
b) second (maxillary) portion of the trigeminal nerve (V)
c) third (mandibular) portion of the trigeminal nerve (V)
d) entire trigeminal nerve (V)
e) mesencephalic nucleus of the trigeminal nerve (V)

2. A 47-year-old female patient presents to her physician with a complaint of double vision when looking to the left, but not when looking to the right. Upon examination, it is found that her left eye does not move laterally. This can be due to a lesion in the:
a) first (ophthalamic) portion of the trigeminal nerve (V)
b) second (maxillary) portion of the trigeminal nerve (V)
c) third (mandibular) portion of the trigeminal nerve (V)
d) abducens nerve (VI)
e) motor portion of the facial nerve (VII)

3. If a 64-year-old male patient has a 1 cm lesion in the caudal pons that affects the abducens nucleus and the surrounding tissue, which of the following symptoms could also be present?
a) a loss of sensation over the ipsilateral forehead and upper eye
b) a loss of motor control to the ipsilateral muscles of mastication

c) a loss of motor control to the ipsilateral muscles of facial expression
d) a loss of hearing on the ipsilateral side
e) a loss of salivary production from the ipsilateral parotid gland

4. A 42-year-old male patient experiences intense sharp pain over his cheek just below his eye when the area is stroked lightly. This heightened sense of touch/pain is referred to as trigeminal neuralgia or tic douloureux. In this patient, the sensitivity is in the:
a) first (ophthalamic) portion of the trigeminal nerve (V)
b) second (maxillary) portion of the trigeminal nerve (V)
c) third (mandibular) portion of the trigeminal nerve (V)
d) entire trigeminal nerve (V)
e) mesencephalic nucleus of the trigeminal nerve (V)

5. If a 77-year-old female patient has a lesion in the rostral pons that affects the medial lemniscus, which of the following symptoms would be present?
a) a loss of sensation over the ipsilateral forehead and upper eye
b) a loss of sensation from the contralateral body below the neck
c) a loss of motor control to the ipsilateral muscles of facial expression
d) a loss of hearing on the contralateral side
e) a loss of tear production from the contralateral lacrimal gland

For more self-assessment questions, visit the companion website at
www.wileyessential.com/neuroanatomy

FURTHER READING

For additional information on the pons, the following textbooks and review articles may be helpful:

Angeles Fernández-Gil M, Palacios-Bote R, Leo-Barahona M, Mora-Encinas JP. 2010. Anatomy of the brain stem: a gaze into the stem of life. *Semin Ultrasound CT MR*, 31(3): 196–219.

Blumenfeld H. 2002. *Neuroanatomy Through Clinical Cases*. Sinauer Associates, Sunderland, Massachusetts.

Felten DL, Shetty A. 2009. *Netter's Atlas of Neuroscience*, 2nd edition. Saunders Elsevier, Philadelphia, Pennsylvania.

Haines DE. 2012. *Neuroanatomy: An Atlas of Structures, Sections and Systems*, 8th edition. Lippincott Williams & Wilkin, Baltimore, Maryland.

Hornung JP. 2003. The human raphe nuclei and the serotonergic system. *J Chem Neuroanat*, 26(4): 331–343.

Moore KL, Dalley AF, Agur AMR. 2014. *Moore Clinically Oriented Anatomy*, 7th edition. Lippincott, Williams & Wilkins, Philadelphia, Pennsylvania.

Moncayo J. 2012. Pontine infarcts and hemorrhages. *Front Neurol Neurosci*, 30: 162–165.

Patestas MA, Gartner LP. 2006. *A Textbook of Neuroanatomy*. Blackwell Publishing, Malden, Massachusetts.

Szabadi E. 2013. Functional neuroanatomy of the central noradrenergic system. *J Psychopharmacol*, 27(8): 659–693.

Urfy MZ, Suarez JI. 2014. Breathing and the nervous system. *Handb Clin Neurol*, 119: 241–250.

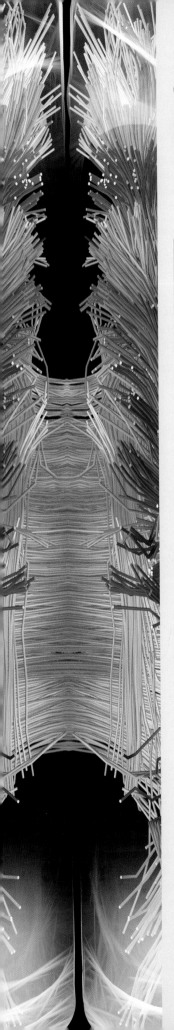

CHAPTER 7
Midbrain

Learning objectives

1. Describe components of the oculomotor and trochlear nerves (III and IV).
2. Describe lesions of the oculomotor and trochlear nerves (III and IV).
3. Identify the nuclei and tracts in cross sections of the midbrain at the level of the superior and inferior colliculus.
4. Identify the clinical symptoms associated with lesions in the midbrain.

Midbrain   96

Tectum
1. Corpora quadrigemina
   a) Superior colliculi (2)
   b) Inferior colliculi (2)
2. Trochlear nerve (IV)
3. Cerebral aqueduct (of Sylvius)

Tegmentum
1. Red nucleus
2. Substantia nigra
3. Cerebral peduncles
   a) Corticospinal tract
   b) Corticobulbar tract
   c) Corticopontine tract
4. Oculomotor nerve (III)

Cross section of the caudal midbrain   97

Tracts
1. Cerebral peduncles
   a) Corticospinal tract
   b) Corticobulbar tract
   c) Corticopontine tract
2. Medial lemniscus
3. Spinothalamic tract
4. Trigeminothalamic tract
5. Medial longitudinal fasciculus
6. Decussation of superior cerebellar peduncles
7. Lateral lemniscus (to inferior colliculus)

Essential Clinical Neuroanatomy, First Edition. Thomas H. Champney.
© 2016 John Wiley & Sons, Ltd. Published 2016 by John Wiley & Sons, Ltd.
Companion website: www.wileyessential.com/neuroanatomy

Nuclei
1. Inferior colliculi
2. Substantia nigra – dopaminergic
3. Trochlear nuclei

Tracts
1. Medial lemniscus
2. Spinothalamic tract
3. Trigeminothalamic tract
4. Medial longitudinal fasciculus
5. Cerebral peduncles
   a) Corticospinal tract
   b) Corticobulbar tract
   c) Corticopontine tract

Nuclei
1. Oculomotor nuclei
2. Red nucleus
3. Substantia nigra – dopaminergic
4. Ventral tegmental area – dopaminergic
5. Periaqueductal gray
6. Superior colliculi

Oculomotor nucleus adjacent to cerebral aqueduct in rostral midbrain

Exits in midline of anterior surface of midbrain

Innervates four extraocular muscles (except lateral rectus and superior oblique muscles)

Autonomic parasympathetic components
1. Nucleus of Edinger-Westphal (near oculomotor nucleus)
2. Follows course of oculomotor nerve (III)

3. Synapse in ciliary ganglion
4. Innervates sphincter pupillae – pupillary constriction
5. Innervates ciliary muscle – accommodation

Exits anterior midbrain, passes between superior cerebellar and posterior cerebral arteries, through cavernous sinus and superior orbital fissure

Lesion produces ptosis ("drooping" eyelid), diplopia, and dilated pupil

Trochlear nucleus adjacent to cerebral aqueduct in caudal midbrain

Exits posteriorly, courses laterally around midbrain, through cavernous sinus

Innervates contralateral superior oblique muscle

Lesion produces loss of superior oblique muscle, diplopia

Midbrain, oculomotor nerve (III) and trochlear nerve (IV) lesions

Parkinson disease – dopamine loss in substantia nigra

Berry (saccular) aneurysm

Superior alternating hemiplegia (Weber's syndrome)

Introduction

In this chapter, the tracts presented in the spinal cord, medulla, and pons will be followed into the **midbrain**. In addition, the cranial nerve nuclei (the oculomotor and trochlear cranial nerves (III and IV)) and other associated nuclei found in the midbrain will be covered. One take home message for the midbrain is that this is a narrow, constricted portion of the upper brain stem through which all axons entering or exiting the thalamus and cortex must pass.

Anatomy of the midbrain

The midbrain is the upper aspect of the brain stem and it can generally be divided into two portions: a posteriorly placed **tectum** and an anteriorly placed **tegmentum** (Figure 7.1). The tectum is found posterior to the **cerebral aqueduct** and contains four "hills", the **corpora quadrigemina**. The corpora quadrigemina can be subdivided into two pairs of "hills", the **superior colliculi** and the **inferior colliculi**. The tegmentum is the portion of the brain stem anterior to the

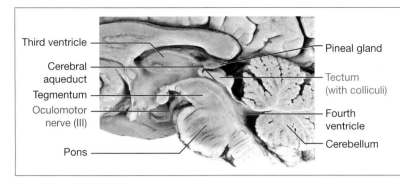

Figure 7.1 A sagittal section of the brain stem with the components of the midbrain highlighted. Note the posteriorly placed tectum and the anteriorly placed tegmentum, with the intervening cerebral aqueduct (of Sylvius).

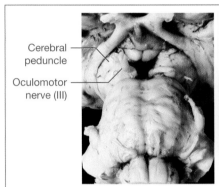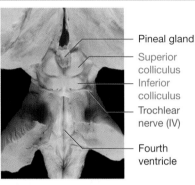

Figure 7.2 Anterior and posterior views of the midbrain. Note the two cranial nerves associated with the midbrain, the oculomotor (III), and trochlear (IV) nerves.

cerebral aqueduct and contains numerous nuclei and tracts, including the **red nucleus**, **substantia nigra**, and **cerebral peduncles**.

When viewed inferiorly/anteriorly, the most noticeable structures in the midbrain are the **cerebral peduncles** that contain the **corticospinal**, **corticobulbar**, and **corticopontine tracts**. Passing medially between the cerebral peduncles, the **oculomotor nerves (III)** can be observed (Figure 7.2). When viewed superiorly/posteriorly, the most noticeable structures in the midbrain are the **corpora quadrigemina** (superior and inferior colliculi). Upon careful examination, the small **trochlear nerve (IV)** can be seen exiting the posterior portion of the midbrain just below the inferior colliculi (Figure 7.2).

Cross section of the caudal midbrain

Two cross sections of the midbrain are usually described: one at the level of the inferior colliculi and the trochlear nerve (IV) (caudal cross section) and one at the level of the superior colliculi and the oculomotor nerve (III) (rostral cross section). Neural tracts are found in both cross sections. The **corticospinal tracts**, for example, are found in the anterior aspect of both cross sections and are referred to as the **cerebral peduncles**. Recall that the corticospinal axons are intermixed with motor axons from the cortex that project to cranial nerve nuclei (**corticobulbar axons**) and motor axons

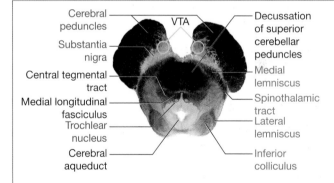

Figure 7.3 A myelin-stained cross section of the caudal midbrain. Note the location of the tracts that pass through the midbrain, along with the specialized nuclei. VTA = ventral tegmental area.

that project to pontine nuclei (**corticopontine axons**) (Figure 7.3).

The tracts found in the caudal midbrain, besides the descending motor tracts, are the three ascending sensory tracts (the **medial lemniscus**, the **trigeminothalamic tract**, and the **spinothalamic tract**) as well as the **medial longitudinal fasciculus**. The sensory tracts are in a similar position as found in the rostral pons – flattened and moving laterally. The medial longitudinal fasciculus is in the same postero-medial position throughout the brain stem. A new set of axons found in the caudal midbrain is a large midline structure – the **decussation of the superior cerebellar peduncles**. The superior cerebellar peduncles leave the cerebellum and then cross over (decussate) to the other side of the midbrain where they ascend to the thalamus or synapse in the large **red nucleus**. In the caudal midbrain, both peduncles are intermingled in a single structure as they cross from one side to the other (much like the center of a large "X").

The nuclei found in the caudal midbrain include the **inferior colliculi** (relay nuclei for hearing) that are in the **tectum** posterior to the **cerebral aqueduct**. Also, the **substantia nigra** ("black substance") is found just posterior to the cerebral peduncles and inferior to the three sensory tracts. These cell bodies are pigmented in normal individuals and hence the name, substantia nigra. These neurons are dopaminergic (use dopamine as a neurotransmitter) and are part of the central motor control system. The last set of nuclei are the **trochlear nuclei** that are adjacent to the medial longitudinal fasciculus (Figure 7.3).

Cross section of the rostral midbrain

The rostral midbrain is quite similar to the caudal midbrain, except that the three sensory tracts (the **medial lemniscus**, the **trigeminothalamic tract**, and the **spinothalamic tract**) have moved laterally in the rostral midbrain, with the medial lemniscus looking like a "stocking cap" on a large centrally placed nucleus (the red nucleus). The **medial longitudinal fasciculus** and the **cerebral peduncles**, on the other hand, have stayed in their usual locations (Figure 7.4).

The nuclei found in the rostral midbrain include the **oculomotor nuclei** found in the postero-medial portion of the tegmentum, just anterior to the medial longitudinal fasciculus. A large centrally located nucleus in the tegmentum is the **red nucleus** that is involved in relaying cerebellar information to the brain stem and spinal cord. Also, the **substantia nigra** is found in the same position as in the caudal midbrain – just posterior to the cerebral peduncles and lateral to the red nucleus. Just medial to the substantia nigra in the anterior region of the tegmentum is another collection of dopaminergic cell bodies, the **ventral tegmental area (VTA)**. This area is involved in emotion and reward mechanisms related to the limbic system. Surrounding the cerebral aqueduct in the tegmentum is a diffuse collection of neuronal cell bodies that mediate pain recognition and defensive behavior, termed the **periaqueductal gray** (similar to the reticular formation in the pons and medulla). In the tectum of the rostral midbrain are the **superior colliculi** (relay nuclei for visual inputs) (Figure 7.4).

Remember to keep in mind that the tracts are made of axons that are passing through these cross sections, so they will be seen in sections above and below the section of interest. If possible, describe the type of fibers and the course they take whenever a neural track is encountered.

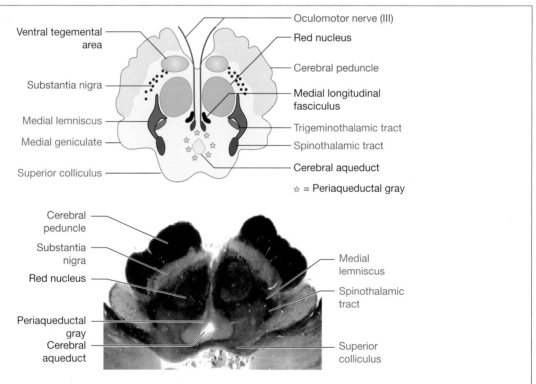

Figure 7.4 A drawing and myelin-stained cross section of the rostral midbrain. Note the location of the ascending sensory tracts and the descending motor tracts.

Clinical box 7.1

There are three major aminergic neurotransmitter systems in the brain: the dopaminergic (dopamine as a neurotransmitter), the noradrenergic (norepinephrine as a neurotransmitter), and the serotonergic (serotonin as a neurotransmitter) system. The cell bodies for each of these systems are found in specific nuclei in the brain stem. The serotonin neurons are in the raphe nuclei, the norepinephrine neurons are in the locus coeruleus, and the dopamine neurons are in the substantia nigra and the ventral tegmental area. Some other aminergic cell bodies are found in the forebrain, but these are the major sites for these systems.

While noting the location and distribution of these specific neuronal systems, it should be kept in mind that many pharmacologic agents (and drugs of abuse) target these specific systems. Drugs that modify serotoninergic actions are used as antidepressants, while dopaminergic compounds can modify attention (for attention deficit disorders). When learning about neuropharmacologic drugs (and drugs of abuse), it is valuable to realize that they modify these entire systems (or components of the systems), which can have the intended effect as well as numerous side effects.

Cranial nerves

There are two cranial nerves associated with the midbrain. These are the **oculomotor nerve** (III) and the **trochlear nerve** (IV).

Oculomotor nerve (III)

The **oculomotor nerve (III)** is a motor nerve that controls muscles in the orbit and parasympathetic innervation of the eye. The skeletal motor component of the oculomotor nerve arises in the **oculomotor nucleus** and passes through the tegmentum of the midbrain to exit out of the anterior surface between the cerebral peduncles. It supplies four muscles of the eye (medial rectus, superior rectus, inferior rectus, inferior oblique) and the levator palpebrae superioris.

The autonomic motor component of the **oculomotor nerve (III)** drives the parasympathetic innervation of both the ciliary muscle and constrictor pupillae muscle of the eye. The preganglionic parasympathetic cell bodies are found in the **nucleus of Edinger-Westphal** (located adjacent to the oculomotor nucleus in the rostral midbrain). The axons course through the midbrain with the oculomotor nerve (III). The axons leave the oculomotor nerve in the orbit to pass along the lateral aspect of the optic nerve to reach the **ciliary ganglion**. The postganglionic parasympathetic axons from this ganglion travel on short ciliary nerves to reach their target organs – the ciliary muscle for accommodation of the lens and the constrictor pupillae muscle to reduce the size of the pupil (Figure 7.5).

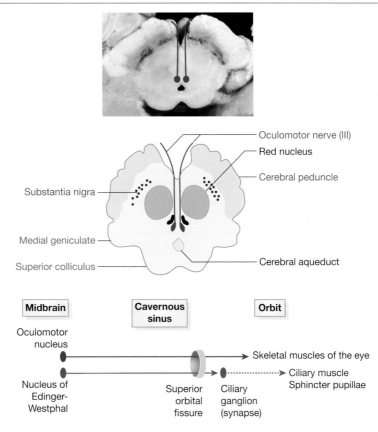

Figure 7.5 A drawing and schematic version of the distribution of the oculomotor nerve (III).

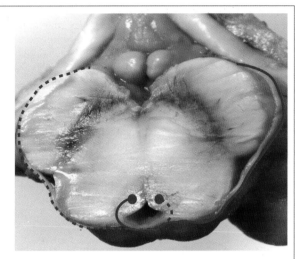

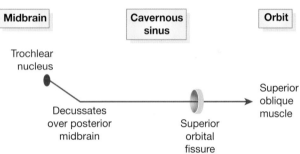

Figure 7.6 A drawing and schematic version of the distribution of the trochlear nerve (IV). Note the early decussation of the nerve fibers, so that the nucleus is contralateral, but the majority of the nerve is ipsilateral to the superior oblique muscle.

The **oculomotor nerve (III)** exits the midbrain between the **cerebral peduncles**, passes through the cranial cavity (between the **superior cerebellar artery** and the **posterior cerebral artery**) to enter the **cavernous sinus**. The nerve leaves the sinus to enter the orbit through the **superior orbital fissure**, where it divides into two branches to supply the muscles of the orbit (Table 7.1). A lesion of the oculomotor nerve produces an ipsilateral motor loss to four of the six muscles of the eye, resulting in a "drooping" eyelid (ptosis), pronounced diplopia, and a dilated pupil that is directed inferiorly and laterally ("down and out") (Figure 7.7).

Trochlear nerve (IV)

The **trochlear nerve (IV)** is a motor nerve that drives one extraocular muscle: the superior oblique muscle. Since the superior oblique muscle courses through a small pulley ("trochlea") in the orbit, the nerve was named the trochlear nerve. The cell bodies for this innervation are found in the **trochlear nucleus** in the caudal midbrain. The axons from the nucleus take a unique course through the tectum to exit the posterior surface of the brain stem (the only cranial nerve to exit posteriorly). The axons decussate and travel around the lateral surface of the midbrain in the subarachnoid space to enter the **cavernous sinus**. They leave the cavernous sinus through the **superior orbital fissure** and innervate the superior oblique muscle (Figure 7.6) (Table 7.1).

A lesion of the trochlear nerve produces diplopia in the ipsilateral eye (since the nerve decussates quickly after leaving the posterior brain stem), while a lesion of the trochlear

Table 7.1   The composition and course of the two cranial nerves associated with the midbrain.

Oculomotor nerve (III):

Motor: Oculomotor nucleus, axons pass through midbrain, exit anterior midbrain medial to cerebral peduncles, pass between superior cerebellar and posterior cerebral arteries, anteriorly through cavernous sinus, enter orbit through superior orbital fissure, innervate levator palpebrae superioris, superior rectus, medial rectus, inferior rectus and inferior oblique muscles.

Autonomic: Nucleus of Edinger-Westphal (preganglionic parasympathetic), axons pass through midbrain, exit anterior midbrain medial to cerebral peduncles, pass between superior cerebellar and posterior cerebral arteries, anteriorly through cavernous sinus, enter orbit through superior orbital fissure, synapse in ciliary ganglion; postganglionic parasympathetic fibers innervate ciliary muscle (accommodation) and sphincter pupillae muscle (constricts pupil).

Trochlear nerve (IV):

Motor: Trochlear nucleus, axons exit posterior midbrain, decussate, pass around lateral border of midbrain, anteriorly through cavernous sinus, enter orbit through superior orbital fissure, innervate superior oblique muscle.

Clinical box 7.2

The midbrain has numerous ascending and descending tracts, as well as specialized nuclei. As emphasized previously, it is a narrow constriction where the majority of fibers exiting or entering the forebrain must pass. This results in a "bottleneck", where a small localized lesion or small loss of blood supply (stroke) can produce large deficits (Moncayo, 2012). Notice the close relationship of the cerebral peduncle (descending motor tracts) with the substantia nigra (a nucleus for central motor control), as well as the ventral tegmental area (dopaminergic cells involved in reward, motivation, and pleasure circuits). Consider how a small vascular loss can impact on the function of these structures.

Recall also that the midbrain flexion rotates the forebrain 90 degrees anteriorly, so that structures that were anterior now become inferior, and structures that were posterior now become superior. The base of the forebrain is now inferior, while the base of the brain stem is anterior.

This completes the anatomical description of the brain stem. It is beneficial to reconstruct the brain stem into a three-dimensional unit by putting together all of the information learned from the previous four chapters. The following figures can help with this task:

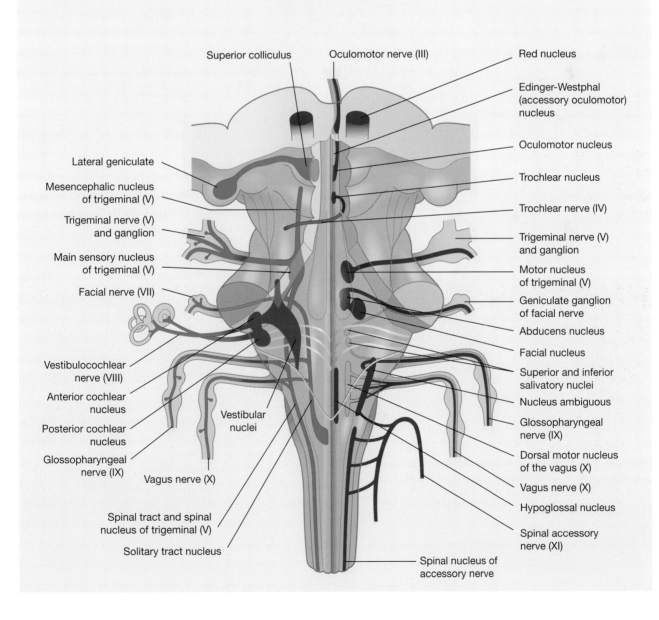

Red nucleus

Oculomotor nerve (III)

Mesencephalic nucleus of trigeminal nerve

Principal sensory nucleus of trigeminal nerve

Trigeminal nerve (V) and ganglion

Motor nucleus of trigeminal nerve

Facial nerve (VII)

Vestibulocochlear nerve (VIII)

Abducens nerve (VI)

Glossopharyngeal nerve (IX)

Hypoglossal nerve (XII)

Vagus nerve (X)

Olive

Accessory nerve (XI)

Spinal tract and spinal nucleus of trigeminal nerve

Edinger-Westphal (accessory oculomotor) nucleus

Oculomotor nucleus

Trochlear nucleus

Trochlear nerve (IV)

Internal genu of facial nerve

Abducens nucleus

Vestibular nuclei

Facial nucleus

Anterior and posterior cochlear nuclei

Superior and inferior salivatory nuclei

Solitary tract nucleus

Posterior (dorsal) nucleus of vagus nerve (X)

Hypoglossal nucleus

Nucleus ambiguous

Spinal nucleus of accessory nerve

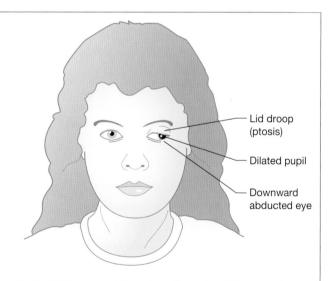

Figure 7.7 The presentation of a patient with a left oculomotor nerve (III) lesion. Note the ptosis of the eyelid, the dilated pupil, and the "down and out" position of the affected eye.

Lid droop (ptosis)

Dilated pupil

Downward abducted eye

nucleus produces a contralateral effect. A patient with a trochlear nerve lesion will present with the head tilted away from the side of the nerve lesion (and slightly flexed) to compensate for the inability of the affected eye to rotate properly (loss of the superior oblique muscle). By keeping the head in this position, the patient does not experience diplopia (Figure 7.8).

Clinical considerations

At this point, it is important to be able to describe the symptoms present if any of these cranial nerves are lesioned (Figures 7.7 and 7.8). In addition, lesions to small portions of the midbrain will produce specific symptoms (Figures 7.7, 7.8, 7.9). A specific biochemical deficit can occur in the substantia nigra that results in decreased dopamine production. This produces typical motor symptoms of Parkinson disease which will be discussed in greater detail in the chapter on central motor control (Chapter 15).

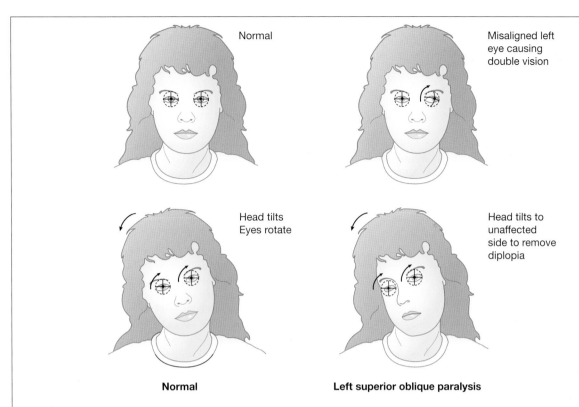

Normal

Misaligned left
eye causing
double vision

Head tilts
Eyes rotate

Head tilts to
unaffected
side to remove
diplopia

Normal   **Left superior oblique paralysis**

Figure 7.8 The presentation of a patient with a left trochlear nerve (IV) lesion. Note the diplopia present in normal viewing and how the diplopia can be relieved by the patient rotating her head to the opposite side to accommodate for the loss of the innervation to the superior oblique muscle.

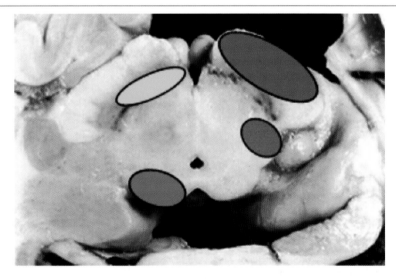

Figure 7.9 Describe the symptoms that would be present in a patient with each of the colored lesions indicated.

Case 1

Mrs Judy Chambers, a 57-year-old, chain-smoking administrative assistant at an accounting firm, begins experiencing headaches and periods where she has double vision. Concerned, she visits her long-time family physician who refers her to a local neurologist, Dr David Eckert. He performs a neurological exam and notices a slight weakness in Mrs Chamber's right eye movements. He suspects there is a problem with her right oculomotor nerve (III).

Dr Eckert suggests that Mrs Chambers has an MRI of her brain stem and orbit to visualize the extent of her third cranial nerve. When viewing her MRI, he believes he sees some compression of her third nerve just after it exits the midbrain. Because of his uncertainty and with his knowledge of the structures in the area of interest, he requests that Mrs Chambers has a vertebral arteriogram to visualize the branches of the vertebral and basilar arteries. When the results of the arteriogram are viewed, Dr Eckert can see a large aneurysm in the right posterior cerebral artery (a **berry or saccular aneurysm**) that would place pressure on the adjacent oculomotor nerve (Figure 7.10).

Dr Eckert suggests that Mrs Chambers has surgery to prevent the aneurysm from rupturing (since it could be fatal). He suggests that she have the aneurysm clipped or a coil inserted into the aneurysm. The coil procedure is less invasive and Mrs Chambers agrees with this approach. The intra-vascular procedure is successful. Mrs Chambers is urged to quit smoking and develop a healthier lifestyle. One year later, she no longer has headaches or double vision, but has not given up smoking.

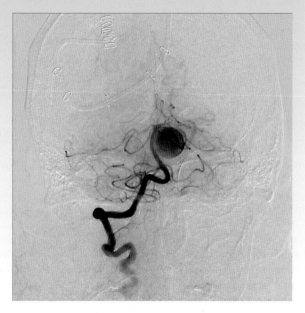

Figure 7.10 A vertebral arteriogram of a large aneurysm in the posterior cerebral artery before treatment.

Case 2

Mr James Adams, a 63-year-old, diabetic carpenter, had just finished working for the day, when he complained of a terrible headache and collapsed. On arrival at the hospital, he regained consciousness and realized that he had no ability to control his muscles on the right side of his body – he could not move his right arm or his right leg. The on-call neurologist in the emergency room, Dr Phil Kagan, did a complete history and physical, along with a neurological exam. Dr Kagan noticed that Mr Adams' sensory abilities were all intact, but that he was unable to exert volitional motor control on the entire right side of his body, including his right extremities and his right tongue, although he could still raise his right eyebrow. Dr Kagan also noted that Mr Adams' left eye was dilated and directed down and out, with a mild drooping of his left eyelid.

After an MRI and cerebral angiography, Dr Kagan informed Mr Adams that he had suffered a small stroke that disabled a majority of his descending motor tracts in his left cerebral peduncle in the midbrain, along with the adjacent cranial nerve (oculomotor III) (**superior alternating hemiplegia** or **Weber's syndrome**) (Figure 7.11). Over the next few hours in the emergency room, Mr Adams regained some motor control in his right lower extremity. After being released from hospital, Mr Adams began physical therapy and six months later he had regained a substantial amount of muscle control, although he did not regain his original strength and coordination. Because of his disability, he retired from his job as a carpenter.

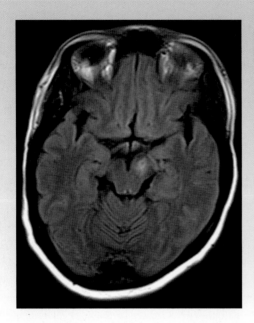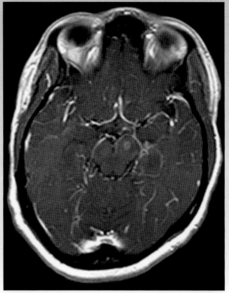

Figure 7.11 Magnetic resonance images of a lesion in the left cerebral peduncle. Note the hyperintense signal in the center of the left cerebral peduncle (pyramid).

Study questions

1. A 52-year-old male patient presents with diplopia. Upon examination, his right eye is directed inferiorly and laterally under a slightly drooping eyelid. Suspecting a cranial nerve lesion, his physician looks for additional symptoms in this patient including:
a) a constricted right pupil due to impaired sympathetic innervation
b) a dilated right pupil due to impaired parasympathetic innervation
c) a dry right eye due to impaired lacrimal secretion
d) impaired action of the right superior oblique muscle
e) impaired action of the right lateral rectus muscle

2. If a 43-year-old female patient presents with a right trochlear nerve (IV) lesion, which of the following symptoms would be present?
a) a constricted right pupil due to impaired sympathetic innervation
b) a dilated right pupil due to impaired parasympathetic innervation
c) a dry right eye due to impaired lacrimal secretion
d) impaired action of the right superior oblique muscle
e) impaired action of the right lateral rectus muscle

3. If a 67-year-old female patient has a lesion in the tectum of her midbrain, which of the following functions would be affected?
a) general sensation from the face, head, and body
b) corticospinal motor function on voluntary skeletal muscles
c) fine motor control with Parkinson-like symptoms
d) mood, memory, arousal, and awareness
e) visual or auditory sensations

4. The cerebral peduncles contain:
a) sensory axons for pain, temperature, and general sensation from the face
b) sensory axons for general sensation from the body below the neck
c) sensory axons for the special senses of vision and hearing
d) cerebellar output axons projecting to the spinal cord
e) corticospinal motor axons to skeletal muscles

5. A 59-year-old female has a lesion in the lateral lemniscus. This would have a direct effect on which of the following midbrain structures?
a) cerebral peduncles
b) red nucleus
c) substantia nigra
d) inferior colliculus
e) superior colliculus

For more self-assessment questions, visit the companion website at
www.wileyessential.com/neuroanatomy

FURTHER READING

For additional information on the midbrain, the following textbooks and review articles may be helpful:

Angeles Fernández-Gil M, Palacios-Bote R, Leo-Barahona M, Mora-Encinas JP. 2010. Anatomy of the brain stem: a gaze into the stem of life. *Semin Ultrasound CT MR*, 31(3): 196–219.

Bae YJ, Kim JH, Choi BS, Jung C, Kim E. 2103. Brainstem pathways for horizontal eye movement: pathologic correlation with MR imaging. *Radiographics*, 33(1): 47–59.

Beitz JM. 2014. Parkinson's disease: a review. *Front Biosci (Schol Ed)*, 6: 65–74.

Blumenfeld H. 2002. *Neuroanatomy Through Clinical Cases*. Sinauer Associates, Sunderland, Massachusetts.

Felten DL, Shetty A. 2009. *Netter's Atlas of Neuroscience*, 2nd edition. Saunders Elsevier, Philadelphia, Pennsylvania.

Haines DE. 2012. *Neuroanatomy: An Atlas of Structures, Sections and Systems*, 8th edition. Lippincott Williams & Wilkin, Baltimore, Maryland.

Moncayo J. 2012. Midbrain infarcts and hemorrhages. *Front Neurol Neurosci.* 30:158–161.

Moore KL, Dalley AF, Agur AMR. 2014. *Moore Clinically Oriented Anatomy*, 7th edition. Lippincott, Williams & Wilkins, Philadelphia, Pennsylvania.

Patestas MA, Gartner LP. 2006. *A Textbook of Neuroanatomy*. Blackwell Publishing, Malden, Massachusetts.

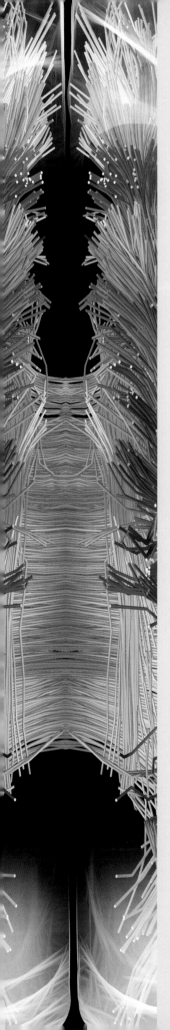

CHAPTER 8
Diencephalon

Learning objectives

1. Describe the main anatomical and functional components of the diencephalon.
2. Identify the ventricular structures of the diencephalon.
3. Identify the external features of the diencephalon.
4. Describe the symptoms of lesions produced in the thalamus and hypothalamus.

Diencephalon anatomy 108

Thalamus
1. Thalamic nuclei – relays to the cortex
2. Massa intermedia
3. Sensory and motor gateway to the cortex

Hypothalamus
1. Infundibulum (pituitary stalk)
2. Mammillary bodies
3. Homeostasis – temperature, energy, metabolism, water balance

Epithalamus
1. Pineal gland – melatonin
2. Stria medullaris
3. Habenula

Third ventricle
1. Choroid plexus – cerebrospinal fluid production
2. Interventricular foramen (of Monro)
3. Cerebral aqueduct (of Sylvius)

Neural tracts 109

Sensory tracts
1. Medial lemniscus
2. Spinothalamic tract
3. Trigeminothlamic tract
4. All terminate in the thalamus, with subsequent projections to the cortex

---

Essential Clinical Neuroanatomy, First Edition. Thomas H. Champney.
© 2016 John Wiley & Sons, Ltd. Published 2016 by John Wiley & Sons, Ltd.
Companion website: www.wileyessential.com/neuroanatomy

Motor tracts
1. Corticospinal tracts
2. Corticobulbar tracts
3. Corticopontine tracts
4. All pass through the internal capsule from the cortex to the cerebral peduncle in the midbrain

Integration tracts
1. Fornix
2. Medial forebrain bundle
3. Stria medullaris
4. Stria terminalis
5. Mamillothalamic tract
6. Thalamocortical fibers (thalamic radiations)

Olfactory (I)
1. Cribriform plate
2. Olfactory bulb

3. Olfactory tract
4. Cortical projections
5. Lesions – anosmia

Optic (II)
1. Ganglion cells of the retina
2. Optic nerve (II)
3. Optic chiasm
4. Optic tract
5. Lateral geniculate (thalamic relay)
6. Optic cortex
7. Lesions – blindness

Hypothalamic tumor

Thalamic pain syndrome

Introduction

The **diencephalon** has two main functions: to mediate the neural input to the cortex and to provide set points for numerous homeostatic mechanisms. The neural mediation takes place in the **thalamus**, while the homeostatic mechanisms are regulated in the **hypothalamus**. Some neuroscientists consider the diencephalon as the "old brain" where basic neural regulation takes place in evolutionarily older species.

The development of the diencephalon is from the original forebrain of the embryo. The forebrain will develop into the telencephalon (the cortical structures), the diencephalon, and the early eye vesicles (Chapter 3).

Neuroanatomy

The diencephalon is made of three components. The largest is the **thalamus**, located in the center of the brain and it contains numerous sensory relay nuclei. The second largest is the **hypothalamus**, located just inferior to the thalamus and it also contains numerous nuclei that are involved in homeostatic mechanisms. The third and smallest area of the diencephalon is the **epithalamus**, which contains the **pineal gland** and the **habenula** (Figure 8.1).

The **thalamus** is composed of two, large, egg-shaped structures connected across the midline by a small bridge known as the **massa intermedia**. Each of the egg-shaped structures contains numerous smaller nuclei which relay information from the periphery to the cortex. For example, sensory information from the body and face are relayed through the ventral posterior lateral and ventral posterior medial nuclei of the thalamus, respectively. Likewise, two projections off the posterior end of the thalamus, the **geniculate nuclei**, are specific relay nuclei for vision (**lateral geniculate**) and audition (**medial geniculate**). While a great deal is known about the specific relay nuclei in the thalamus and their projections, this level of detail is not necessary for clinical diagnosis. Generally, if a lesion or stroke occurs in the thalamus then major dysfunction occurs (Satpute *et al.*, 2013; Schmahmann, 2003).

The thalamus is subdivided into numerous, small, well-demarcated nuclei that act as relay points for cortical information (thalamocortical fibers). Virtually all sensory information must pass through the thalamus before reaching the cortex (olfactory sensation is an exception). Motor information from the basal ganglia and cerebellum to the cortex is also relayed through thalamic nuclei, as is information from the limbic system. Finally, information that leaves the cortex is also a major input to the thalamus (corticothalamic fibers). All of these inputs to the thalamus result in a major regulatory role of the thalamus on cortical function (Figure 8.2).

The **hypothalamus** is a bilateral structure located on either side of the third ventricle, just inferior to the thalamus, and contains numerous nuclei involved in **homeostasis** (the balance of normal physiologic function in a changing environment). For example, there are specific nuclei that regulate circadian rhythms, food intake, water intake, metabolism, temperature regulation, and reproductive function. All of these nuclei are found in a relatively small region in the inferior

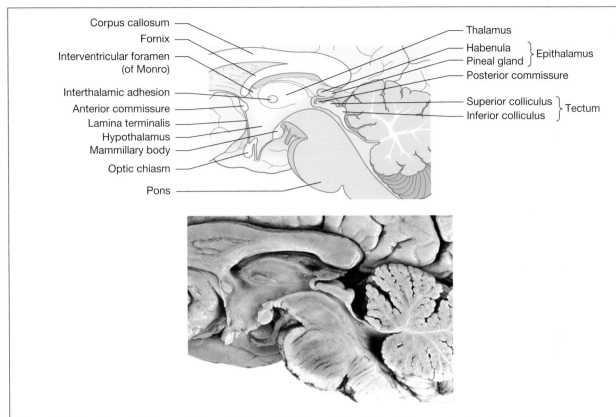

Corpus callosum
Fornix
Interventricular foramen (of Monro)
Interthalamic adhesion
Anterior commissure
Lamina terminalis
Hypothalamus
Mammillary body
Optic chiasm
Pons

Thalamus
Habenula } Epithalamus
Pineal gland
Posterior commissure
Superior colliculus } Tectum
Inferior colliculus

Figure 8.1 A drawing and photograph of a sagittal view of the diencephalon. Note the three parts of the diencephalon: the hypothalamus, the thalamus, and the epithalamus.

aspect of the diencephalon. The hypothalamus has numerous neural connections with other parts of the nervous system. This includes connections with the autonomic nervous system (parasympathetic and sympathetic regulation of heart rate, blood pressure, and digestion) as well as the limbic system (emotional responses). A number of these nuclei also communicate directly with the pituitary gland by means of a neural connection, the infundibulum or pituitary stalk. Other nuclei communicate indirectly with the pituitary gland by releasing small hormones into a dedicated hypothalamo-hypophyseal portal venous system. The pituitary releases numerous hormones into the general circulation to modify growth, metabolism, reproductive function, and other endocrine functions.

The hypothalamus can be subdivided into medial nuclei (adjacent to the third ventricle) and more lateral nuclei. Within these subdivisions, there are specific nuclei distributed throughout the rostral-caudal plane. Rostral (anterior) nuclei are associated with regulation of circadian rhythms, parasympathetic function, and heat dissipation. Caudal (posterior) nuclei are associated with sympathetic function and heat conservation. The lateral portion of the hypothalamus contains a "hunger" center, while the medial hypothalamus contains a "satiety" center. However, the control of food intake and eating behavior, which is still not completely understood, is very complex and is not solely limited to these hypothalamic regions (Figure 8.2).

The **epithalamus** is a small area located posteriorly and superiorly to the thalamus. Its main contribution is the **pineal gland**, a source of the hormone **melatonin** which is involved in sleep and circadian rhythm regulation. The epithalamus also contains the habenula and the stria medullaris that are involved in limbic system communication.

The diencephalon also contains a portion of the ventricular system. The **third ventricle** is found at the center of the diencephalon with the massa intermedia passing through it. It is connected anteriorly to the lateral ventricles through the **interventricular foramina** (of Monro). It is connected posteriorly to the cerebral aqueduct in the midbrain. Within the third ventricle, cerebrospinal fluid is produced by tufted layers of ependymal cells called **choroid plexus** (Figure 8.3).

Neural tracts

Motor nerve tracts from the cortex to the periphery pass lateral to the diencephalon through a structure termed the **internal capsule**. These tracts are descending from cortical areas as the corticospinal, corticobulbar, and corticopontine tracts, and intermingle to form the **cerebral peduncles** in the midbrain.

The majority of sensory nerve tracts, on the other hand, end within the thalamic nuclei of the diencephalon. Therefore,

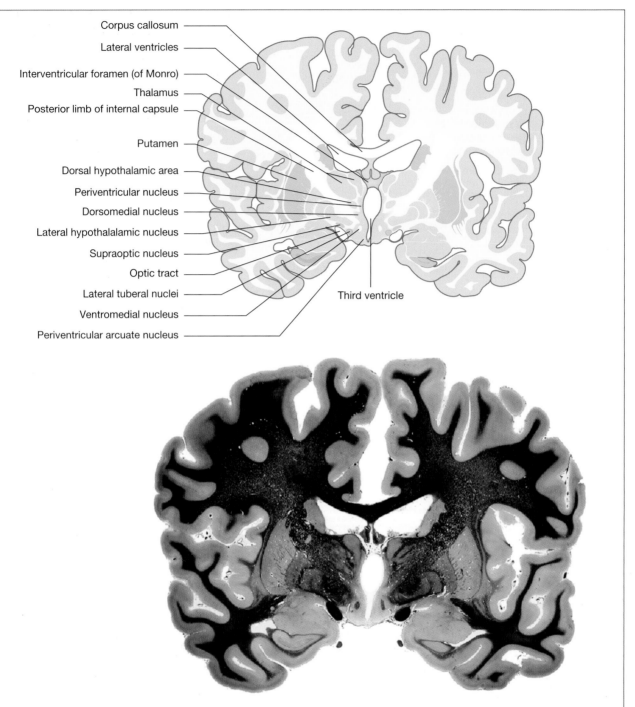

Corpus callosum

Lateral ventricles

Interventricular foramen (of Monro)

Thalamus

Posterior limb of internal capsule

Putamen

Dorsal hypothalamic area

Periventricular nucleus

Dorsomedial nucleus

Lateral hypothalalamic nucleus

Supraoptic nucleus

Optic tract

Lateral tuberal nuclei

Ventromedial nucleus

Periventricular arcuate nucleus

Third ventricle

Figure 8.2   A drawing and myelin-stained photograph of a coronal view of the diencephalon. Note the location of the hypothalamic and thalamic nuclei.

the sensory tracts that were followed through the spinal cord and brain stem, such as the **medial lemniscus**, the **spinothalamic tract**, and the **trigeminothalamic tract**, all terminate in thalamic nuclei. From there, the specific sensations will be relayed through the internal capsule to specific areas of the cortex by third or fourth order neurons.

There are numerous white matter tracts that originate or pass through the diencephalon. These connect the nuclei in the thalamus and hypothalamus with other diencephalic nuclei as well as with other central nervous system structures. The **fornix** is a prominent white matter tract that connects the hippocampus (limbic system) with the hypothalamus. It can be

Clinical box 8.1

The thalamus is subdivided into anterior, medial, or lateral groups of nuclei. These groups of nuclei can be further subdivided into dorsal or ventral portions, as well as anterior or posterior divisions. Each of these small subdivisions has specific inputs and specific outputs that are well characterized, but are beyond the scope of clinically relevant neuroanatomy. Generally, the anterior nuclear group is involved in relays within the limbic system, involving emotions, memory, and learning. The medial nuclear group is involved in integration of sensory and emotional information. The larger, lateral nuclear group has many specific nuclei for sensory, motor, and integrative information. For example, the nucleus that acts as a relay for the medial lemniscus and spinothalamic tracts (sensory information from the contralateral side of the body) is the **ventral posterior lateral** (VPL) nucleus of the thalamus, while the nucleus that acts as a relay for the trigeminal system (sensory information from the face) is the **ventral posterior medial** (VPM) nucleus of the thalamus.

Because of the numerous roles and interconnectivity of the thalamic nuclei and the small space they occupy in the diencephalon, tumors or strokes in this region tend to be very debilitating, with major functional disturbances (Schmahmann, 2003; Satpute *et al.*, 2013). For example, the loss of the ventral posterior medial and lateral nuclei will produce a loss of sensation from the head and body on the contralateral side. This loss can be preceded by altered sensations (tingling or burning) (**parasthesias**), which, in some cases, can lead to the sensation of excruciating pain (**thalamic pain syndrome**). In addition, normal, non-painful stimuli can produce painful responses (**allodynia**) due to altered function in these thalamic nuclei.

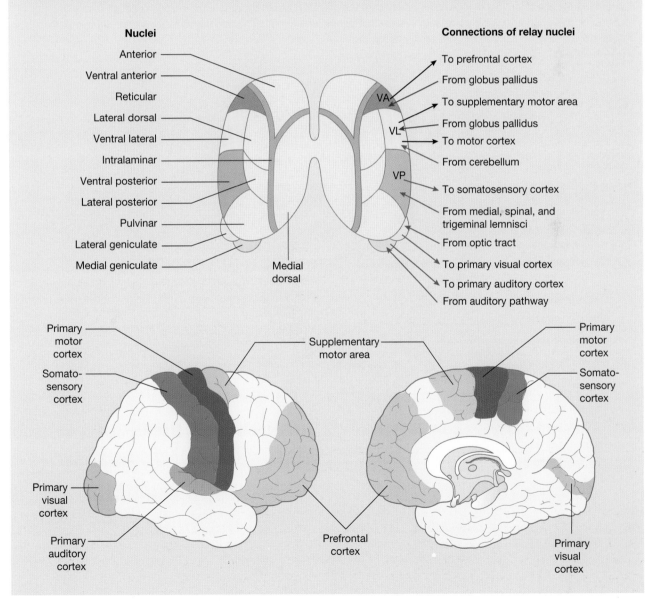

Clinical box 8.2

The hypothalamus is composed of many small, function-specific nuclei located on both sides of the third ventricle. The input, outputs, and function of these nuclei has been well characterized. The rostral (anterior) nuclei are the nuclei associated with optic chiasm. The preoptic nuclei regulate reproductive function by controlling hormone release from the anterior pituitary. These nuclei are morphologically different in males compared to females; they are **sexually dimorphic**. The nuclei caudal (posterior) to the preoptic nuclei are the nuclei above the optic chiasm. These are a varied set of nuclei that set circadian rhythms (suprachiasmatic nuclei), increase heat loss (anterior hypothalamic nuclei), and conserve water (paraventricular and supraoptic nuclei). The paraventricular and supraoptic nuclei produce hormones that are stored and released from the posterior pituitary. **Anti-diuretic hormone** (ADH, vasopressin) acts in the collecting ducts of the kidney to concentrate the urine and conserve water, while **oxytocin** is involved in parturition, lactation, and social trust/bonding. Individuals with lesions or tumors in the posterior pituitary exhibit **diabetes insipidus**, leading to **polyuria** (frequent urination) with a dilute urine as well as **polydipsia** (frequent thirst).

Further caudal (posterior) is another set of nuclei (the arcuate nuclei in the tuberal region) that control hormone release from the anterior pituitary by releasing small function specific hormones into a localized portal system. This tuberal region also contains the dorsomedial, ventromedial and lateral hypothalamic nuclei that modify food intake through "**satiety**" or "**hunger**" centers, respectively (Figure 8.2). Interestingly, lesions to these nuclei in animal models can markedly alter food intake as well as behavior of the animal. Lateral hypothalamic lesions produce a lack of interest in eating and drinking, along with passive behaviors, while medial hypothalamic lesions produce overeating, leading to obesity and extremely aggressive behaviors.

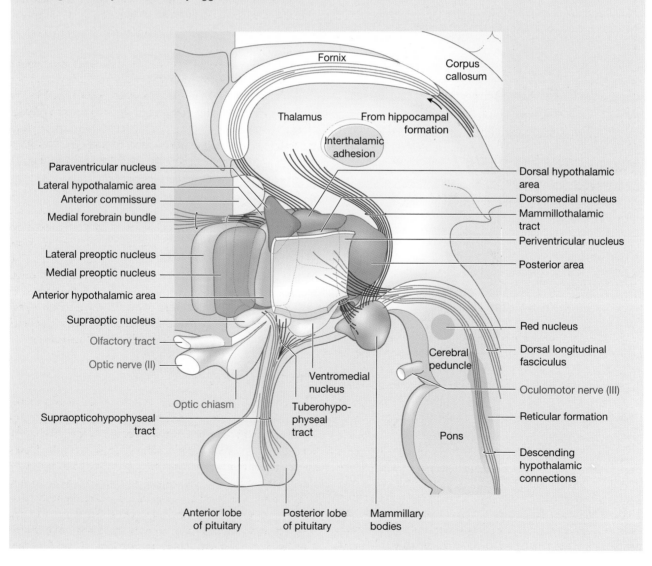

The most caudal (posterior) set of nuclei are the mammillary and posterior hypothalamic nuclei. The combined mammillary nuclei bulge inferiorly from the hypothalamus to produce the **mammillary bodies** on the inferior surface of the brain. These nuclei interact with the limbic system to modify emotions and will be discussed in more detail in that chapter. The posterior hypothalamic nuclei respond to a decrease in **body temperature** by preventing heat loss (constriction of peripheral blood vessels) and increasing heat production (increased thyroid hormone activity and shivering). As noted above, the anterior hypothalamic nuclei modify body temperature by increasing heat loss (peripheral vasodilation and sweating), so these two sets of nuclei (anterior and posterior) act as a thermostat to maintain body temperature at a specific set point (Flouris, 2011). This is an excellent example of the hypothalamic role in maintaining homeostasis. A lesion in the anterior hypothalamus can lead to an increase in body temperature, due to the unopposed effects of the posterior hypothalamus. A lesion in the posterior hypothalamus, however, produces a lack of control of body temperature, since the axons from the anterior hypothalamus pass through the posterior hypothalamus, leading to a loss of function from both sets of nuclei.

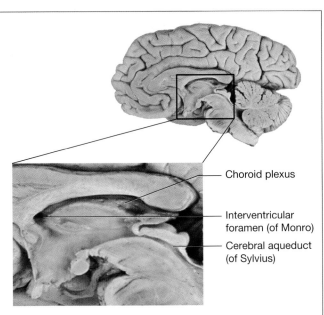

Choroid plexus

Interventricular foramen (of Monro)

Cerebral aqueduct (of Sylvius)

Figure 8.3 A photograph of the ventricular structures associated with the diencephalon including the interventricular foramen (of Monro), the third ventricle, the choroid plexus, and the cerebral aqueduct (of Sylvius).

observed arching postero-laterally from the hippocampus to the infero-medially placed mammillary bodies supplying the mammillary nuclei and other hypothalamic nuclei (Figure 8.1). Its function will be discussed in greater detail in the chapter on the limbic system. The **medial forebrain bundle** is a collection of axons that are entering or exiting the hypothalamus. Many of the neural connections between the hypothalamus and other neural structures are contained in this tract, including the important pathways that regulate autonomic function. The **stria medullaris** and **stria terminalis** are pathways connecting the hypothalamus with nearby structures. They are both found on the superior surface of the thalamus, with the stria terminalis located laterally. The stria medullaris is a bi-directional pathway between the hypothalamus and the habenula (of the epithalamus), while the stria terminalis runs from the amygdala to the hypothalamus. The **mammillothalamic tracts** are self-descriptive; they run from the mammillary nuclei to the anterior nucleus of the thalamus and are involved in limbic system function. Finally, the **thalamocortical fibers** (thalamic radiations) are axons leaving the thalamus, destined for the cortex, that spread out as they leave the thalamus to enter the internal capsule.

It should be apparent that the close configuration of numerous nuclei, along with many white matter tracts in both the thalamus and hypothalamus, can lead to major deficits if a lesion occurs in either of these regions. It is important to recognize that a tumor or stroke in these areas can impact on both the nuclei present as well as the fibers of passage, sometimes making it difficult to diagnose the actual site of the lesion.

Cranial nerves

While the remaining two cranial nerves to be discussed do not arise directly from the diencephalon, they are, in some ways, related to structures within the diencephalon. The **olfactory nerve (I)** is unique in that it does not relay through the thalamus prior to sending information to the cortex. It actually has a direct connection to the cortex. The **optic nerve (II)** relays vision from the eye and interacts with nuclei in both the thalamus and the hypothalamus (Table 8.1).

Olfactory nerve (I)

The olfactory nerves (I) are special sensory, small bipolar nerves found in the nasal mucosa that project through small openings in the ethmoid bone (the **cribriform plate**) to reach the **olfactory bulb**. The second order neurons in the olfactory bulb project through the **olfactory tract** to synapse in olfactory areas of the cortex, including the amygdala and entorhinal cortex (Figure 8.4). This may be why specific odors can quickly elicit powerful memories and emotions. Obviously, lesions in the olfactory nerve would produce a loss of smell (**anosmia**), which also diminishes a patient's ability to taste foods. One of the first

Table 8.1 The composition and course of the two cranial nerves associated with the diencephalon.

Olfactory nerve (I):

<u>Sensory:</u> Olfactory mucosa receptor cells, first order axons pass through cribriform plate, synapse in olfactory bulb; second order axons travel in olfactory tract, project to orbitofrontal cortex and amygdala.

Optic nerve (II):

<u>Sensory:</u> Retinal photoreceptor cells, axons of retinal bipolar cells project to retinal ganglion cells, ganglion cell axons project through optic nerve (II), optic canal, optic chiasm and optic tract to lateral geniculate nuclei, then through optic radiations to occipital cortex.

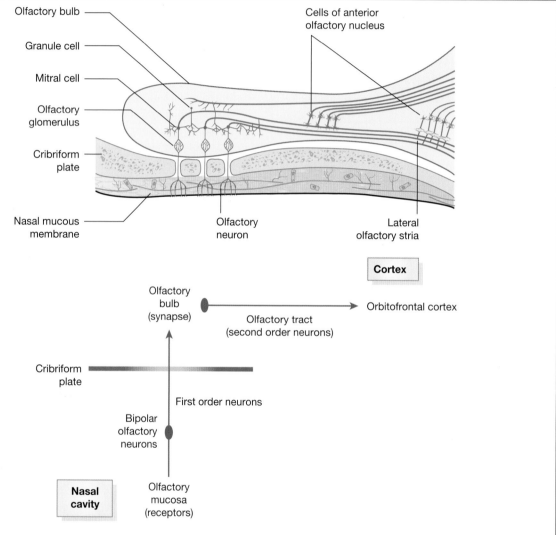

Figure 8.4 A drawing and schematic version of the distribution of the olfactory nerves (I).

deficits associated with dementia is a loss of smell and these patients will complain of "bland" tasting food (Doty and Kamath, 2014). They will add salt or other spices to their food to heighten the flavor. Further details on the olfactory nerve are covered in Chapter 14 on olfaction and taste.

Optic nerve (II)

The optic nerve (II) contains special sensory axons that arise from the **ganglion cells** of the retina and travel through the **optic canal** to leave the orbit and enter the cranium. The right and left optic nerves join together at the **optic chiasm**

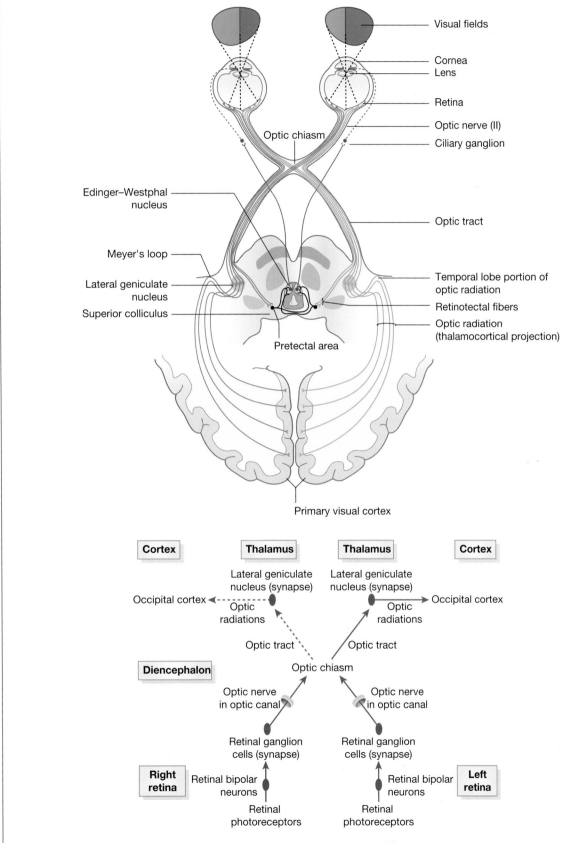

Figure 8.5 A drawing and schematic version of the distribution of the optic nerves (II).

and then leave as right and left **optic tracts**. The tracts contain different axons than the nerves, with visual information from the left visual field in the right optic tract and visual information from the right visual field in the left optic tract. Some of the axons leave the optic tract to enter the **hypothalamus**, providing light and dark information to the suprachiasmatic nucleus to set the daily circadian rhythms. The majority of axons in the optic tracts project to the **lateral geniculate** (a sensory relay nucleus of the thalamus) which then project onto the primary visual cortex in the occipital lobe. A few of the axons project to the **superior colliculus** and the tectum of the midbrain to provide visual information for pupillary light reflexes, as well as head, neck, and eye coordination (Figure 8.5). A lesion in the optic nerve produces blindness in that eye, which also produces problems with depth of field vision (Duong *et al.*, 2008). Further details about the optic nerve are covered in Chapter 12 on the visual system.

Clinical considerations

Case 1

Mr William Brooks, a 47-year-old mechanical engineer who smokes two packs of cigarettes per day, begins experiencing night sweats, a racing heart rate and an increase in appetite associated with an increase in body weight. A few months later, he begins to have a loss of vision. This symptom brings him into the hospital, where the emergency room physician takes a detailed history and physical. Hypothesizing that Mr Brooks has a tumor compressing the optic nerve, the physician arranges for a consultation with a neurologist and a neurosurgeon. After examining an MRI of Mr Brooks' brain, the neurologist and neurosurgeon consult with Mr Brooks. They describe the location of a tumor in his hypothalamus that is placing pressure on the optic nerve (Figure 8.6). After discussing many options, Mr Brooks decides to have localized radiation exposure along with brain surgery to remove the tumor.

The results of the radiation and surgery are successful, although Mr Brooks has permanent changes in his metabolism due to the damage caused in his hypothalamus by the tumor. He no longer has visual deficits associated with the tumor, but, six months later, he is diagnosed with a small cell carcinoma of the lung that, sadly, proves fatal less than a year later. Unbeknownst to Mr Brooks, the small cell carcinoma was probably the source for his **hypothalamic tumor**.

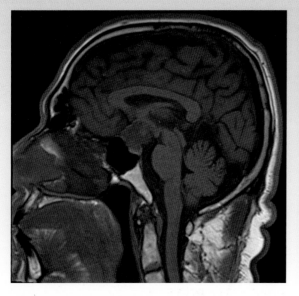 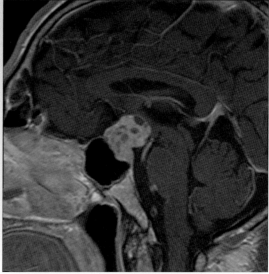

Figure 8.6 Magnetic resonance images of a large hypothalamic tumor. Note the hyperintense signal in the second contrast-enhanced image.

Case 2

Ms Carrie Thomas, a 48-year-old pharmacist who is diabetic and smokes one pack of cigarettes per day, wakes one morning with tingling and a "pins and needles" sensation from the entire right side of her body and her head. After one hour, with no relief from the symptoms, she goes to the local emergency room where her history and physical exams are collected by a young resident, Dr Jordan Keller. After consideration of the results and consultation with the resident neurologist, Dr Keller suspects that Ms Thomas has had a small stroke in her thalamus. Ms Thomas accepts the recommendation for a CT of her head and a small ischemic thalamic stroke is identified. She is told there is little that can be done and is given aspirin (to act as a pain reliever and anticoagulant) to limit the scope of the damaged tissue. Her symptoms wax and wane over a three to four-week period and eventually she develops a more consistent, deep throbbing pain on the right side of her body. This pain is not alleviated with standard pain relievers.

She returns to the emergency room and, after a consultation with a neurologist, she is told that she may have **thalamic pain syndrome** (Dejerine-Roussy syndrome). Over a six-month period, while still suffering from the deep throbbing pain, Ms Thomas is given a number of pharmacologic treatments to help alleviate the pain, including antidepressants, anticonvulsants, and opiates. None of these are completely successful, but Ms Thomas has the best success (and fewest side effects) with an anticonvulsant. During this same time frame, she has quit smoking, exercises more, and attempts to control her diabetes. These lifestyle changes, along with the drug treatments, help limit the pain, but she is continually aware of background pain on the right side of her body.

Study questions

1. A unilateral lesion in the left thalamus of a 75-year-old male patient would directly produce:
a) skeletal motor deficits on the right side of the patient
b) skeletal motor deficits on the left side of the patient
c) sensory losses from the right side of the patient
d) sensory losses from the left side of the patient
e) bilateral autonomic motor losses in the patient

2. The thalamic relay for vision is found in the:
a) anterior thalamus
b) lateral thalamus
c) medial thalamus
d) medial geniculate
e) lateral geniculate

3. A 66-year-old male patient with a lesion in the hypothalamus has major deficits in:
a) skeletal muscle motor control
b) general sensation input to the cortex
c) homeostatic control of basal metabolic rate
d) visual acuity
e) tonotopic hearing ability

4. A 64-year-old male patient's increased blood pressure (hypertension) causes expansion of the ophthalmic artery in the optic canal. This expansion places pressure on an accompanying nerve that can eventually produce:
a) blindness in the eye
b) loss of motor control to the superior oblique muscle
c) loss of motor control to the lateral rectus muscle
d) loss of pupillary constriction
e) anosmia

5. All of the following sensory modalities are relayed through the thalamus except:
a) general sensation from the body
b) general sensation from the face
c) pain and temperature from the face
d) hearing
e) smell

For more self-assessment questions, visit the companion website at
www.wileyessential.com/neuroanatomy

FURTHER READING

For additional information on the diencephalon, the following textbooks and review articles may be helpful:

Blumenfeld H. 2002. *Neuroanatomy Through Clinical Cases*. Sinauer Associates, Sunderland, Massachusetts.

Doty RL, Kamath V. 2014. The influences of age on olfaction: a review. *Front Psychol*, 5: 20 (1–20).

Duong DK, Leo MM, Mitchell EL. 2008. Neuro-ophthalmology. *Emerg Med Clin North Am*, 26(1): 137–180.

Felten DL, Shetty A. 2009. *Netter's Atlas of Neuroscience*, 2nd edition. Saunders Elsevier, Philadelphia, Pennsylvania.

Flouris AD. 2011. Functional architecture of behavioural thermoregulation. *Eur J Appl Physiol*, 111(1): 1–8.

Haines DE. 2012. *Neuroanatomy: An Atlas of Structures, Sections and Systems*, 8th edition. Lippincott Williams & Wilkin, Baltimore, Maryland.

Moore KL, Dalley AF, Agur AMR. 2014. *Moore Clinically Oriented Anatomy*, 7th edition. Lippincott, Williams & Wilkins, Philadelphia, Pennsylvania.

Patestas MA, Gartner LP. 2006. *A Textbook of Neuroanatomy*. Blackwell Publishing, Malden, Massachusetts.

Satpute S, Bergquist J, Cole JW. 2013. Cheiro-Oral syndrome secondary to thalamic infarction: a case report and literature review. *Neurologist*, 19(1): 22–25.

Schmahmann JD. 2003. Vascular syndromes of the thalamus. *Stroke*, 34: 2264–2278.

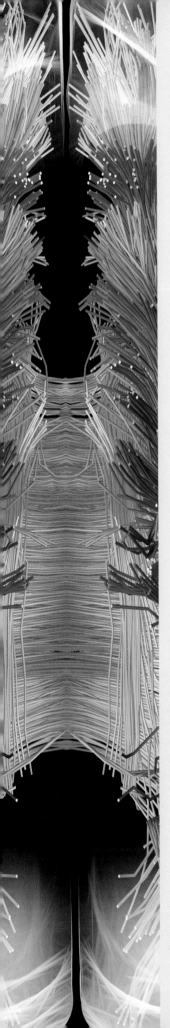

CHAPTER 9
Telencephalon

Learning objectives

1. Describe the anatomical and functional components of the telencephalon.
2. Identify the ventricular structures of the telencephalon.
3. Identify the external features of the telencephalon.

Essential Clinical Neuroanatomy, First Edition. Thomas H. Champney.
© 2016 John Wiley & Sons, Ltd. Published 2016 by John Wiley & Sons, Ltd.
Companion website: www.wileyessential.com/neuroanatomy

Introduction

The **telencephalon** is the largest portion of the brain and consists of the **cerebral cortex**, the **basal ganglia**, and portions of the **limbic system**. The telencephalon has high-level sensory, motor, and integrative components. In addition, the telencephalon contains the regions for long-term memory storage, emotional expression, personality, and decision-making processes.

This chapter will provide a brief overview of the development and anatomy of the telencephalon, while the more detailed functional aspects of the telencephalon will be covered in subsequent chapters on central motor control (Chapter 15), the limbic system (Chapter 16), and cortical integration (Chapter 17). The goal of this chapter is to be able to identify the structures described and appreciate their relationships with adjacent anatomical structures.

Development

As detailed in Chapter 3, the development of the telencephalon occurs from the primitive region referred to as the **forebrain**. The forebrain consists of the **diencephalon**, the **optic vesicles**, and **telencephalic vesicles**. The telencephalic vesicles are lateral outgrowths of the third ventricle and are referred to as the lateral ventricles in adults. The forebrain has the largest growth potential of the central nervous system, with the telencephalon being the largest and most complex (Geschwind and Rakic, 2013). As the telencephalon develops, it over grows both the diencephalon and portions of the midbrain and hindbrain. Therefore, when observing the brain, the majority of surface area is composed of telencephalic structures.

Cerebral cortex

The largest portion of the telencephalon is the **cerebral cortex**, which is the most superficial portion of the brain and is most noticeable by its large **sulci** and **gyri**. The cerebral cortex has been subdivided into five major regions. The most anterior or frontal portion of the cortex is referred to as the **frontal cortex** and is bounded posteriorly by the **precentral gyrus** and the **central sulcus**. The central sulcus and the **postcentral gyrus** act as the anterior boundary of the **parietal cortex**. Posterior to the parietal cortex is the pyramidal-shaped **occipital cortex**. Inferiorly and laterally placed (inferior to the **lateral fissure**), is the **temporal cortex** (Figure 9.1). If the lateral fissure is spread

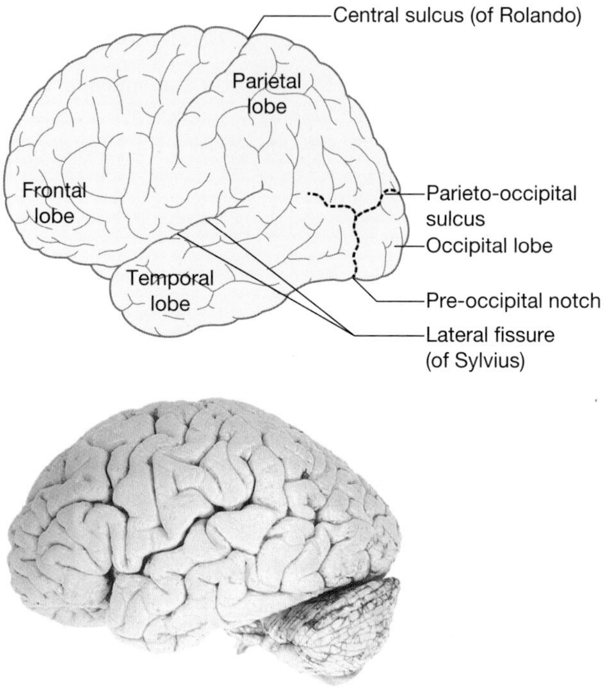

Figure 9.1 A drawing and photograph of the major regions of the cerebral cortex. Note the central sulcus, with the precentral and postcentral gyrus on either side.

open, a more deeply residing portion of the cortex can be observed, the **insular cortex**. Each of these five regions of cortex has a separate function, while also integrating functions from the other regions. The anterior frontal cortex is associated with higher-level thought processes and emotional/personality expression; while the posterior frontal cortex is involved in organizing and driving skeletal muscle function. The parietal cortex is associated with processing incoming tactile sensory information and distributing it to other portions of the cortex. The occipital cortex is responsible for integrating and distributing visual information, while the temporal cortex is responsible for integrating and distributing auditory information. The insular cortex deals with integrating and distributing complex emotions and conscious desires.

Each of these regions of the cortex interacts with the other regions by means of interneurons that pass through white matter structures just deep to the cortical layers. One of the large white matter structures, the **internal capsule**, is used to bring

Clinical box 9.1

The gyri and the sulci of the cortex are quite similar between brains. The gyri have been named based on their location. Specific gyri have specific functions: most notably the precentral gyrus as the motor strip for skeletal muscle control; the postcentral gyrus for tactile sensory input; the superior temporal gyrus for primary auditory input; and the occipital gyrus for primary visual input.

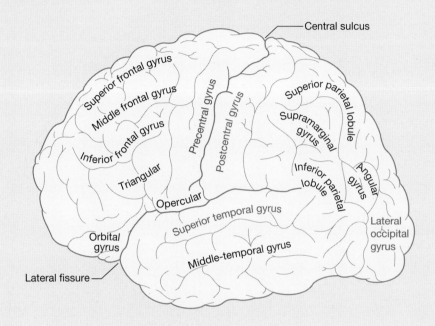

The functional aspects of the precentral and postcentral gyri can be further subdivided based on the location for muscle control or sensory input, respectively. These specific somatotopic distribution patterns are referred to as a **homunculus** and will be covered in more detail in the chapter on sensory and motor tracts (Chapter 11).

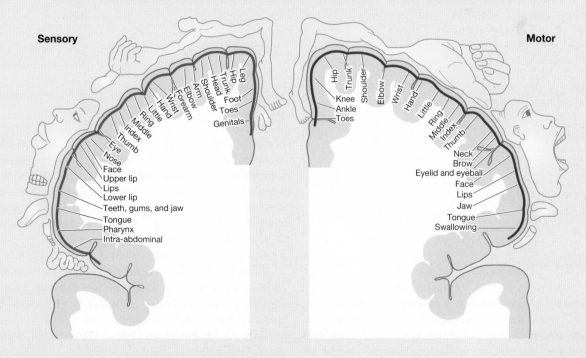

Likewise, specific auditory tones and visual fields are distributed in their respective gyri. The cerebral cortex is highly organized for specific tasks as shown on the following figure.

Clinical box 9.1 (continued)

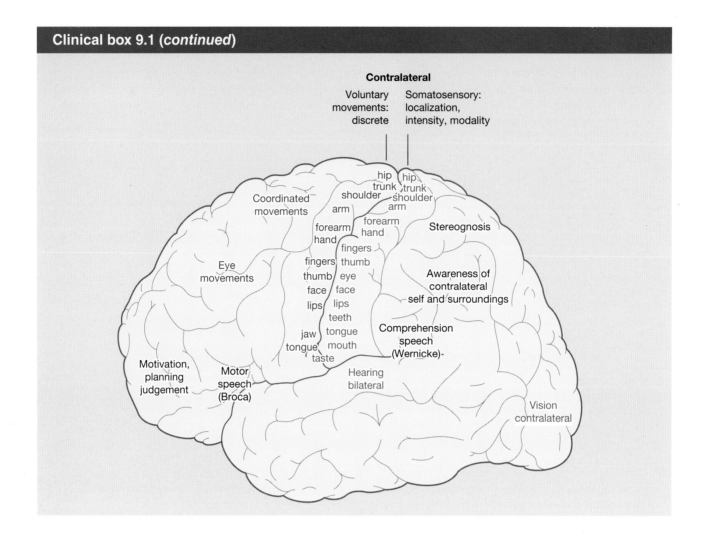

sensory information into the cortex and distribute motor information out of the cortex. Smaller white matter structures, such as the **external capsule**, are used to integrate information around the same hemisphere of the brain. To integrate information between hemispheres of the brain, another large white matter structure, the **corpus callosum**, is utilized. There are also small white matter interconnections (the **anterior and posterior commissures**) that provide specific interhemispheric communication (Figures 9.2 and 9.3). Therefore, all regions of the cortex on both sides of the brain communicate with each other by way of these white matter structures.

Corpus callosum

When a midsagittal section of the brain is viewed, the large white matter **corpus callosum** is easily observed (Figure 9.4). This structure is the major means of communication between the two hemispheres of the brain. When it is bisected or lesioned, the right half of the brain is unaware of what the left half of the brain is processing. Patients with this disorder are referred to as split brain patients and present with unique

symptoms. The case study at the end of this chapter describes this disorder in more detail.

Basal ganglia

Beneath the layers of the frontal and parietal cortex and lateral to the **thalamus** and **internal capsule** are specific telencephalic nuclei, referred to as the **basal ganglia**. Recall that this is poor nomenclature since ganglia should reside outside of the central nervous system. The basal ganglia are motor relay nuclei in charge of producing smooth and precise muscle activity. They work in conjunction with the cerebellum to regulate complex motor output.

The basal ganglia are made of three distinct nuclei: the **caudate**, the **putamen**, and the **globus pallidus**. Two other regions are associated with the basal ganglia, the **subthalamic nucleus** and the **substantia nigra**. The caudate and the putamen together are referred to as the **striatum**, while the putamen and globus pallidus are referred to as the **lenticular nuclei**. Note that the putamen is part of both the striatum and the lenticular nuclei.

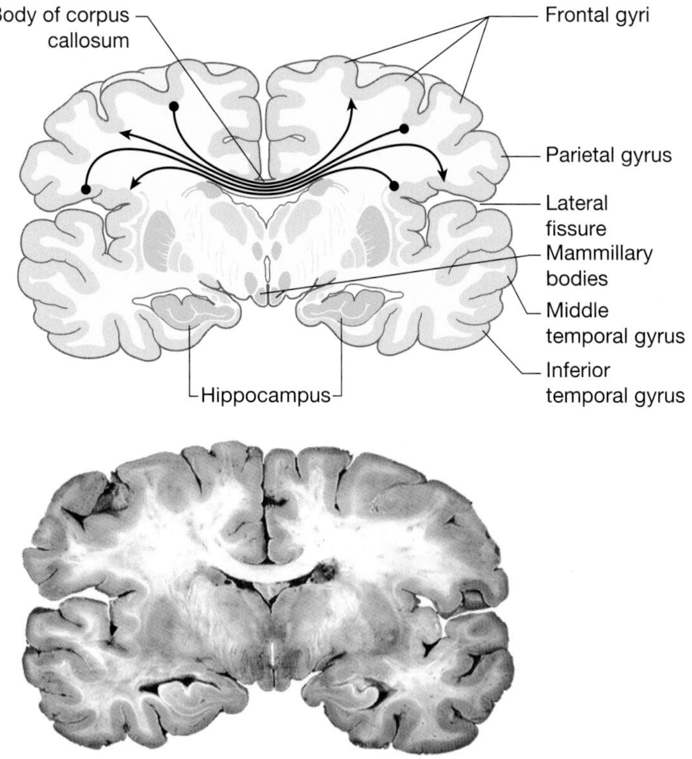

Figure 9.2 A drawing and photograph of two closely related coronal (frontal) sections of the brain. Note the gyri and sulci as well as the major white matter tracts.

Utilizing all three views (sagittal, horizontal, and coronal), identify the distribution of these components. Note that the caudate begins at the anterior end of the putamen (as the head) and then arches superiorly and laterally to extend into the temporal lobe (as the tail) (Figure 9.5). The tail of the caudate ends at the **amygdala** in the anterior pole of the temporal lobe. Therefore, in an anterior coronal section, the putamen and caudate will be closely related, while in a posterior coronal section, the caudate can be found superior to the putamen (Figure 9.6). On a horizontal section, the head of the caudate and putamen are closely related, while the tail of the caudate is found posteriorly (Figure 9. 7). In a coronal section of the brain, just medial to the putamen, two "crescent moon" shaped structures are found: the external and internal segments of the globus pallidus (Figure 9.6). In this view, the putamen and globus pallidus look like three "lenses", hence their combined name the **lenticular nuclei**. In a horizontal section, the globus pallidus is found medial to the putamen, but lateral to the internal capsule and the thalamus. Lateral to the putamen is the small white matter tract, the external capsule (Figure 9.7). Note on the coronal view that the subthalamic nucleus is inferior to the thalamus and infero-medial to the globus pallidus. The substantia nigra is inferior and posterior to the subthalamic nucleus in the upper portion of the midbrain.

The complete role of the basal ganglia in motor function and its dysfunction in specific clinical disorders (Parkinsonism, Huntington's chorea) is discussed in greater detail in Chapter 15 on central motor control.

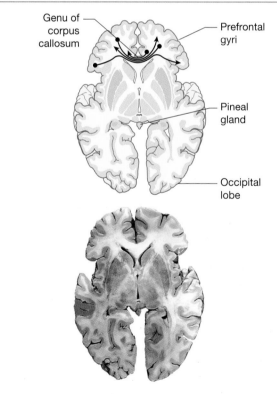

Figure 9.3 A drawing and photograph of two closely related horizontal sections of the brain. Note the gyri and sulci as well as the major white matter tracts.

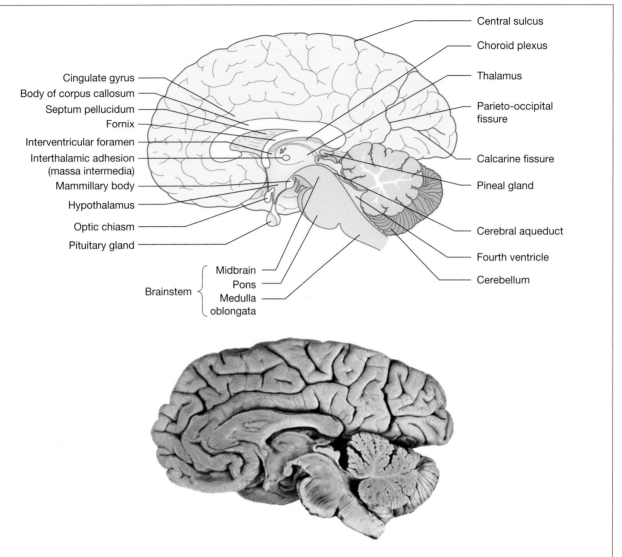

Cingulate gyrus
Body of corpus callosum
Septum pellucidum
Fornix
Interventricular foramen
Interthalamic adhesion (massa intermedia)
Mammillary body
Hypothalamus
Optic chiasm
Pituitary gland

Central sulcus
Choroid plexus
Thalamus
Parieto-occipital fissure
Calcarine fissure
Pineal gland
Cerebral aqueduct
Fourth ventricle
Cerebellum

Brainstem
Midbrain
Pons
Medulla oblongata

Figure 9.4 A drawing and photograph of a sagittal section of the brain. Note the gyri and sulci as well as the major white matter tracts including the corpus callosum.

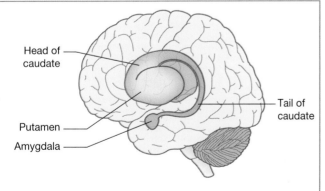

Head of caudate
Tail of caudate
Putamen
Amygdala

Figure 9.5 A drawing of a lateral view of the brain with the putamen and caudate nucleus superimposed to show their distribution.

Amygdala and hippocampus

The **amygdala** and **hippocampus** are found beneath the layer of the temporal cortex in the temporal lobe of the brain. The amygdala is the most anterior of these two structures, with the hippocampus extending posteriorly and superiorly (Figure 9.8). These two structures, along with other deeply placed cortical nuclei, make up a functional system in the brain referred to as the **limbic system**. These nuclei are involved in emotional processing and memory consolidation and are referred to in greater detail in Chapter 16 on the limbic system.

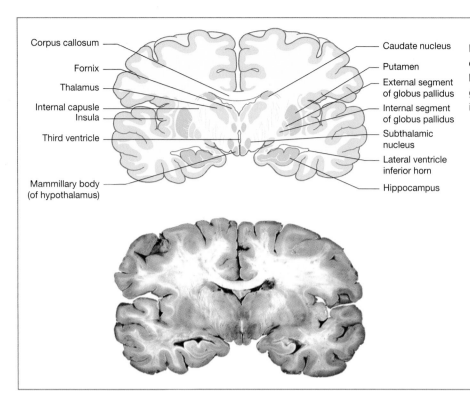

Figure 9.6 A drawing and photograph of a coronal (frontal) section of the brain. Note the components of the basal ganglia and their relationships to the internal capsule and thalamus.

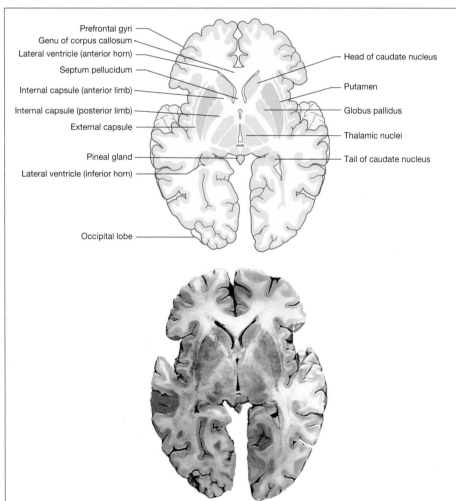

Figure 9.7 A drawing and photograph of a horizontal section of the brain. Note the components of the basal ganglia and their relationships to the internal capsule and thalamus.

Lateral ventricles

As was discussed previously, the **lateral ventricles** are the ventricular outgrowths of the telencephalon and have a wide distribution in the depths of the cortex. These ventricles extend posteriorly into the occipital lobe and laterally into the temporal lobe, as well as in the deep portions of the frontal and parietal lobes. **Cerebrospinal fluid** produced in the lateral ventricles by the **choroid plexus** drains into the third ventricle via the **interventricular foramen** (of Munro) (Figure 9.9). Recall that the lateral ventricles are blind ended cul-de-sacs in which the only drainage point is through the interventricular foramen. Therefore, any blockage of the foramen can produce an increase in ventricular pressure and size compressing the adjacent cortical tissue.

The main goal of this chapter is to identify and localize the components of the telencephalon: the cerebral cortex with it lobes, gyri, and sulci; the basal ganglia; the structures associated with the limbic system; and the large white matter tracts coursing through the brain. The functional aspects of these structures will be covered in more detail in subsequent chapters.

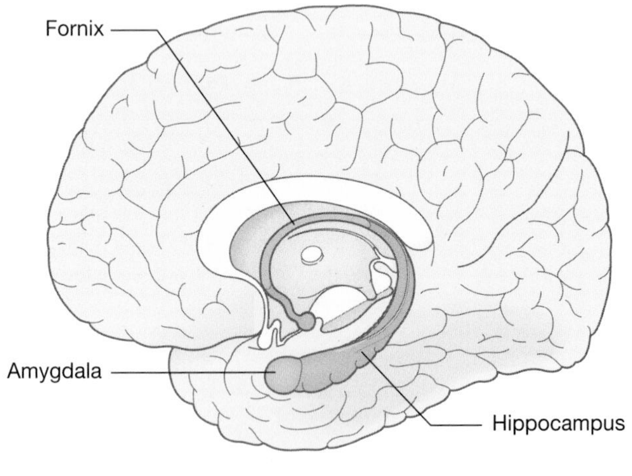

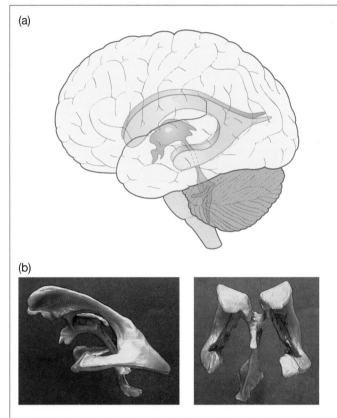

Figure 9.9 (a) A drawing of the brain with the distribution of the lateral ventricles superimposed. (b) A "cast" of the ventricles with the surrounding brain tissue removed. Note the "C" shaped lateral ventricles, the midline third ventricle with the opening for the mass intermedia, and the cerebral aqueduct. The red material represents the choroid plexus.

Fornix

Amygdala

Hippocampus

Figure 9.8 Sagittal view of the brain with the brain stem removed. Note the amygdala (orange), hippocampus (purple), and fornix (blue) superimposed to show their distribution.

Clinical box 9.2

Over one hundred years ago, Korbinian Brodmann, a neuroanatomist, histologically examined the regions of the cortex and found specific differences in these regions (Zilles and Amunts, 2010; Loukas, *et al.*, 2011). He numbered each region of cortex that was histologically different and produced a cortical map, with over 50 different areas delineated. This was long before any known functions were attributed to the specific regions and it was only decades later that researchers applied specific functions to these numbered regions. **Brodmann's areas**, as they are known today, are used to denote specific areas of cortex that have specific functions. For example, the strip of cortex anterior to the central sulcus is referred to as the **precentral gyrus** or Brodmann's area 4 and is functionally attributed to the skeletal motor output of the corticospinal tract. Likewise, the strip of cortex posterior to the central sulcus (referred to as the **postcentral gyrus** or Brodmann's area 3 (along with 1 and 2)) is functionally attributed to the somatosensory input from the thalamus.

Clinical box 9.2 (*continued*)

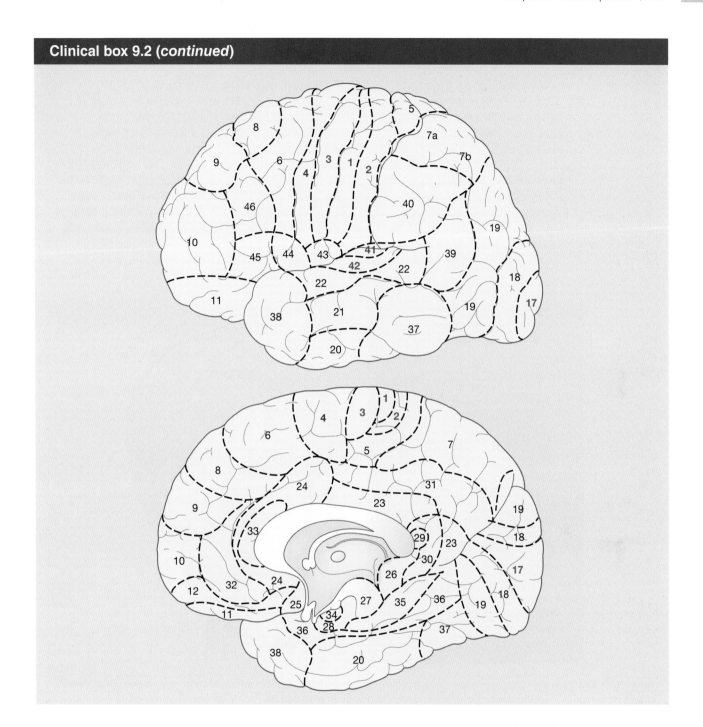

Clinical considerations

One of the unique features of the cerebral cortex is its ability to reroute function when portions of the cortex are damaged. This ability to produce redundant circuits is clinically beneficial in that lesions of small areas of the cortex can be bypassed without sacrificing functional ability. Compare this ability with the nuclei and tracts of the brain stem in which no redundancy is present. Therefore, a lesion of the brain stem can be much more devastating then a similar sized lesion of the cortex.

Case 1

This case study details the true account of a railroad foreman, Phineas Gage, who, in 1848, accidently had an iron tamping rod blasted through his skull. The rod entered beneath his left eye and exited out of the top of his skull (Figure 9.10). This caused severe damage to his left frontal cortex. Within a short time frame, he was speaking clearly and the effects of the wound appeared to be limited to the loss of vision in his left eye and a partial paralysis of his left facial muscles. Six months later, he was well enough to work, although he did not return to the railroad. He had a number of jobs, including as a stagecoach driver in Chile, before returning to the United States in 1859 when his health began to deteriorate. After his death in 1860, his skull and the iron tamping rod were placed in an anatomical museum associated with Harvard Medical School.

Mr Gage's case has been written about extensively, with details on the extent of the wound and the personality changes that occurred. This was one of the first cases to describe personality changes associated with loss of the frontal cortex. The extent of Mr Gage's personality changes is still being debated in the literature, but the fact that the loss of the frontal cortex produced personality changes provides good evidence for the functional role of this area of the cortex.

(a)　　　　　　　　　　　　　　　　(b)

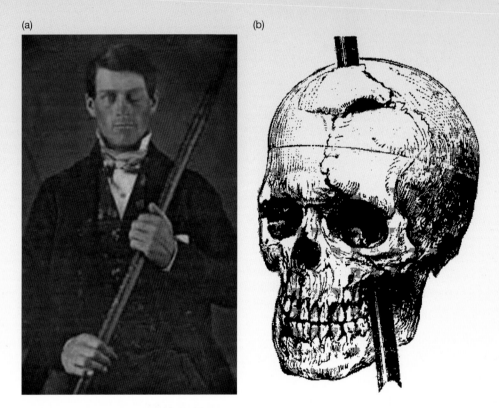

Figure 9.10 An archival photograph of Phineas Gage, a railroad worker who lost a portion of his frontal cortex and experienced personality changes. Sources: (a) From the collection of Jack and Beverly Wilgus; (b) From Harlow JM. *Publ Mass Med Soc* (1868), 2: 327–347.

Case 2

At the age of 25, Mr Jacob Wilson had an operation to surgically separate his two cerebral hemispheres to relieve intractable epileptic seizures. The surgery, a **corpus callosotomy**, was successful in reducing Mr Wilson's seizures (Figure 9.11), but it produced a situation where information from one hemisphere of his brain could not be accessed by the other hemisphere (a split brain).

After recovery from the surgery, Mr Wilson underwent a number of neurological tests indicating that there was loss of transfer of information from one hemisphere to the other. However, most individuals and even trained physicians have difficulty determining that Mr Wilson has a split brain, since he is able to develop strategies to compensate for this loss. Using patients like the fictional Mr Wilson, insights into the function of each hemisphere were found. Dr Roger Sperry won a Noble Prize in 1981 for his research on hemispheric specialization using split brain patients as his subjects.

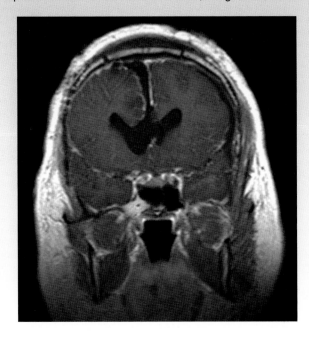

Figure 9.11 A coronal (frontal) magnetic resonance image of a patient with a corpus callosotomy. Note the loss of connectivity between the hemispheres at the base of the falx cerebri.

Study questions

1. A 47-year-old male patient has a lesion that impacts on his final coordination of motor output signals. A physician would expect to find the lesion in the:
a) frontal cortex
b) parietal cortex
c) temporal cortex
d) occipital cortex
e) insular cortex

2. If a blockage occurs in one of the interventricular foramen, which of the following structures would be susceptible to increased pressure hydrocephalus?
a) lateral ventricle
b) third ventricle
c) fourth ventricle
d) cerebral aqueduct
e) central canal

3. A 46-year-old male patient presents with symptoms that lead his physician to conclude that a lesion has occurred in his limbic system. Therefore, a lesion could have occurred in the:
a) caudate nucleus
b) putamen

c) globus pallidus
d) hippocampus
e) subthalamic nucleus

4. A 45-year-old female patient is diagnosed with the inability of one cortical hemisphere to communicate with the other cortical hemisphere (a split brain). A cortical structure involved in her disorder is the:
a) caudate nucleus
b) amygdala
c) corpus callosum
d) internal capsule
e) external capsule

5. A 45-year -old female patient has a gunshot wound to her head that impacts on her ability to interpret sounds and words. A physician would expect to find the lesion in the:
a) frontal cortex
b) parietal cortex
c) temporal cortex
d) occipital cortex
e) insular cortex

For more self-assessment questions, visit the companion website at
www.wileyessential.com/neuroanatomy

FURTHER READING

For additional information on the telencephalon, the following textbooks and review articles may be helpful:

Blumenfeld H. 2002. *Neuroanatomy Through Clinical Cases.* Sinauer Associates, Sunderland, Massachusetts.

Coutlee CG, Huettel SA. 2012. The functional neuroanatomy of decision making: prefrontal control of thought and action. *Brain Res*, 1428: 3–12.

Felten DL, Shetty A. 2009. *Netter's Atlas of Neuroscience*, 2nd edition. Saunders Elsevier, Philadelphia, Pennsylvania.

Garcia-Larrea L. 2012. Insights gained into pain processing from patients with focal brain lesions. *Neurosci Lett*, 520(2): 188–191.

Geschwind DH, Rakic P. 2013. Cortical evolution: judge the brain by its cover. *Neuron*, 80(3): 633–647.

Haines DE. 2012. Neuroanatomy: *An Atlas of Structures, Sections and Systems*, 8th edition. Lippincott Williams & Wilkin, Baltimore, Maryland.

Krubitzer L, Dooley JC. 2013. Cortical plasticity within and across lifetimes: how can development inform us about phenotypic transformations? *Front Hum Neurosci*, 7(620): 1–14.

Loukas M, Pennell C, Groat C, Tubbs RS, Cohen-Gadol AA. 2011. Korbinian Brodmann (1868–1918) and his contributions to mapping the cerebral cortex. *Neurosurgery*, 68(1): 6–11.

Moore KL, Dalley AF, Agur AMR. 2014. *Moore Clinically Oriented Anatomy*, 7th edition. Lippincott, Williams & Wilkins, Philadelphia, Pennsylvania.

Patestas MA, Gartner LP. 2006. *A Textbook of Neuroanatomy*. Blackwell Publishing, Malden, Massachusetts.

Zilles K, Amunts K. 2010. Centenary of Brodmann's map – conception and fate. *Nat Rev Neurosci*, 11(2): 139–145.

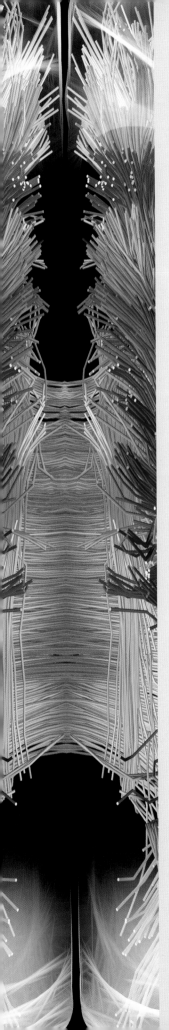

CHAPTER 10
Cerebellum

Learning objectives

1. Describe the main functions of the cerebellum.
2. Describe the organization of the cerebellum.
3. List the anatomic and functional inputs to the cerebellum.
4. Describe the anatomy and circuitry of the cerebellar cortex.
5. Describe the structure and function of the cerebellar deep nuclei.
6. List the anatomic and functional outputs from the cerebellum.
7. Describe cerebellar dysfunction.

Essential Clinical Neuroanatomy, First Edition. Thomas H. Champney.
© 2016 John Wiley & Sons, Ltd. Published 2016 by John Wiley & Sons, Ltd.
Companion website: www.wileyessential.com/neuroanatomy

Introduction

The cerebellum is a uniquely specialized structure at the posterior end of the brain. It has been referred to as the "little brain". It has three primary connections with the rest of the central nervous system: the superior, middle, and inferior cerebellar peduncles. Even when viewed grossly, the cerebellum is quite different than the rest of the brain. It has tightly folded outer layers (**folia**) with centrally oriented white matter (Figure 10.1). The highly branched folia allow for a large increase in the surface area of the cerebellum, increasing the amount of gray matter present.

The main function of the cerebellum is coordination of skeletal muscle action in concert with the cerebral cortex and the basal ganglia. In regulating skeletal muscle action, the cerebellum helps to modify motor neuron activity and, in this

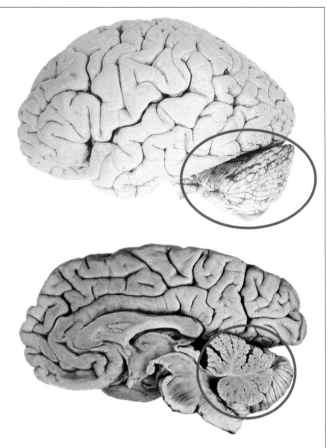

Figure 10.1 A lateral and sagittal view of the cerebellum. Note the highly branched folia increasing the surface area of gray matter.

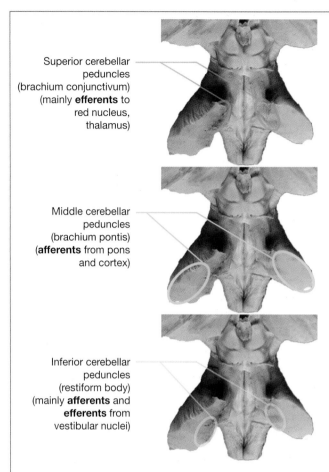

Superior cerebellar peduncles (brachium conjunctivum) (mainly **efferents** to red nucleus, thalamus)

Middle cerebellar peduncles (brachium pontis) (**afferents** from pons and cortex)

Inferior cerebellar peduncles (restiform body) (mainly **afferents** and **efferents** from vestibular nuclei)

Figure 10.2 A posterior view of the brain stem with the cerebellum removed. Note the three peduncles that connect the cerebellum to the brain stem and their contents.

manner, provides error correction for ongoing motor activity. The cerebellum also helps to maintain posture, balance, and muscle tone. In addition, the cerebellum is involved in motor memory activities, such as bicycle riding or dancing, in which many muscles must work in synchrony. Other functions for the cerebellum have been hypothesized, including memory consolidation, but these functions have not been well studied (Buckner, 2013; Reeber, *et al.*, 2013). Further details of the cerebellum's involvement in motor action will be described in Chapter 15 on central motor control.

The main goal of this chapter is to describe the cerebellar anatomy, the cellular anatomy of the cerebellum, and the pathways into and out of the cerebellum. This will provide a good overview of the cerebellum and its interactions with the rest of the central nervous system.

Cerebellar anatomy

The cerebellum is attached to the brain stem in the pons by three distinct connections. The **superior cerebellar peduncle** (brachium conjunctivum) is a major outflow (efferent) pathway to structures such as the red nucleus and thalamus. The **middle cerebellar peduncle** (brachium pontis) is a major inflow (afferent) pathway to the cerebellum from the cortex

and pontine nuclei. The **inferior cerebellar peduncle** (restiform body) contains both afferent and efferent pathways, primarily from the vestibular nuclei (Figure 10.2).

When examining the functional layout of the cerebellar cortex, three regions are apparent: the midline structure (the **vermis**), the **intermediate portion** adjacent to the vermis, and the **lateral portion**. The vermis is responsible for motor control of the trunk musculature and some of the proximal muscles of the extremities. The intermediate part of the cerebellum is responsible for motor control of the distal muscles of the extremities. The lateral part of the cerebellum is responsible for motor planning of the extremities. For example, consciously modifying muscle activity in the abdomen when dancing would involve the vermis. On the other hand, consciously modifying muscle activity in the hand when catching a ball would involve the intermediate portion of the cerebellum, with some involvement from the lateral portion in motor planning. A final and fourth portion of the cerebellum is the **flocculonodular lobe**, a small lobe that runs from medial to lateral on the inferior surface of the cerebellum. This lobe is primarily responsible for balance and vestibulo-ocular reflexes (Figure 10.3).

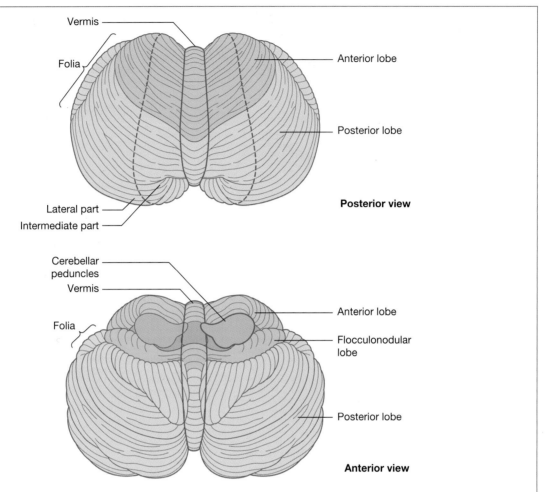

Figure 10.3 A superior and inferior view of the cerebellum highlighting the functional aspects of the cerebellar cortex. Note that the lateral portion of the cortex is involved in motor planning, the intermediate portion is involved in muscle regulation in the distal extremities, and the medial portion (vermis) is involved in muscle regulation in the trunk and proximal extremities. A separate portion, the flocculonodular lobe, is involved in balance and vestibular/vision coordination.

The outputs from these regions of the cerebellum must pass through **deep cerebellar nuclei** before leaving the cerebellum. These deep cerebellar nuclei consolidate information from the cerebellum prior to sending out their axons. The deep cerebellar nuclei are arranged such that each nucleus interacts with a specific part of the cerebellum. The most lateral of the deep cerebellar nuclei are the **dentate nuclei** and they interact with the lateral cerebellar cortex. Two nuclei that are just medial to the dentate nucleus are collectively referred to as the **interposed nuclei** and are made of the **emboliform** and **globose** nuclei. These nuclei interact with the intermediate portion of the cerebellar cortex. The most medial of the deep cerebellar nuclei are the **fastigial nuclei** and they interact with the vermis and the flocculonodular lobe (Figure 10.4). Therefore, when executing motor planning activity in the lateral cerebellar cortex, the dentate nuclei are the final output pathway from the cerebellum. Likewise, when balance is modified by the flocculonodular lobe, the final output from the cerebellum would be through the fastigial nuclei.

Cerebellar input pathways

The inputs to the cerebellum come from virtually all areas of the central nervous system. These include inputs from the spinal cord, providing information on limb position, joint angle, muscle length, and tension (proprioception). In addition, the cerebellum receives input from the vestibular system, the auditory system, and the visual system. These systems provide multi-modal sensory input to the cerebellum. The cerebellum also receives descending motor input from the cerebral cortex and brain stem nuclei. All of these inputs provide the cerebellum with a "view" of the outside world that it can incorporate into appropriate motor activity.

When describing inputs into the cerebellum, three particular regions can be described. The first is the **spinocerebellum** (the spinal cord input to the cerebellum) and these inputs project to the vermis and the intermediate part of the cerebellum. As you recall, these regions of the cerebellum control the trunk and extremity musculatures. The input from the spinal cord to

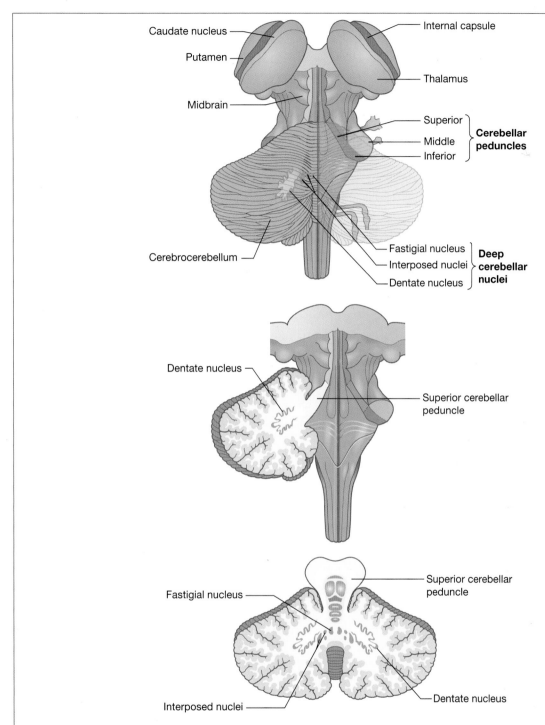

Figure 10.4 A shadow and oblique view of the cerebellum highlighting the deep cerebellar nuclei. Note the three sets of nuclei: the laterally placed dentate nuclei, the intermediate interposed (globose and emboliform) nuclei, and the medially placed fastigial nuclei, which respectively correspond to the three zones of the cerebellar cortex.

the cerebellum can come by numerous pathways. The two most prominent pathways are the **posterior (dorsal) spinocerebellar tract** and the **anterior (ventral) spinocerebellar tract** (Figure 10.5). The posterior spinocerebellar tract is an ipsilateral spinal cord projection to the cerebellum by way of the inferior

cerebellar peduncle. It provides proprioceptive information from the spinal cord to the cerebellum. The anterior spinocerebellar tract is also an ipsilateral spinal cord input into the cerebellum, but it takes a unique course through the spinal cord to reach the cerebellum. This tract is actually a double decussated

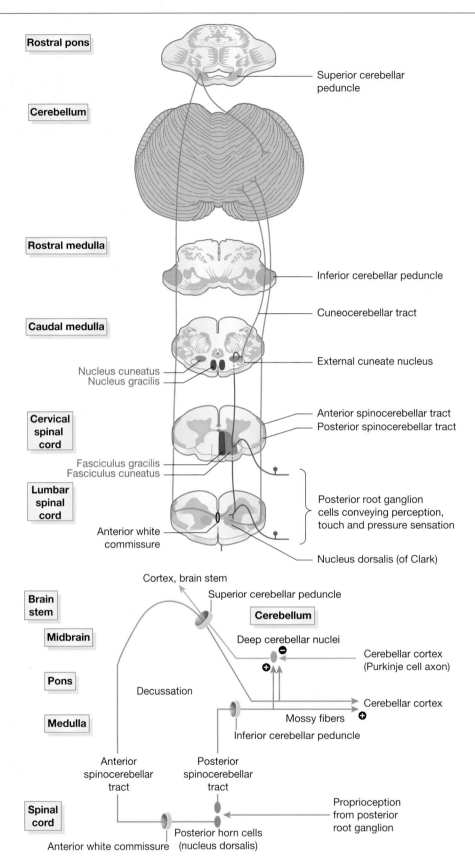

Figure 10.5 A drawing and schematic of the spinocerebellar tracts. Note the double decussation of the anterior spinocerebellar tract and no decussation of the posterior spinocerebellar tract, leading to ipsilateral input to the cerebellum from the peripheral proprioceptors. Also, the anterior spinocerebellar tract enters the cerebellum through the superior cerebellar peduncle, while the posterior spinocerebellar tract enters the cerebellum through the inferior cerebellar peduncle.

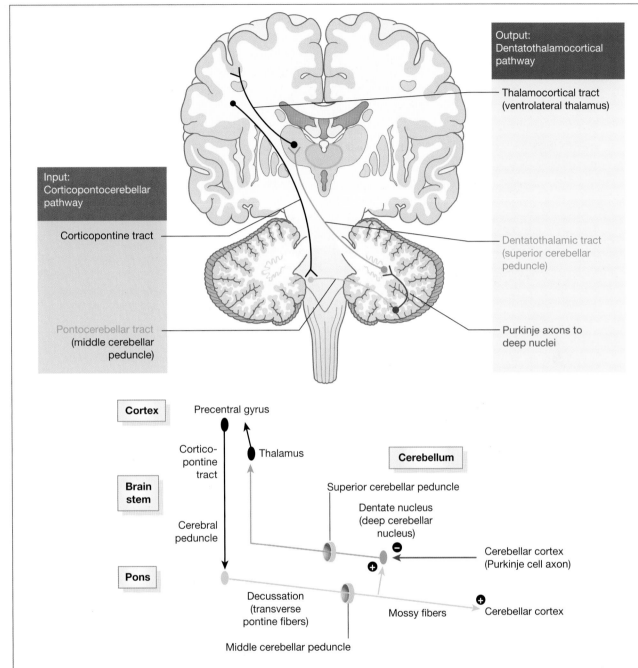

Input:
Corticopontocerebellar
pathway

Corticopontine tract

Pontocerebellar tract
(middle cerebellar
peduncle)

Output:
Dentatothalamocortical
pathway

Thalamocortical tract
(ventrolateral thalamus)

Dentatothalamic tract
(superior cerebellar
peduncle)

Purkinje axons to
deep nuclei

Cortex

Precentral gyrus

Cortico-
pontine
tract

Thalamus

Cerebellum

Brain
stem

Superior cerebellar peduncle

Dentate nucleus
(deep cerebellar
nucleus)

Cerebral
peduncle

Cerebellar cortex
(Purkinje cell axon)

Pons

Decussation
(transverse
pontine fibers)

Mossy fibers

Cerebellar cortex

Middle cerebellar peduncle

Figure 10.6 A drawing and schematic of the corticopontine, pontocerebellar, and dentatothalamic tracts. Note the decussation of input and output fibers so that the cerebellum is contralateral to the cortex. Also, the input to the cerebellum is through the middle cerebellar peduncle, while the output from the cerebellum is through the superior cerebellar peduncle.

pathway, such that it crosses over when it enters the spinal cord, ascends on the contralateral side and then crosses back over to enter the cerebellum through the superior cerebellar peduncle. Since it decussates twice, it remains an ipsilateral pathway. This pathway provides modified proprioceptive information to the cerebellum by way of interneurons within the spinal cord.

A second major input into the cerebellum is via the cerebral cortex and is the **cerebrocerebellar** input. This pathway

originates in the cerebral cortex and descends to the pons, where it synapses. The pontine nuclei send fibers across the pons to enter the contralateral cerebellum through the middle cerebellar peduncle. Therefore, the cortical and pontine input into the cerebellum is contralateral (Figure 10.6). These fibers project to the lateral portion of the cerebellum and, as you recall, are involved in the regulation of complex motor planning.

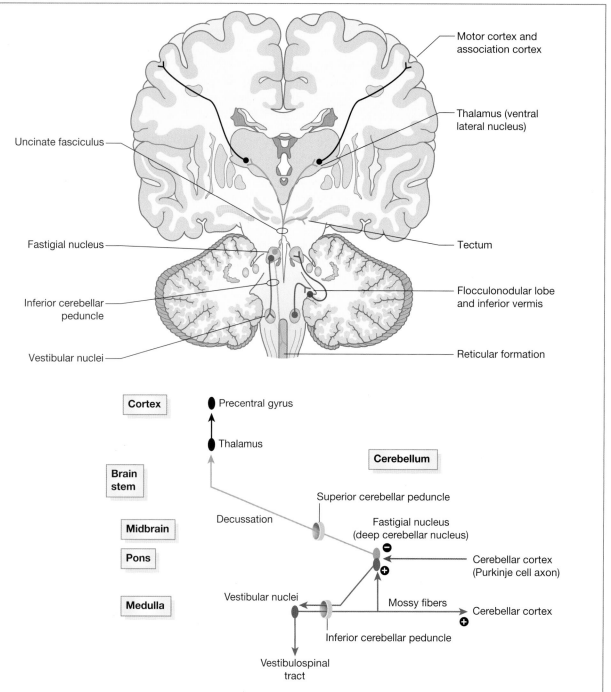

Figure 10.7 A drawing and schematic of the vestibulocerebellar tracts. Note the ipsilateral input and output to the cerebellum from the vestibular nuclei coursing through the inferior cerebellar peduncle.

The third major input into the cerebellum is via the vestibular nuclei and is the **vestibulocerebellar** input. These fibers arise from the vestibular nuclei and enter the cerebellum via the inferior cerebellar peduncle to project to the flocculonodular lobe of the cerebellum (Figure 10.7).

A final, specialized input to the cerebellum is from the inferior olive in the medulla oblongata. These olivary fibers are **climbing fibers** which project to both the deep cerebellar nuclei and to the cerebellar cortex. These fibers are part of a regulatory loop that helps to modify cerebellar activity. This loop consists of fibers projecting from the cerebellum to the **red nucleus** in the midbrain; then fibers projecting from the red nucleus to the **inferior olive**; and finally the inferior olive fibers (climbing fibers) project back to the cerebellum (Figure 10.8).

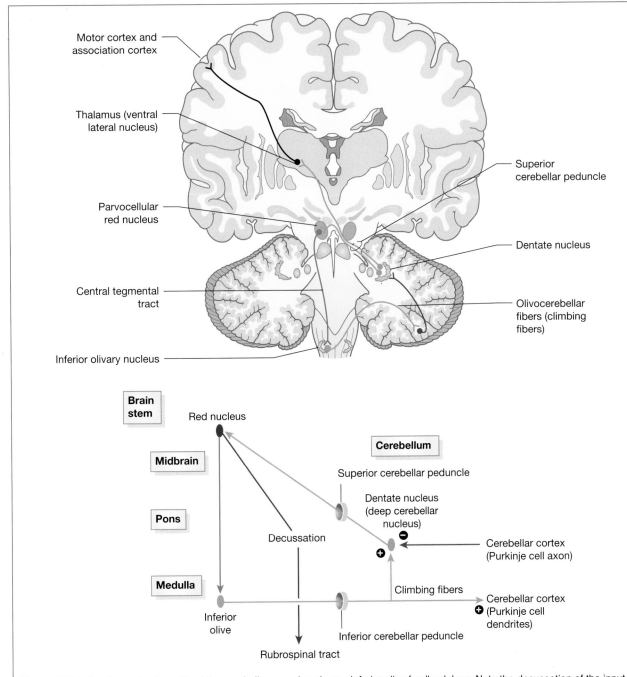

Figure 10.8 A drawing and schematic of the cerebellum – red nucleus – inferior olive feedback loop. Note the decussation of the input and output tracts, so that the red nucleus and inferior olive are contralateral to the cerebellum. Also, note that the descending rubrospinal tract decussates, so that it is ipsilateral to the cerebellum.

Cerebellar cortex histology

When examining the histology of the cerebellar cortex, three distinct layers are observed. The outer layer is the **molecular layer** which has a low density of cellular nuclei. A single-celled middle layer contains large multipolar neurons termed Purkinje cells and this constitutes the **Purkinje cell layer**. An inner layer is the **granule cell layer** that has a high density of

cellular nuclei. Deep to this layer is the white matter of the cerebellum, which contains axons ascending to the cortex as well as axons descending from the cortex to the **deep cerebellar nuclei**.

There are two input pathways to the cerebellar cortex: **mossy fibers**, which contain the majority of the inputs to the cerebellum, and specialized fibers, referred to as **climbing fibers** (which arise from the inferior olive). The climbing fibers

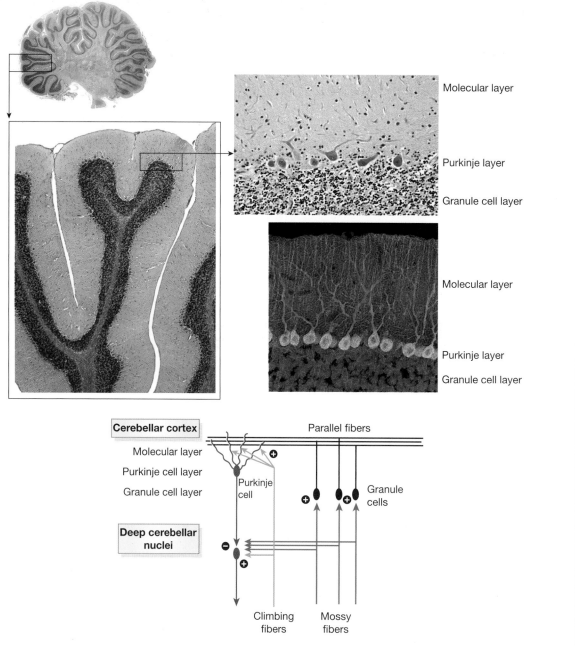

Figure 10.9 A histologic and schematic view of the cerebellar cortex. Note the three layers of the cortex with the prominent Purkinje cells in the middle layer. Also, note the interactions between the incoming mossy and climbing fibers, the neurons within the cortex, and the outgoing Purkinje cell axon. Sources: Science Photo Library/Dr Gladden Willis; Science Photo Library/Thomas Deerinck; Science Photo Library/ Steve Gschmeissner; Dr Keith Wheeler.

send positive (excitatory) branches to the **deep cerebellar nuclei**, other branches that wrap the dendrites of the Purkinje cell and branches to Golgi cells in the granular layer of the cerebellar cortex. The climbing fibers were named based on their anatomical configuration around the dendrites of the Purkinje cells, since they appear like ivy wrapping around the trunk of a tree. All other inputs to the cerebellar cortex from the cerebral cortex, the spinal cord, and the vestibular system

are referred to as **mossy fibers**. The mossy fibers send positive (excitatory) branches to the deep cerebellar nuclei, to **granule cells**, and to **Golgi cells** (Figure 10.9).

The internal circuitry of the cerebellar cortex centers around the **Purkinje cell**, since the Purkinje cell is the final output pathway from the cerebellar cortex. It is the only descending pathway from the cerebellar cortex and it provides a negative (inhibitory) signal to the deep cerebellar nuclei.

Clinical box 10.1

The neural interactions in the cerebellar cortex are quite complex. The inputs to the cortex come from excitatory mossy and climbing fibers, while the only output from the cerebellar cortex comes from the Purkinje cells (as an inhibitory output). **Climbing fibers** arise from the inferior olivary nucleus and synapse on the Purkinje cell dendrites directly – like ivy wrapping around tree branches. The **mossy fibers** come from numerous sources throughout the central nervous system, including the cerebral cortex, the vestibular nuclei, and the spinal cord. All of these input fibers are excitatory and send collateral branches to the deep cerebellar nuclei on their way to the cerebellar cortex.

There are many interneurons in the cerebellar cortex (granule cells, basket cells, stellate cells, Golgi cells) that modify Purkinje cell output. The dendrites of the Purkinje cells are arranged in a "fan-like" fashion (dense and wide in one plane, while narrow in the other plane). Many **parallel fibers** from **granule cells** run perpendicular to the fan of the Purkinje cell dendrites. **Basket cells** interact between the parallel fibers and send axons to the Purkinje cell body. **Golgi cells** act as feedback neurons from the parallel fibers to the granule cell's body. **Stellate cells** are small interneurons found within the parallel fibers in the molecular layer of the cerebellar cortex. This complex arrangement of cell bodies and axons in the cerebellar cortex produces zones of activated Purkinje cells and zones of quiet Purkinje cells.

The Purkinje cells send an inhibitory output to the deep cerebellar nuclei (a small set of fibers go directly to the vestibular nuclei). It is the balance of inhibitory signals from the Purkinje cells versus the excitatory signals from the climbing and mossy fiber collaterals that dictate the activity of the deep cerebellar nuclei. The **deep cerebellar nuclei** are the final common pathway for signals leaving the cerebellum.

While these interactions are quite well known, there is little clinical significance to their function. In most clinical conditions, specific regions of the cerebellum are damaged, including the cortex and deep nuclei. Therefore, it is much more relevant to know the specific inputs to the cerebellum, which regions of the cerebellum perform which functions, and the specific outputs from the cerebellum.

Within the layers of the cerebellar cortex there are complex axonal interactions between the mossy and climbing fibers as well as three types of interneurons: the **Golgi cells**, **basket cells**, and **stellate cells**. These interactions produce variable stimulation of Purkinje cells, such that certain zones of cells are stimulated or inhibited. Since the final pathway from the cerebellar cortex is via the descending axon of the Purkinje cell, it is important to understand that these interneurons modify the dendritic activity of the Purkinje cell and determine whether the Purkinje cell body produces an inhibitory output or not. This is a highly complex neuronal interaction that is scientifically interesting, but is not clinically relevant.

Cerebellar output pathways

The negative (inhibitory) descending output from the Purkinje cell axon inhibits the deep cerebellar nuclei. Recall that the mossy and climbing fibers provided excitatory stimulation to the same deep cerebellar nuclei, such that a competition occurs between the inhibitory Purkinje cell axons and the excitatory mossy and climbing fibers. This balance of inhibitory versus stimulatory activity regulates the final output from the deep cerebellar nuclei to the central nervous system. Therefore if the deep cerebellar nuclei are damaged, output from the cerebellum is compromised.

The deep cerebellar nuclei project to three main targets. The first target is the **red nucleus** in the midbrain, which has a reciprocal projection to the **inferior olive** and then back to the cerebellum, producing a feedback regulatory mechanism (Figure 10.8). Recall that the red nucleus also has descending fibers in the **rubrospinal tract**, so that output information from the cerebellum is directed to the spinal cord as well. The second target of the deep cerebellar nuclei are projections to the **thalamus** and then on to the **cerebral cortex**. These projections provide motor planning to the cortex before the final motor output is sent to the skeletal muscles (Figure 10.6). The third target of the deep cerebellar nuclei are projections to the **vestibular nuclei** in a feedback mechanism that modifies vestibular activity (Figure 10.7).

Recall that the majority of the fibers leaving the cerebellum pass through the superior cerebellar peduncle. These fibers cross in the midbrain so that output from the left cerebellum is projected to the right cortex. This means that the left cerebellum will ultimately have impact on the left side of the body due to a double decussation of motor control. Lesions of one side of the cerebellum will usually produce ipsilateral effects. However, midline lesions of the cerebellum (the vermis/flocculonodular lobe) will impact on midline trunk musculature and balance/equilibrium. This typically occurs bilaterally (not ipsilaterally).

To understand how the cerebellum interacts with the basal ganglia and the motor cortex to regulate complex skeletal muscle activity, Chapter 15 on central motor control can be helpful. Generally, the cerebellum provides input to the cortex for motor planning (on muscle tone, balance, orientation in space) as well as ongoing error correction for current muscular activity. One way to understand the functions of the cerebellum is to witness the activity of patients with cerebellar lesions. As patients with cerebellar lesions attempt various motor activities, the role of the cerebellum becomes apparent (Yu, *et al.*, 2015).

Clinical considerations

Cerebellar problems usually occur due to toxicity (alcoholism, overdose of lithium, or anticonvulsants), genetic disorders, or traumatic experiences (stroke, accidents). One of the major disturbances observed with cerebellar dysfunction is **ataxia**. Ataxia is an uncoordinated movement disorder which can be characterized as an unsteady gait or uncoordinated movement of the limbs involving intention tremors (Winchester, *et al.*, 2013). One mechanism to test for cerebellar dysfunction is to ask a patient to touch his nose and then to touch your finger. Try this multiple times as you move your finger and see if the patient can smoothly follow. If the patient cannot move his finger smoothly and correctly to touch yours, then there may be cerebellar dysfunction. Another way to test for cerebellar function is to ask a patient to perform a rapidly alternating movement such as flipping their hands from one side to the other. If a patient is unable to perform this task, the patient would have **dysdiadochokinesia**. Infants that have cerebellar dysfunction tend to have a decrease in muscle tone, referred to as **hypotonia**. Some patients with cerebellar disorders can also have involuntary eye movements. For example, the eyes can move rapidly in one direction (to the left) and then can return slowly back in the opposite direction (to the right). This is **nystagmus** and it can occur for a number of reasons, including vestibular or cerebellar defects. It can also be seen in a normal individual who is spun rapidly on a stool and then stopped abruptly. This individual's eyes will display nystagmus for a short period of time.

Clinical box 10.2

The blood supply to the cerebellum is from three primary sources, the **superior cerebellar artery**, the **anterior inferior cerebellar artery**, and the **posterior inferior cerebellar artery**. They supply specific regions of the cerebellum and, if lost due to stroke or trauma, will present with region specific deficits. These arteries also supply the cerebellar peduncles as well as parts of the brain stem, so there can be non-cerebellar (lateral brain stem) symptoms present when these vessels are compromised. Likewise, if the blood supply to one of the peduncles is lost, this can produce cerebellar deficits due to loss of input or output fibers, even though the cerebellum itself is not affected.

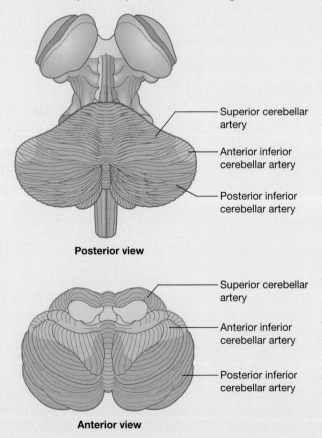

Superior cerebellar artery

Anterior inferior cerebellar artery

Posterior inferior cerebellar artery

Posterior view

Superior cerebellar artery

Anterior inferior cerebellar artery

Posterior inferior cerebellar artery

Anterior view

Case 1

During a physical examination with his new physician, Mr Phil Walker, a 64-year-old lawyer, is observed to have muscle weakness in his lower extremities and difficulty getting from a sitting position to a standing position. Once standing, he has a wide stance gait and appears to have difficulties with balance (standing with his feet together and his eyes closed). His physician, Dr Gary McChamber, obtains a detailed history from Mr Walker with the salient feature that Mr Walker consumes six to eight cocktails every evening after work. He mentions that this does not interfere with his working or social life. Dr McChamber collects blood for tests to rule out metabolic disturbances, along with infectious causes, such as Lyme disease or Legionella.

A few weeks later, Dr McChamber meets with Mr Walker and discusses the results and his interpretations. He suggests that Mr Walker has **alcoholic cerebellar degeneration** (Jaatinen and Rintala, 2008) due to his long-term alcohol intake (Figure 10.10). While there are few treatments available, Dr McChamber suggests that Mr Walker cease his alcohol use and that he make sure he has good nutrition (especially thiamine). He suggests that moderate exercise with physical therapy could help prevent any further loss and may even reverse some of the loss.

One year later, Dr McChamber sees Mr Walker during his annual examination. Mr Walker's symptoms have remained the same. Mr Walker admits that he has not given up alcohol, although he has improved his nutrition and has had some help with physical therapy.

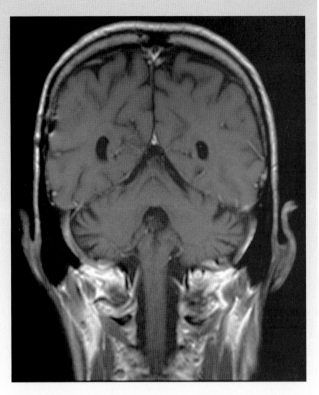

Figure 10.10 A frontal (coronal) magnetic resonance image of a patient with cerebellar degeneration. Note the increased space between the folia of the cerebellum.

Case 2

Mrs Judith Jones notices that her six-month-old daughter, Jennifer, does not appear to be developing as quickly as other children her age. She also notices that Jennifer's head appears larger than normal. She mentions this to her pediatrician, Dr Jeff Brown. He conducts a physical and neurological exam on Jennifer and concludes that she has a rare congenital disorder that affects development of the cerebellum (**Dandy-Walker syndrome**) (Spennato, et al., 2011). Genetic tests and magnetic resonance imaging confirm Dr Brown's diagnosis (Figure 10.11).

A magnetic resonance image of Jennifer's head indicates an enlargement in her ventricles, especially the fourth ventricle. Dr Brown suggests to Mrs Jones that Jennifer has a ventricular shunt placed between her fourth ventricle and her peritoneal cavity to reduce the hydrocephalus present and to limit any other neurological damage. Dr Brown supplies information to Jennifer's parents about the genetic disorder. The Jones' discuss the implications of the syndrome and agree to the shunt surgery for Jennifer.

Jennifer is monitored carefully over the next few years of her development. She has moderate developmental delays in motor activities, such as crawling and walking, but appears to have normal intellectual development.

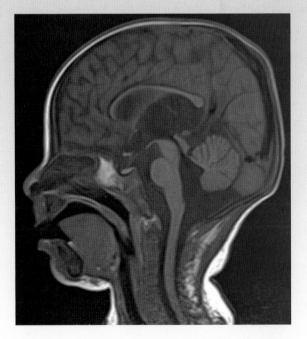

Figure 10.11 A sagittal magnetic resonance image of a child with Dandy-Walker syndrome. Note the poorly developed cerebellum and the enlarged ventricles, especially the fourth ventricle.

Study questions

1. Climbing fibers originate from the _____
and are _____ to the deep cerebellar nuclei.
a) red nucleus, excitatory
b) red nucleus, inhibitory
c) inferior olive, excitatory
d) inferior olive, inhibitory
e) pontine nuclei, excitatory
f) pontine nuclei, inhibitory

2. The output from the cerebellar cortex to the deep
cerebellar nuclei is through the:
a) granule cell axons
b) Golgi cell axons
c) basket cell axons
d) stellate cell axons
e) Purkinje cell axons

3. A 65-year-old female has a lesion in the left
cerebellum that produces deficits on the:
a) ipsilateral, left side
b) contralateral, left side
c) ipsilateral, right side
d) contralateral, right side

4. The cortical input to the cerebellum travels
through the _____ while the cerebellar
output to the cortex travels through the

_____.
a) inferior cerebellar peduncle, middle cerebellar peduncle
b) middle cerebellar peduncle, superior cerebellar peduncle
c) inferior cerebellar peduncle, superior cerebellar peduncle
d) middle cerebellar peduncle, inferior cerebellar peduncle
e) superior cerebellar peduncle, middle cerebellar peduncle
f) superior cerebellar peduncle, inferior cerebellar peduncle

5. A 56-year-old male has a lesion in the lateral
cerebellar cortex that produces deficits in:
a) midline trunk motor activity
b) distal extremity motor activity
c) planned motor activity
d) visual field acuity
e) tonotopic auditory reception

For more self-assessment questions, visit the companion website at
www.wileyessential.com/neuroanatomy

FURTHER READING

For additional information on the cerebellum, the
following textbooks and review articles may be helpful:

Blumenfeld H. 2002. *Neuroanatomy Through Clinical
Cases.* Sinauer Associates, Sunderland, Massachusetts.

Buckner RL. 2013. The cerebellum and cognitive function:
25 years of insight from anatomy and neuroimaging.
Neuron, 80(3): 807–815.

Felten DL, Shetty A. 2009. *Netter's Atlas of Neuroscience*,
2nd edition. Saunders Elsevier, Philadelphia,
Pennsylvania.

Habas C, Guillevin R, Abanou A. 2010. In vivo structural
and functional imaging of the human rubral and inferior
olivary nuclei: A mini-review. *Cerebellum*, 9(2): 167–173.

Haines DE. 2012. *Neuroanatomy: An Atlas of Structures,
Sections and Systems*, 8th edition. Lippincott Williams
& Wilkin, Baltimore, Maryland.

Jaatinen P, Rintala J. 2008. Mechanisms of ethanol-induced
degeneration in the developing, mature, and aging
cerebellum. *Cerebellum*, 7(3): 332–347.

Moore KL, Dalley AF, Agur AMR. 2014. *Moore Clinically
Oriented Anatomy*, 7th edition. Lippincott, Williams
& Wilkins, Philadelphia, Pennsylvania.

Patestas MA, Gartner LP. 2006. *A Textbook of Neuroanatomy*.
Blackwell Publishing, Malden, Massachusetts.

Reeber SL, Otis TS, Sillitoe RV. 2013. New roles for the
cerebellum in health and disease. *Front Syst Neurosci*,
7 (83): 1–11.

Spennato P, Mirone G, Nastro A, Buonocore MC,
Ruggiero C, Trischitta V, *et al.*, 2011. Hydrocephalus
in Dandy-Walker malformation. *Childs Nerv Syst*,
27(10):1665–1681.

Winchester S, Singh PK, Mikati MA. 2013. Ataxia. *Handb
Clin Neurol*, 112: 1213–1217.

Yu F, Jiang QJ, Sun XY, Zhang RW. 2015. A new case of
complete primary cerebellar agenesis: clinical and
imaging finding in a living patient. *Brain*, 138: in press.

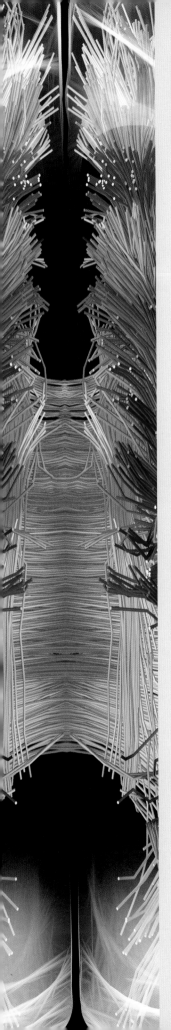

CHAPTER 11
Spinal tracts

Learning objectives

1. Identify the ascending tracts in the spinal cord.
2. Describe the components of the posterior columns and medial lemniscus.
3. Describe the symptoms in patients with lesions in the posterior columns.
4. Identify the components of the spinothalamic (anterolateral) tract.
5. Describe the functions of the spinothalamic tract.
6. Describe the symptoms in patients with lesions in the spinothalamic tract.
7. Identify the descending tracts in the spinal cord.
8. Identify the components of the corticospinal tract.
9. Describe upper motor neuron and lower motor neuron pathways.
10. Describe the symptoms in patients with lesions in the corticospinal tract.

Ascending tract: general sensation (fine touch, vibration sense, proprioception)   147

Function
1. Fine touch – Meissner corpuscles
2. Vibration sensation – Pacinian corpuscles
3. Position sense – muscle spindles, Golgi tendon organs
4. Stereognosis – recognize an object by touch, without visual cues

Pathway for body (posterior (dorsal) columns and medial lemniscus)
1. Myelinated, rapidly conducting axons enter via posterior (dorsal) root ganglion/dorsal root (first order neurons)
2. Ascend in posterior (dorsal) columns (no synapse)
   a) Below T6, ascend in fasciculus gracilis (medial)
   b) Above T6, ascend in fasciculus cuneatus (lateral)
3. In the caudal medulla
   a) Fibers in fasciculus gracilis synapse in nucleus gracilis
   b) Fibers in fasciculus cuneatus synapse in nucleus cuneatus
4. Second order neurons cross over in medulla oblongata
5. Ascend in contralateral medial lemniscus
6. Synapse in thalamus (VPL)
7. Third order neurons ascend through internal capsule to cerebral cortex (postcentral gyrus)

Essential Clinical Neuroanatomy, First Edition. Thomas H. Champney.
© 2016 John Wiley & Sons, Ltd. Published 2016 by John Wiley & Sons, Ltd.
Companion website: www.wileyessential.com/neuroanatomy

Pathway for face (trigeminal system)
1. Myelinated, rapidly conducting axons enter via trigeminal nerve/trigeminal ganglion (first order neurons)
2. Synapse in main sensory ganglion of trigeminal
3. Second order neurons cross over (decussate) in pons
4. Ascend in contralateral trigeminothalamic tract
5. Synapse in thalamus (VPM)
6. Third order neurons ascend through internal capsule to cerebral cortex (postcentral gyrus)

1. Lesion in spinal cord – ipsilateral loss of sensation below lesion
2. Lesion in brain stem, thalamus, cortex – contralateral loss of sensation
3. Two-point discrimination

Function
1. Pain – free, unmyelinated nerve endings in skin
2. Temperature – free, unmyelinated nerve endings in skin

Pathway for body (spinothalamic tract/anterolateral tract)
1. Enter via posterior (dorsal) root ganglion/ dorsal root (first order neurons)
2. Synapse in posterior (dorsal) horn
3. Second order neurons cross over at the spinal cord level of entry (anterior white commissure)
4. Ascend in contralateral spinothalamic tract (anterolateral)
5. Synapse in the thalamus (VPL)
6. Third order neurons ascend through internal capsule to cerebral cortex (postcentral gyrus)

Pathway for face (trigeminal system)
1. Myelinated, rapidly conducting axons enter via trigeminal nerve/trigeminal ganglion (first order neurons)
2. Descend in spinal tract of trigeminal
3. Synapse in nucleus of spinal tract of trigeminal
4. Second order neurons cross over (decussate) in pons/medulla oblongata
5. Ascend in contralateral trigeminothalamic tract
6. Synapse in thalamus (VPM)
7. Third order neurons ascend through internal capsule to cerebral cortex (postcentral gyrus)

1. Dermatomal overlap
2. Tract lesions produce contralateral loss, due to early crossing over
3. Homunculus distribution on postcentral gyrus

Anterior spinocerebellar tract – double decussated, ipsilateral cerebellum

Posterior spinocerebellar tract – ipsilateral cerebellum

Pathway – corticospinal tract
1. Arise in cerebral cortex (precentral gyrus/ premotor cortex) (upper motor neurons)
2. Descend through internal capsule, cerebral peduncle in midbrain
3. Cross over in caudal medulla (decussate) becoming the lateral corticospinal tract
4. Descend through spinal cord (contralateral side)
5. Synapse in anterior (ventral) horn on anterior (ventral) horn cells (3%), or on interneurons
6. Lower motor neurons pass through anterior (ventral) root to spinal nerve to supply skeletal muscles

Pathway – corticobulbar tract
1. Arise in cerebral cortex (precentral gyrus/ premotor cortex) (upper motor neurons)
2. Descend through internal capsule, cerebral peduncle in midbrain
3. Synapse in motor nuclei associated with cranial nerves (V, VII, IX, X, and XII)
4. Lower motor axons pass through cranial nerves to skeletal muscles

1. Upper motor neuron lesions
   a) Spasticity
   b) Hypertonia
   c) Increased deep tendon reflexes
   d) Muscle weakness
   e) Babinski test
2. Lower motor neuron lesions
   a) Fibrillations
   b) Fasciculations

c) Muscle weakness/wasting/atrophy
d) Hypotonia
e) Decreased deep tendon reflexes

Descending tract: cerebellar input

Pathway – corticopontine tract

1. Arise in cerebral cortex (precentral gyrus/premotor cortex)
2. Descend through internal capsule, cerebral peduncle in midbrain
3. Synapse on pontine nuclei (corticopontine axons)
4. Cross over (decussate) in the pons (transverse pontine fibers), enter the cerebellum in the middle cerebellar peduncle (pontocerebellar fibers – mossy fibers)

Descending tract: rubrospinal tract

Pathway

1. Arise in red nucleus in midbrain (from cerebellum and cerebral cortex)
2. Axons to inferior olive in medulla oblongata – feedback loop to cerebellum
3. Axons cross over (decussate) in midbrain, descend to upper cervical spinal cord – function is not clear

Descending tract: anterior corticospinal tract

Pathway

1. Arise in cerebral cortex (precentral gyrus/premotor cortex) (upper motor neurons)
2. Descend through internal capsule, cerebral peduncle in midbrain

3. Do not cross over (decussate) in caudal medulla – remain ipsilateral
4. Descend through anterior columns of spinal cord (ipsilateral)
5. Synapse bilaterally in anterior (ventral) horn cells
6. Lower motor neurons pass through ventral root to spinal nerve to supply trunk skeletal muscles

Descending tracts: sensory input to motor nuclei in anterior horn

Pathways

1. Reticulospinal tract – postural movements, autonomic control, pain modulation
2. Vestibulospinal tract – balance input to motor neurons
3. Tectospinal tract – visual input to cervical motor neurons

Clinical considerations

Spinal cord lesions

Case studies

Brown Séquard syndrome

Syphilitic myelopathy (tabes dorsalis)

Study questions

Introduction

The neuroanatomy of the central nervous system has been covered in the previous ten chapters. The following chapters will utilize this neuroanatomical information to present the sensory systems, the motor system, and other functional aspects of the nervous system. These chapters should add functional and clinical context to the specific neuroanatomy that has already been presented.

Since the anatomy of the spinal cord has been previously discussed, this chapter will focus on the distribution of the tracts through the spinal cord and their function. Ascending and descending tracts will be covered, along with the clinical aspects associated with loss of these tracts.

Ascending (sensory) tracts

There are a number of sensory modalities that are brought from the periphery through the spinal cord to the cortex or cerebellum. The sensations of touch, vibration, proprioception (space/position sense based on muscle tension), and stereognosis (ability to recognize shapes by feel) are carried via the **posterior columns** of the spinal cord. The sensations of pain and temperature are carried by a different pathway within the spinal cord: the **spinothalamic tract** (or the anterolateral pathway). Finally, the proprioceptive information is also sent directly to the cerebellum via the **spinocerebellar tracts**.

Posterior (dorsal) columns

The well-recognized sensation of touch (along with vibration and proprioception) is carried from peripheral receptors in the skin to the spinal cord by way of long sensory axons whose cell bodies reside in the posterior (dorsal) root ganglion. The central projection of these axons continues in the posterior root and into the posterior horn of the spinal cord. Some branches of these axons may synapse in the posterior horn to provide a rapid reflex arc through motor neurons in the anterior (ventral) horn, while other axons ascend in the posterior columns to deliver the somatosensory information to the cortex (and the awareness of the individual). These ascending branches enter into the **fasciculus gracilis** or **fasciculus cuneatus** of the posterior columns. Those sensory axons from the lower extremity (generally below the T6 vertebral level), ascend in the fasciculus gracilis (medially), where they synapse in the **nucleus gracilis** within the medulla oblongata. Those sensory axons from the upper extremity ascend in the fasciculus cuneatus (laterally), where they synapse in the **nucleus cuneatus** within the medulla. These axons are considered **first order axons** and, as mentioned previously, have their cell bodies in the posterior (dorsal) root ganglion. Recall that the posterior root ganglion does not contain synapses; it is merely a repository for the cell bodies of the pseudounipolar neurons.

The **second order sensory neurons** that arise from the nucleus gracilis or nucleus cuneatus decussate across the caudal medulla oblongata and ascend through the brain stem in the contralateral **medial lemniscus**. These somatosensory fibers maintain a distinct orientation (somatotopy) within the medial lemniscus, such that fibers from the lower extremity are arranged together and fibers from the upper extremity are arranged together. The second order neurons in the medial lemniscus begin in a more medial orientation, then move anteriorly and laterally as they ascend through the brain stem. These axons eventually terminate in the **thalamus**, specifically the ventral posterior lateral nucleus.

The **third order sensory neurons** that arise in the thalamus ascend through the **internal capsule** to end in the **postcentral gyrus** of the cerebral cortex. This is where the conscious sensation of touch is localized. It is important to recognize that the first order neurons in the spinal cord are ipsilateral, while the second order and third order neurons in this pathway are contralateral (Figures 11.1, 11.2). This has important clinical significance since lesions in the spinal cord or brain stem produce different sensory losses.

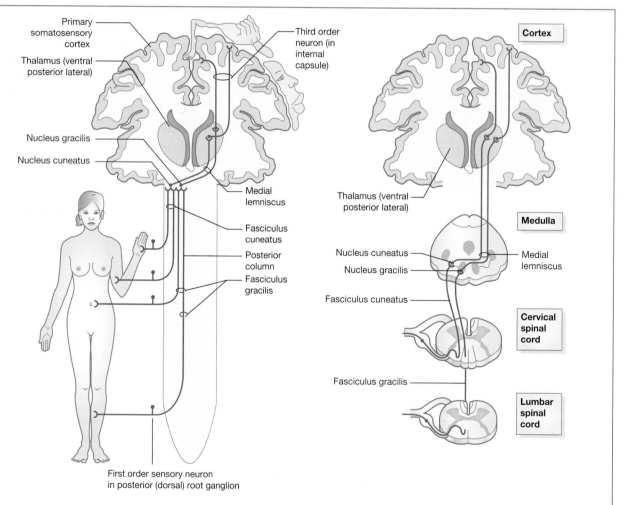

Figure 11.1 A diagramatic and cross-sectional view of the posterior column sensory pathways (fine touch and proprioception) from the spinal cord through the brain stem to the cortex. Note the decussation in the caudal medulla.

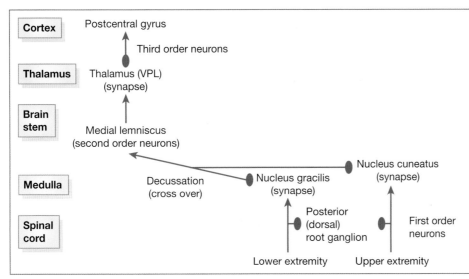

Figure 11.2 Schematic view of the posterior column sensory pathways (fine touch and proprioception) from the spinal cord through the brain stem to the cortex. Note the decussation in the caudal medulla.

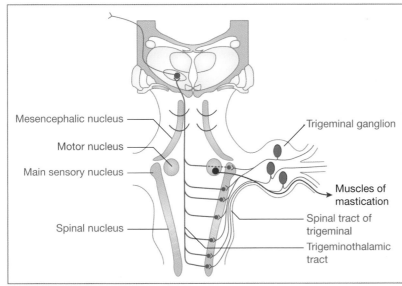

Figure 11.3 Diagramatic view of the trigeminal sensory pathways from the face and head (fine touch, proprioception, pain, and temperature) from the spinal cord through the brain stem to the cortex. Note the fine touch and proprioceptive fibers synapse in the main sensory nucleus, while the pain and temperature fibers synapse in the spinal nucleus of the trigeminal. Note that the decussation occurs throughout the pons and medulla in the brain stem. The sensory components from the facial nerve (VII), glossopharyngeal nerve (IX), and vagus nerve (X) use this same pathway, with their first order axons synapsing in the main sensory and spinal nucleus of the trigeminal.

The sensation of touch from the face follows a similar pathway. Peripheral receptors in the skin of the face are activated. First order peripheral sensory axons with cell bodies in the **trigeminal ganglion** project into the pons and synapse in the **main sensory trigeminal nucleus**. Second order axons decussate across the pons and ascend in the **trigeminothalamic tract** (or trigeminothalamic lemniscus) to synapse in the **thalamus**, specifically the ventral posterior medial nucleus. In similar fashion, the third order sensory neurons from the thalamus ascend in the **internal capsule** to end in the **postcentral gyrus** of the cerebral cortex. The touch sensation components of the other cranial nerves (facial (VII), glossopharyngeal (IX), and vagus (X)) have their first order sensory cell bodies (pseudounipolar neurons) in ganglia associated with the nerves and send central processes into the **main sensory trigeminal nucleus** where they synapse. The second order and third order neurons follow the same pathway as the trigeminal components (trigeminothalamic tract, thalamus (VPM), and postcentral gyrus) (Figures 11.3, 11.4 as well as 6.11, 6.12).

The proprioceptive fibers from the muscles of the jaw are unique in that their first order cell bodies (pseudounipolar) are found in the brain stem (pons and midbrain) in the **mesencephalic nucleus of the trigeminal (V)** (not in a peripheral ganglion). These first order fibers provide the sensory proprioceptive portion of a reflex arc for the jaw muscles. These fibers terminate centrally in the **main sensory trigeminal nucleus** as well as sending collateral branches to the **motor nuclei of the trigeminal** (bilaterally) to mediate the jaw reflex.

One aspect of general touch sensation is the ability for two-point discrimination. This means that some portions of the skin are highly sensitive to touch discrimination, while others are less sensitive. For example, on the back, an individual may be unable to distinguish two separate pinpricks even though they are separated by ½ inch. On the other hand, individuals can easily separate two pinpricks on the finger with much finer discrimination. The loss of two-point discrimination over a specific dermatomal region of the body can be indicative of a posterior column lesion (Figure 11.5).

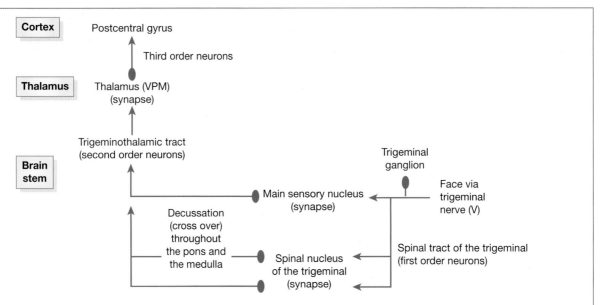

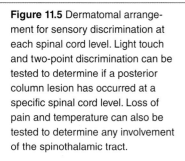

Figure 11.4 Schematic view of the trigeminal sensory pathways from the face and head (fine touch, proprioception, pain, and temperature) from the spinal cord through the brain stem to the cortex. Note the fine touch and proprioceptive fibers synapse in the main sensory nucleus, while the pain and temperature fibers synapse in the spinal nucleus of the trigeminal. Note that the decussation occurs throughout the pons and medulla oblongata in the brain stem. The sensory components from the facial nerve (VII), glossopharyngeal nerve (IX), and vagus nerve (X) use this same pathway with their first order axons synapsing in the main sensory and spinal nucleus of the trigeminal.

Figure 11.5 Dermatomal arrangement for sensory discrimination at each spinal cord level. Light touch and two-point discrimination can be tested to determine if a posterior column lesion has occurred at a specific spinal cord level. Loss of pain and temperature can also be tested to determine any involvement of the spinothalamic tract.

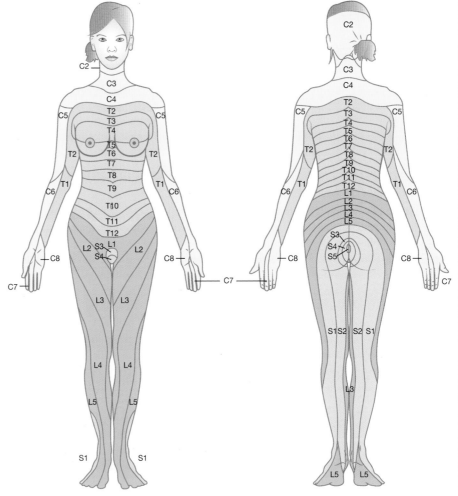

Recall that "all good second order sensory axons decussate" so that second and third order neurons are contralateral to their sensory input, while first order neurons are ipsilateral. At this point, it should be apparent that lesions in the posterior columns of the spinal cord will produce ipsilateral tactile deficits below the level of the lesion. For example, if a patient has a traumatic injury to the posterior columns of the spinal cord at the level of the fourth thoracic spinal segment, then all tactile sensation from the lower extremity and the abdomen will be lost on the ipsilateral side. One method to ensure understanding of this pathway is to be able to describe the clinical deficits that would be seen in patients with lesions at various points along this pathway. This concept will be highlighted in the clinical correlation section.

Spinothalamic tract

The sensations of pain and temperature from the skin (as well as itch, interestingly) arise as free nerve endings within the skin and are carried by pseudounipolar neurons through the peripheral nerves, with their cell bodies in the posterior (dorsal) root ganglion. The central projections of these **first order neurons** pass through the posterior root and into the posterior horn of the spinal cord, where they synapse. The **second order neurons** arise in the posterior horn and, as all good second order sensory neurons do, they decussate. These fibers decussate across the **anterior white commissure** of the spinal cord and ascend in the contralateral **spinothalamic tract** (spinothalamic lemniscus, anterolateral pathway). The second order sensory neurons in the spinothalamic tract ascend through the lateral region of the spinal cord and brain stem to synapse in the **thalamus**, specifically the ventral posterior lateral thalamus. The **third order neurons** ascend through the **internal capsule** to project to the **postcentral gyrus** of the cortex, bringing pain and temperature sensations from specific anatomical regions of the skin (somatotopic distribution) (Figures 11.6, 11.7).

The sensations of pain and temperature (and itch) from the skin of the face also arise as free nerve endings and are carried by pseudounipolar neurons in the trigeminal nerve with

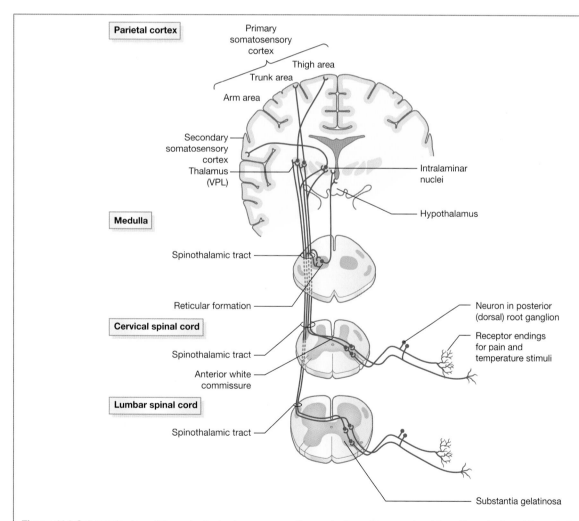

Figure 11.6 Schematic view of the spinothalamic sensory pathways (pain and temperature) from the spinal cord through the brain stem to the cortex. Note the decussation in the anterior white commissure in the spinal cord.

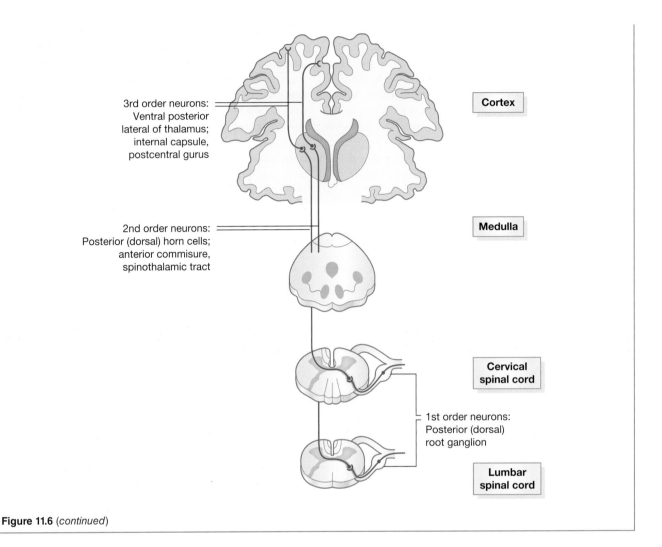

3rd order neurons:
Ventral posterior
lateral of thalamus;
internal capsule,
postcentral gurus

Cortex

2nd order neurons:
Posterior (dorsal) horn cells;
anterior commisure,
spinothalamic tract

Medulla

Cervical
spinal cord

1st order neurons:
Posterior (dorsal)
root ganglion

Lumbar
spinal cord

Figure 11.6 (*continued*)

Figure 11.7 Schematic view of the anterolateral column sensory pathways (pain and temperature) from the spinal cord through the brain stem to the cortex. Note the decussation in the anterior white commissure in the spinal cord.

Cortex — Postcentral gyrus

Third order neurons

Thalamus — Thalamus (VPL) (synapse)

Brain stem — Spinothalamic tract (second order neurons)

Spinal cord

Anterior white commissure

Decussation (cross over)

Posterior (dorsal) horn (synapse)

First order neurons — Posterior (dorsal) root ganglion

Body wall and extremities

their cell bodies in the **trigeminal ganglion**. These first order sensory axons enter the pons through the trigeminal nerve and, uniquely, descend through the pons and medulla as the **spinal tract of the trigeminal**. At various points in the pons and medulla, these axons synapse on cell bodies within the **spinal nucleus of the trigeminal**. As soon as they synapse, the second order sensory neurons decussate across the brain stem and ascend in the **trigeminothalamic tract** to the thalamus (ventral posterior medial nucleus). The third order neurons follow the same pathway from the **thalamus** through the **internal capsule** to the **postcentral gyrus** of the cortex. The pain and temperature sensation components of the other cranial nerves (facial (VII), glossopharyngeal (IX), and vagus (X)) have their first order sensory cell bodies (pseudounipolar neurons) in associated ganglia, which send central processes into the **spinal tract of the trigeminal** to synapse at the **spinal nucleus of the trigeminal**. The second order axons decussate and follow the same pathway as the trigeminal components (trigeminothalamic tract, thalamus (VPM), and third order neurons to the postcentral gyrus) (Figures 11.3, 11.4).

The distribution of somatosensory information (touch, pain, and temperature) on the postcentral gyrus is arranged anatomically via a specific somatotopic distribution referred to as a sensory **homunculus**. Therefore, when observing a coronal section of the postcentral gyrus, distinct regions of the gyrus receive specific anatomical somatosensory input (Figure 11.8). Understanding the homuncular distribution of somatosensory inputs to the postcentral gyrus is clinically relevant, since a small ischemic lesion of the cortex can produce specific somatosensory losses related to the extent of the lesion. Notice how sensory input from the hand is next to the sensory input from the face; therefore, a small lesion could produce this unique loss of sensation. Recall that portions of the cortex are supplied by branches of the anterior and middle cerebral

Clinical box 11.1

In the spinal cord and brain stem, the sensations of pain and temperature are carried separately from the sensations of touch, vibration, and proprioception. Therefore, patients can have a loss of one type of sensation but not a loss of the other. In a posterior column lesion, the patient would have no loss of pain or temperature, only touch and vibration. If, however, a patient had a lesion of the spinothalamic tract, the patient would not feel pain or temperature on the contralateral side of the body (due to the early decussation of the second order fibers).

An interesting clinical consideration is a compressive loss of the **anterior white commissure** in the spinal cord due to a widening of the central canal (**syringomyelia**) (Roy, *et al.*, 2011). A lesion at this point would produce a bilateral deficit in pain and temperature at the specific spinal cord levels affected since the fibers from both sides are decussating at that point. Interestingly, this loss would not impact on pain or temperature sensation above or below these spinal levels since the more laterally placed spinothalamic tract would still be intact. Again, to ensure understanding of these pathways, you should be able to describe deficits observed in patients with lesions at numerous points along the pathways.

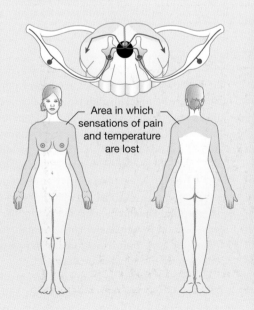

Area in which sensations of pain and temperature are lost

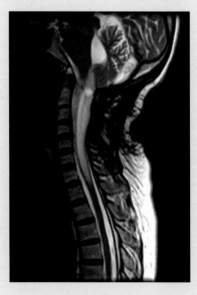

Figure 11.8 A drawing of the somatotopic distribution of sensory fibers in the somatosensory postcentral gyrus of the cortex (sensory homunculus). Note that this distribution is for general sensation, pain, and temperature. There is no separation of these sensory modalities at the level of the cortex.

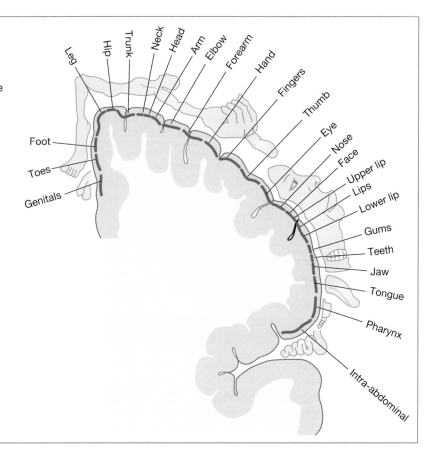

arteries (Chapter 2). If a patient lost the anterior cerebral artery supply to the left postcentral gyrus, what sensory deficits would be observed?

Spinocerebellar pathway

The **spinocerebellar tracts** receive proprioceptive information from first order sensory neurons, but, instead of relaying this information to the cortex, separate fibers provide this information to the cerebellum. These pathways provide unconscious proprioceptive information to the ipsilateral cerebellum. Fibers in the **posterior (dorsal) spinocerebellar tract** remain ipsilateral within the spinal cord as they ascend into the cerebellum through the inferior cerebellar peduncle. In comparison, the fibers in the **anterior (ventral) spinocerebellar tract** decussate across the spinal cord at their level of entry (through the anterior white commissure), ascend up the contralateral spinal cord and brain stem to enter the cerebellum through the superior cerebellar peduncle. These fibers then decussate back into the ipsilateral cerebellum. Therefore, this pathway contains a double decussation which leads to an ipsilateral representation in the cerebellum (Figure 11.9). These pathways were previously described in Chapter 10 on the cerebellum (Figure 10.5). There are other less prominent spinocerebellar pathways, but the important concept to keep in mind is that the inputs are ipsilateral and provide unconscious proprioception to the cerebellum.

Descending tracts

There are five descending tracts in the spinal cord; the most important is the corticospinal tract. This tract carries the bulk of upper motor neurons for control of skeletal muscle function. The other descending tracts carry information from higher levels of the central nervous system to the spinal cord for integrative coordination of muscular activity (Table 11.1).

Corticospinal tract

The **corticospinal tract** arises primarily from large multipolar neurons in the **precentral gyrus** of the cortex (primary motor cortex), with additional axons arising from the supplementary motor cortex and the parietal cortex. The axons descend in the **internal capsule** through the **cerebral peduncles** of the midbrain. These fibers (referred to as **upper motor neurons**) continue through the pons and the **pyramids** of the medulla where they decussate (pyramidal decussation) and form the **lateral corticospinal tract** in the opposite side of the spinal cord. The fibers descend in the lateral corticospinal tract, eventually to synapse on large motor neurons in the anterior horn of the spinal cord or on spinal interneurons.

The **lower motor neurons** arise from the anterior horn, exit through the anterior (ventral) root and spinal nerve to supply skeletal muscles associated with that spinal level. All of

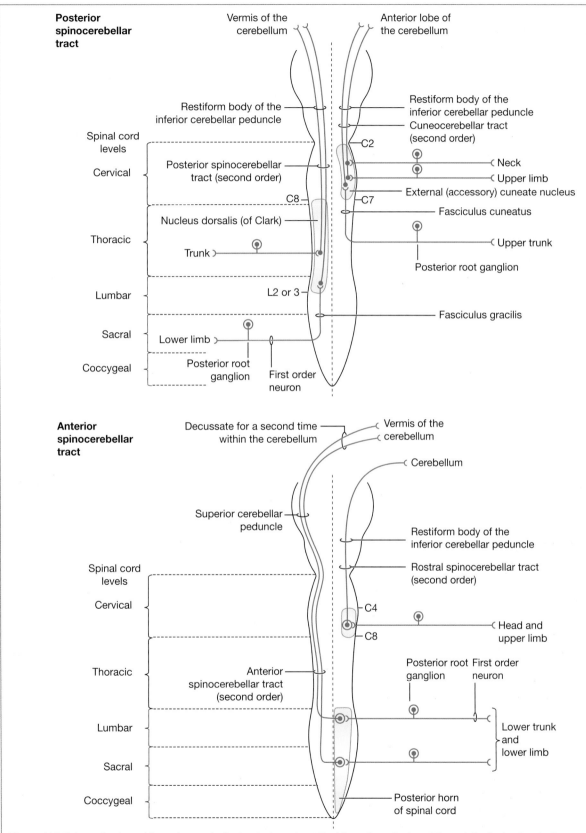

Posterior spinocerebellar tract

Vermis of the cerebellum

Anterior lobe of the cerebellum

Restiform body of the inferior cerebellar peduncle

Restiform body of the inferior cerebellar peduncle

Cuneocerebellar tract (second order)

C2

Neck

Spinal cord levels

Cervical

Posterior spinocerebellar tract (second order)

Upper limb

External (accessory) cuneate nucleus

C8

C7

Fasciculus cuneatus

Nucleus dorsalis (of Clark)

Thoracic

Upper trunk

Trunk

Posterior root ganglion

Lumbar

L2 or 3

Fasciculus gracilis

Sacral

Lower limb

Coccygeal

Posterior root ganglion

First order neuron

Anterior spinocerebellar tract

Decussate for a second time within the cerebellum

Vermis of the cerebellum

Cerebellum

Superior cerebellar peduncle

Restiform body of the inferior cerebellar peduncle

Spinal cord levels

Rostral spinocerebellar tract (second order)

Cervical

C4

C8

Head and upper limb

Posterior root ganglion

First order neuron

Thoracic

Anterior spinocerebellar tract (second order)

Lumbar

Lower trunk and lower limb

Sacral

Coccygeal

Posterior horn of spinal cord

Figure 11.9 Schematic view of the spinocerebellar tracts (proprioception) from the spinal cord through the brain stem to the cerebellum. Note the double decussation of the anterior spinocerebellar tract, once in the spinal cord and then again in the cerebellum to supply the ipsilateral cerebellum.

Table 11.1 Name and function of the ascending and descending tracts in the spinal cord and the brain stem. Note the sensory tracts are in green, while the motor tracts are in red.

Spinal cord tracts

Posterior (dorsal) columns – ascending tracts (sensory: fine touch, proprioception)

Fasciculus gracilis – lower extremity ipsilateral
Fasciculus cuneatus – upper extremity ipsilateral

Lateral columns – ascending and descending tracts

Lateral corticospinal tract – descending (motor: skeletal muscle ipsilateral, upper motor neurons)
Rubrospinal tract – descending (motor: cerebellum to skeletal muscle)
Spinothalamic (anterolateral) tract – ascending (sensory: pain and temperature contralateral)
Posterior (dorsal) spinocerebellar – ascending (sensory: proprioception to cerebellum)
Anterior (ventral) spinocerebellar – ascending (sensory: proprioception to cerebellum)

Anterior (ventral) columns – descending tracts

Anterior corticospinal tract – descending (motor: trunk skeletal muscle bilateral)
Vestibulospinal tract – descending (sensory: vestibular, balance to motor neurons)
Reticulospinal tract – descending (pain gating, autonomic to motor neurons)
Tectospinal tract – descending (sensory: visual to cervical motor neurons)

Brain stem tracts

Ascending tracts

Medial lemniscus (sensory: fine touch and proprioception from contralateral body, second order)
Spinothalamic tract (sensory: pain and temperature from contralateral body, second order)
Trigeminothalamic tract (sensory: fine touch, proprioception, pain and temperature from contralateral head, second order)
Spirocerebellar tracts (sensory: proprioception to cerebellum)

Descending tracts

Cerebral peduncles, corticospinal, medullary pyramids (motor: skeletal muscle contralateral, upper motor neurons)
Rubrospinal tract (motor: cerebellum to skeletal muscle, upper motor neurons)

Vestibulospinal tract – descending (sensory: vestibular, balance to motor neurons)
Reticulospinal tract – descending (pain gating, autonomic to motor neurons)
Tectospinal tract – descending (sensory: visual to cervical motor neurons)

the lower motor neurons are on the same side of the body (ipsilateral) to the muscles they innervate. In contrast, the upper motor neurons from the precentral gyrus of the cortex to the medulla oblongata are on the opposite side of the brain from the skeletal muscles they innervate (contralateral), while the spinal portion of the upper motor neurons (lateral corticospinal tract) are on the ipsilateral side of the body (due to the decussation of the axons in the medulla oblongata) (Figures 11.10, 11.11, 11.12).

Corticobulbar tract

The upper motor neurons that project to cranial nerve nuclei for skeletal motor innervation of the face, jaw, tongue, and throat are referred to as **corticobulbar neurons** (or corticonuclear neurons). These neurons have a similar course as the corticospinal neurons from the **precentral gyrus of the cortex** through the **internal capsule** and the **cerebral peduncles** of the midbrain. Within the brain stem, these neurons synapse on the cranial nerve nuclei associated with: the muscles of mastication (motor nucleus of trigeminal V); the muscles of facial expression (facial nucleus VII); the muscles of the palate, pharynx, and larynx (nucleus ambiguous for cranial nerves IX and X); and the muscles of the tongue (hypoglossal nucleus XII) (Figures 11.13, 11.14).

The majority of these corticobulbar fibers project bilaterally to the cranial nerve nuclei with two prominent exceptions. Innervation to the hypoglossal nucleus (cranial nerve XII) is only unilateral, such that upper motor neuron lesions produce contralateral deficits, while lower motor neuron lesions produce ipsilateral deficits. Also, the facial nerve (VII) has some unilateral innervation. The muscles of the face below the eye are innervated unilaterally by corticobulbar fibers, such that upper motor neuron lesions will affect the contralateral facial muscles below the eye, with no effect on the muscles of the forehead. On the other hand, a lower motor neuron lesion will result in the loss of motor activity ipsilaterally from the entire side of the face (Figure 11.15).

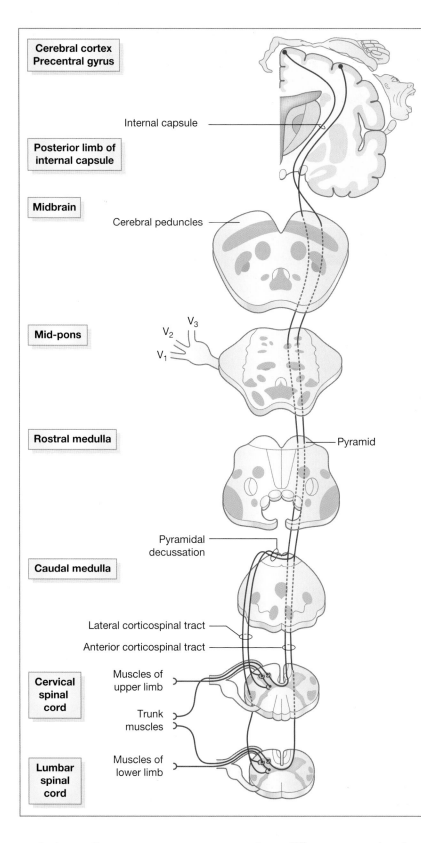

Cerebral cortex Precentral gyrus

Internal capsule

Posterior limb of internal capsule

Midbrain

Cerebral peduncles

Mid-pons

V_3
V_2
V_1

Rostral medulla

Pyramid

Pyramidal decussation

Caudal medulla

Lateral corticospinal tract

Anterior corticospinal tract

Cervical spinal cord

Muscles of upper limb

Trunk muscles

Lumbar spinal cord

Muscles of lower limb

Figure 11.10 A view of the descending voluntary motor pathways (corticospinal tracts) from the cortex through the brain stem to the spinal cord. Note the decussation of the upper motor neurons in the caudal medulla oblongata.

Lesions of upper motor neurons produce different symptoms than lesions of lower motor neurons (Table 11.2). When lower motor neurons are lost, the skeletal muscles are not innervated, so random contractions from muscle fascicles can take place (**fasciculations** (coarse contractions)). The muscles begin to atrophy, show signs of weakness, and develop a decrease in muscle tone (**hypotonia**), as well as a decrease in deep tendon reflexes (**hyporeflexia**). With

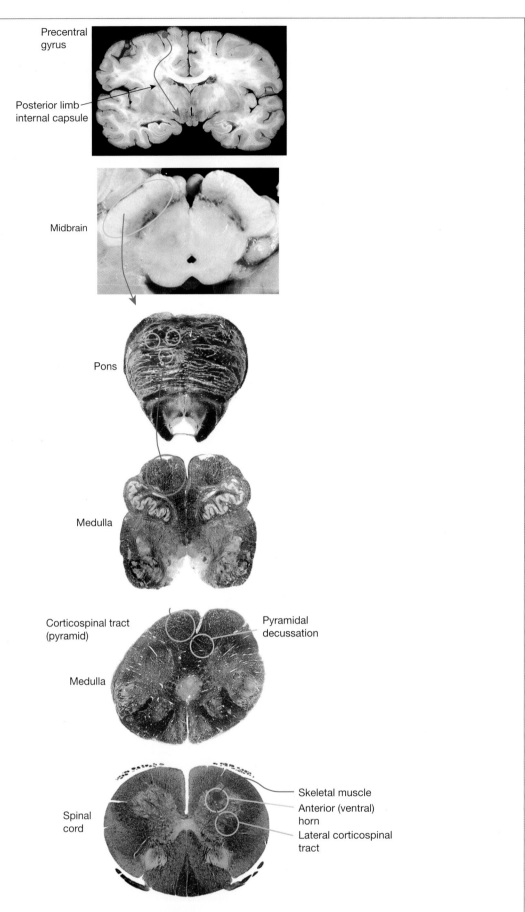

Figure 11.11 A view of the descending voluntary motor pathways (corticospinal tracts) from the cortex through the brain stem to the spinal cord in fresh tissue (upper two) and myelin stained tissue (lower four). Note the decussation of the upper motor neurons in the caudal medulla oblongata.

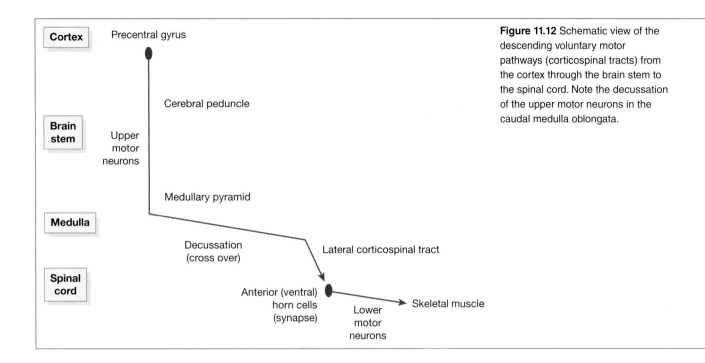

Figure 11.12 Schematic view of the descending voluntary motor pathways (corticospinal tracts) from the cortex through the brain stem to the spinal cord. Note the decussation of the upper motor neurons in the caudal medulla oblongata.

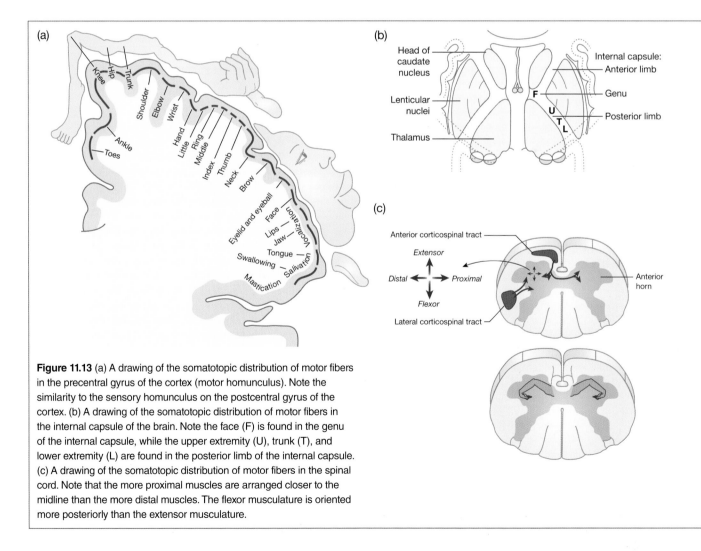

Figure 11.13 (a) A drawing of the somatotopic distribution of motor fibers in the precentral gyrus of the cortex (motor homunculus). Note the similarity to the sensory homunculus on the postcentral gyrus of the cortex. (b) A drawing of the somatotopic distribution of motor fibers in the internal capsule of the brain. Note the face (F) is found in the genu of the internal capsule, while the upper extremity (U), trunk (T), and lower extremity (L) are found in the posterior limb of the internal capsule. (c) A drawing of the somatotopic distribution of motor fibers in the spinal cord. Note that the more proximal muscles are arranged closer to the midline than the more distal muscles. The flexor musculature is oriented more posteriorly than the extensor musculature.

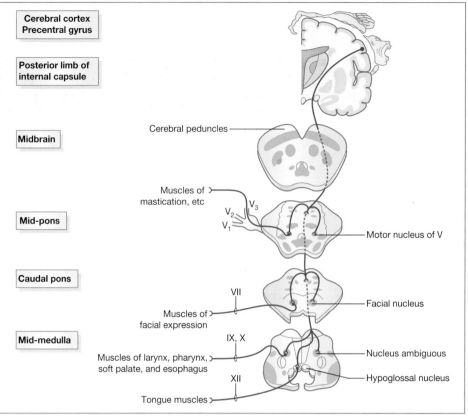

Figure 11.14 Drawing of the descending motor pathways (corticobulbar tracts) from the cortex through the brain stem to the cranial nerve nuclei controlling the skeletal muscles of the jaw (trigeminal V), the muscles of the face (facial VII), the muscles of the pharynx and larynx (glossopharyngeal IX and vagus X), and the muscles of the tongue (hypoglossal XII). Note the bilateral projection of the upper motor neurons to the majority of these cranial nerve nuclei. Two notable exceptions exist: the lower portion of the facial nerve (VII) is contralateral, not bilateral and the hypoglossal nerve (XII) to the tongue is contralateral, not bilateral.

Cerebral cortex
Precentral gyrus

Posterior limb of internal capsule

Midbrain

Cerebral peduncles

Mid-pons

Muscles of mastication, etc

V₂ V₃
V₁

Motor nucleus of V

Caudal pons

VII

Muscles of facial expression

Facial nucleus

Mid-medulla

IX, X

Muscles of larynx, pharynx, soft palate, and esophagus

Nucleus ambiguous

XII

Hypoglossal nucleus

Tongue muscles

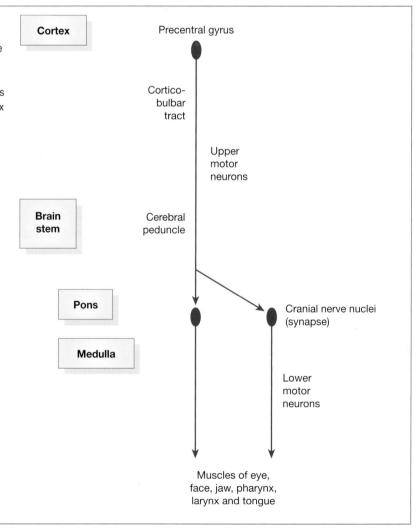

Figure 11.15 Schematic view of the descending motor pathways (corticobulbar tracts) from the cortex through the brain stem to the cranial nerve nuclei controlling the skeletal muscles of the eye (oculomotor III, trochlear IV, and abducens VI), the muscles of the jaw (trigeminal V), the muscles of the face (facial VII), the muscles of the pharynx and larynx (glossopharyngeal IX and vagus X), and the muscles of the tongue (hypoglossal XII). Note the bilateral projection of the upper motor neurons to the majority of these cranial nerve nuclei. Two notable exceptions exist: the lower portion of the facial nerve (VII) is contralateral, not bilateral and the hypoglossal nerve (XII) to the tongue is contralateral, not bilateral.

Cortex

Precentral gyrus

Cortico-bulbar tract

Upper motor neurons

Brain stem

Cerebral peduncle

Pons

Cranial nerve nuclei (synapse)

Medulla

Lower motor neurons

Muscles of eye, face, jaw, pharynx, larynx and tongue

Table 11.2 Clinical deficits observed after an upper motor neuron or lower motor neuron lesion. Note the differences in muscle tone and the response of deep tendon reflexes.

Upper motor neuron lesions

1. no atrophy
2. no fasciculations
3. muscle weakness
4. hypertonia
5. increased deep tendon reflexes

Lower motor neuron lesions

1. fibrillations - rapid contractions of muscle fibers
2. fasciculations - course form of involuntary muscle contractions
3. muscle weakness/wasting
4. hypotonia
5. decreased deep tendon reflexes

upper motor neuron lesions, muscle weakness can be present, but the muscle does not exhibit random contractions and only atrophies after long periods without use. Initially, after upper motor neuron lesions, the muscles of the patient display hypotonia and hyporeflexia, but, after a period of time, the muscles will have increased tone (hypertonia) and increased deep tendon reflexes (hyperreflexia). This is known as **spasticity**. An additional marker of upper motor neuron lesions is observed when a blunt object is run up the sole of the foot from the heel to the toes. In an individual with an upper motor neuron lesion, the toes will spread out (**Babinski sign**) while, in a normal individual, the toes will curl under. A normal child that has not begun walking can also demonstrate a positive Babinski sign, since the upper motor neurons have not begun to functionally modify lower motor neuron activity.

As was mentioned with the sensory neurons, there is a somatotopic distribution (**homunculus**) of the motor control of skeletal muscles. This motor homunculus is found on the precentral gyrus of the cortex and an orderly somatotopic distribution continues as the fibers descend through the cerebral peduncles, pyramids of the brain stem and into the spinal cord (Figure 11.16).

Corticopontine tracts

Paralleling the corticobulbar tract through the internal capsule and upper brain stem are the **corticopontine fibers** that descend from the cortex and synapse in the pons to provide information to the cerebellum via the decussating **pontocerebellar fibers** (Figure 11.17). Recall that these fibers decussate and ascend in the contralateral middle cerebellar peduncle as mossy fibers to provide cortical input to the opposite side of the cerebellum (Chapter 10).

Rubrospinal tract

The **rubrospinal tract** is a descending tract that begins in the red nucleus of the midbrain, decussates quickly and descends in the contralateral brain stem and spinal cord. In the spinal cord, it is found in close proximity to the lateral corticospinal tract (Figure 11.18). The function of the rubrospinal tract in humans is believed to be minimal, perhaps modifying tone in upper extremity flexor muscles. It has been suggested that the rubrospinal tract can take over function after damage in the lateral corticospinal tract.

Anterior (ventral) columns

The anterior columns contain four small descending tracts: the anterior corticospinal tract, the reticulospinal tract, the vestibulospinal tract, and the tectospinal tract. The combined role of these tracts is to maintain postural balance, along with the orientation of the head and neck with the trunk musculature (Table 11.1).

The **anterior corticospinal tracts** are a subdivision of the pyramidal motor system. As you recall, the majority of fibers in the pyramidal tracts decussate in the caudal medulla to become the lateral corticospinal tract. A small number of these axons do not decussate and descend in the spinal cord as the anterior corticospinal tracts (Figure 11.10). These fibers bilaterally innervate alpha motor neurons that control trunk musculature where coordination between the muscles on both sides of the body is important. It has been suggested that these tracts can also help to regain function after loss of the lateral corticospinal tract.

The **reticulospinal tracts** arise from the reticular formation of the pons and medulla and descend ipsilaterally through the spinal cord (Figure 11.18). Their main function is to provide

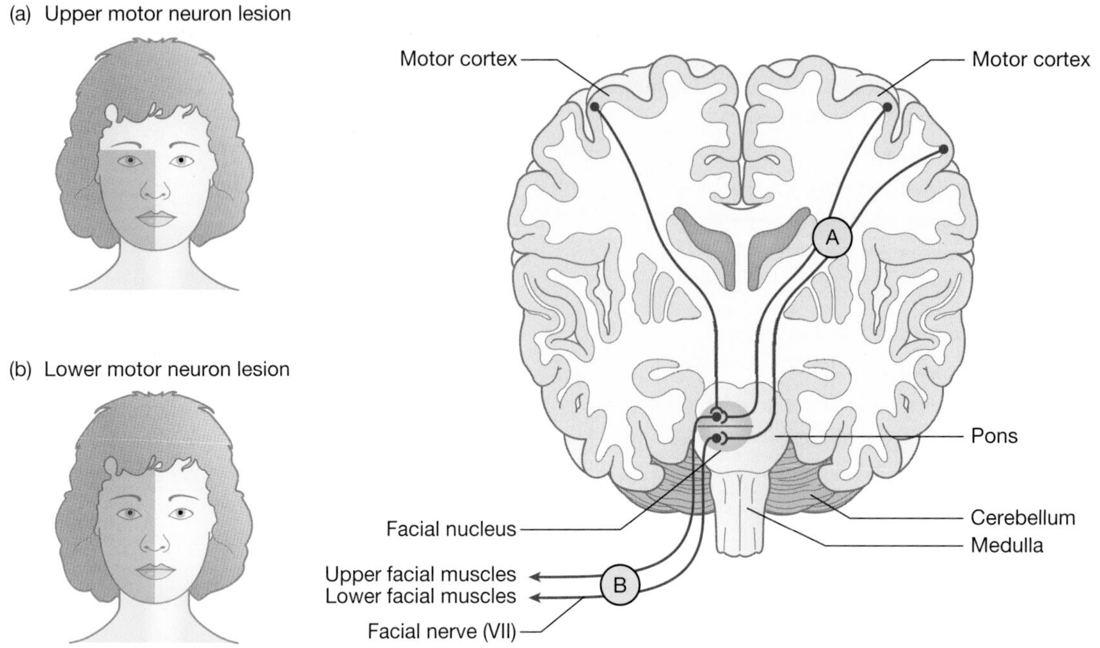

(a) Upper motor neuron lesion

(b) Lower motor neuron lesion

Motor cortex

Motor cortex

A

Pons

Cerebellum

Medulla

Facial nucleus

Upper facial muscles

Lower facial muscles

B

Facial nerve (VII)

Figure 11.16 Schematic view of the corticobulbar tract controlling the muscles of the face (facial VII). Note the bilateral projection of the upper motor neurons to the facial muscles superior to the eye, while the upper motor neurons to the facial muscles inferior to the eye are only contralateral, not bilateral. Therefore, lesion "A" (upper motor neuron lesion) produces a loss of contralateral facial muscles below the eye, while lesion "B" (lower motor neuron lesion) produces a loss of ipsilateral facial muscles from the entire side of the face.

Clinical box 11.2

The somatotopic distribution of axons in both the ascending sensory tract and the descending motor tracts is highly organized. In the ascending sensory tracts, there is a specific somatotopic arrangement of fibers in the posterior columns, in the medial meniscus, and in the internal capsule – as well as the homunculus distribution on the postcentral gyrus (Figure 11.8). Likewise there is a somatotopic distribution in the spinothalamic tract for pain and temperature, as well as a specific distribution in the trigeminothalamic tract.

The descending motor tracts also contain a somatotopic distribution, beginning with the homunculus on the precentral gyrus (Figure 11.13a), continuing in the internal capsule (Figure 11.13b), the cerebral peduncles, the medullary pyramids, and the lateral corticospinal tract. The lower motor neurons in the anterior horn of the spinal cord are also somatotopically distributed (Figure 11.13c).

This indicates the extreme specificity of distribution of axons throughout the central nervous system. This should be kept in mind when examining any tracts or nuclei, since a partial lesion of a tract or nuclei will impact on the specifically distributed axons or cell bodies in the lesion. For example, a small lesion in the internal capsule will have very specific effects on sensory information to the cortex and motor control from the cortex.

Clinical box 11.3

There are diseases and disorders that specifically affect sensory, upper, and lower motor neurons. **Amyotrophic lateral sclerosis** (Lou Gehrig's disease or motor neuron disease) (Robberecht and Philips, 2013), for example, affects both upper and lower motor neurons. The cause of this disease is unknown, although there may be a genetic component. This disease usually occurs in middle age or older adults and specifically targets large motor neurons in the cortex, brain stem, and spinal cord. Therefore, both the upper motor neurons in the cortex as well as the lower motor neurons in the brain stem and spinal cord are involved. Affected individuals experience muscle weakness in many muscle groups (usually beginning in the limbs and progressing proximally). They may also experience difficulties in swallowing or breathing. The diagnosis for this disease is usually one of exclusion – determining that other diseases or conditions are not involved. Patients with amyotrophic lateral sclerosis exhibit signs of both upper and lower motor neuron involvement (Table 11.2), including upper motor neuron signs of increased reflexes, Babinski sign, and spasticity, along with lower motor neuron signs of fasciculations, muscle wasting, and atrophy. There is no cure and only limited treatment options (riluzole) for this disease. The prognosis is poor, with most patients living less than five years after the onset of the disease.

Poliomyelitis is caused by the poliovirus that specifically infects the lower motor neurons in the spinal cord (and, more rarely, in the brain stem) which leads to muscle weakness and flaccid paralysis. The infected neurons are usually found in the lumbosacral region of the spinal cord and this leads to lower motor neuron disease in the lower extremities. If the neurons regulating respiration in the brain stem are affected, this can require the use of mechanical ventilation. President Franklin Delano Roosevelt was affected by polio and had muscular disabilities in his lower extremities. At the beginning of the last century, thousands of individuals became infected with polio each year. In the 1950s, a vaccine for polio was developed and modifications of the vaccine have been used around the world to eradicate polio. Polio is no longer a threat to human health (Nathanson and Kew, 2010). However, individuals who had polio as children can have a more rapid decline in motor function in old age, since they have fewer healthy lower motor neurons (**post-polio syndrome**).

Viruses can also infect sensory neurons, and the chickenpox virus (**varicella zoster**) is a good example. An individual infected with varicella will have chickenpox, usually as a child. After the acute phase of the pox ends, the virus can reside in sensory and autonomic ganglia. In later life, the virus can be reactivated and produce inflammation and pain along the route of the infected sensory neurons (**shingles**) (herpes zoster) (Bader, 2013). These affected individuals will have pain and irritation along the specific dermatome of the infected nerve. Recently, vaccines against varicella and shingles have been developed that limit the outbreak or reoccurrence of this disease.

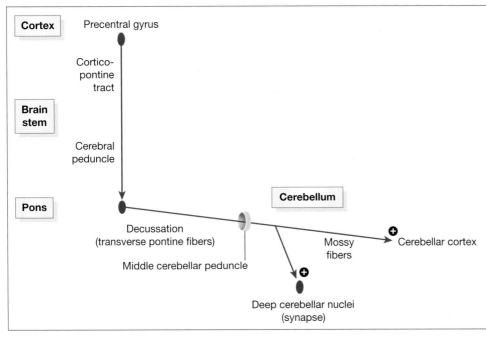

Figure 11.17 Schematic view of the descending motor pathways (corticopontine tracts) from the cortex through the brain stem to the pontine nuclei. Note that the pontocerebellar fibers decussate in the pons to enter the cerebellum through the contralateral middle cerebellar peduncle.

descending autonomic and pain modulation information to the spinal cord, but they also help supply coordinated postural movements.

The **vestibulospinal tracts** arise from the vestibular nuclei and are descending sensory tracts that provide balance and spatial information to the spinal cord (Figure 11.19). They act on spinal cord neurons for proper control of head and neck musculature in balance and posture. A loss of these tracts can produce disorientation and postural instability.

The **tectospinal tracts** arise from the superior colliculus in the midbrain and are descending sensory tracts that provide visual spatial orientation to the spinal cord. These axons

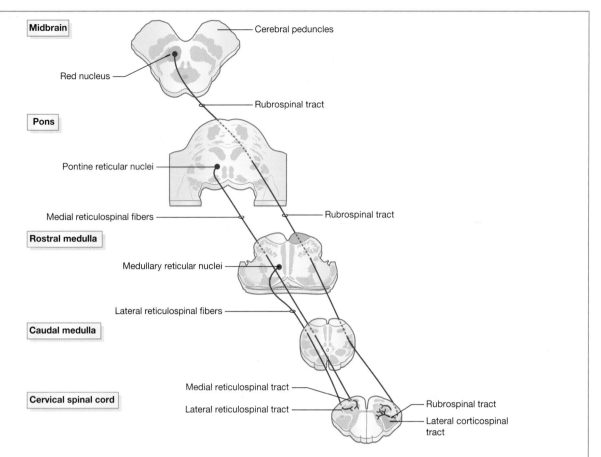

Figure 11.18 Schematic view of the rubrospinal tract and reticulospinal tracts from the midbrain through the brain stem to the spinal cord. Note the decussating fibers of the rubrospinal tract and its relation to the lateral corticospinal tract. Also note that the reticulospinal tracts remain ipsilateral (they do not decussate).

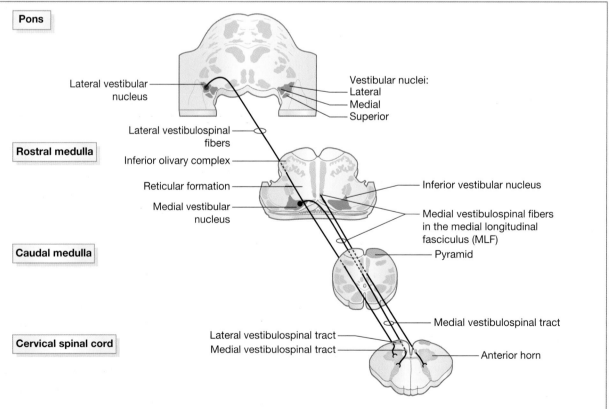

Figure 11.19 Schematic view of the vestibulospinal tracts from the pons to the spinal cord. Note the ipsilateral descending axons of both vestibulospinal tracts.

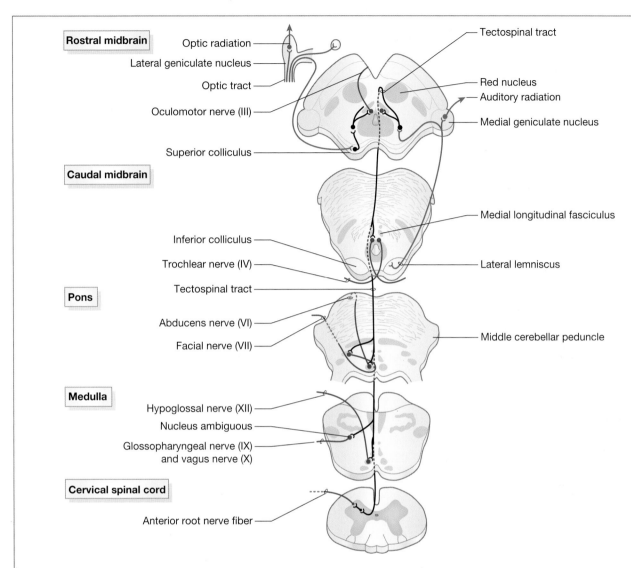

Rostral midbrain
- Optic radiation
- Lateral geniculate nucleus
- Optic tract
- Oculomotor nerve (III)
- Superior colliculus

Caudal midbrain

- Tectospinal tract
- Red nucleus
- Auditory radiation
- Medial geniculate nucleus

- Inferior colliculus
- Trochlear nerve (IV)
- Tectospinal tract

Pons

- Medial longitudinal fasciculus
- Lateral lemniscus

- Abducens nerve (VI)
- Facial nerve (VII)

- Middle cerebellar peduncle

Medulla
- Hypoglossal nerve (XII)
- Nucleus ambiguous
- Glossopharyngeal nerve (IX) and vagus nerve (X)

Cervical spinal cord
- Anterior root nerve fiber

Figure 11.20 Schematic view of the tectospinal tract from the midbrain through the brain stem to the cervical spinal cord. Note the decussation in the midbrain.

decussate in the midbrain to act on contralateral motor neurons in the upper spinal cord, mediating head and neck musculature (Figure 11.20). This allows for proper head and neck postural reflexes based on visual information.

Clinical considerations

Examine each of the figures of the spinal cord, brain stem, or cortex and identify which functions would be lost with each of the indicated lesions ("Pin the tail on the lesion"; Figures 11.21, 11.22, 11.23, 11.24, 11.25, 11.26, 11.27, 11.28, 11.29). While these are neuroanatomically distinct lesions, be aware that this is not the normal clinical presentation of neural loss. Ischemic loss or tumors will affect larger areas with multiple tracts and nuclei often involved. Remember to consider both fiber tracts of passage as well as neuronal cell bodies that may be present. When identifying

lesions, there are six points to consider: 1) identify the region of the lesion (spinal cord, brain stem); 2) identify the actual structures lesioned (corticospinal tract, medial lemniscus); 3) identify if there is a sensory, motor, or sensory and motor deficit; 4) identify whether there are contralateral and/or ipsilateral deficits; 5) identify the type of fibers lesioned and/or cells lesioned; and 6) describe how a patient would present with the lesion.

Spinal cord injury produces lasting disabilities in many patients. The spinal cord can be "bruised" (contusion); it can be compressed (externally by a herniated disc or internally by syringomyelia), it can be traumatically hemisected or completely transected. Consider the clinical ramifications of each of these spinal cord injuries. Does the patient lose sensory or motor function? Is this a loss at specific spinal segments or does this produce a complete loss inferior to the site of the injury?

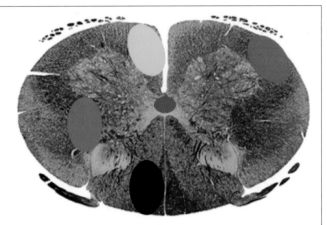

Figure 11.21 Describe the symptoms that would be present in a patient with each of the colored lesions indicated in this myelin-stained spinal cord cross section.

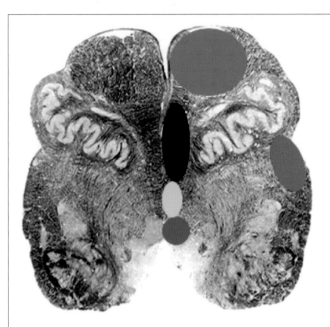

Figure 11.23 Describe the symptoms that would be present in a patient with each of the colored lesions indicated in this myelin-stained rostral medulla oblongata cross section.

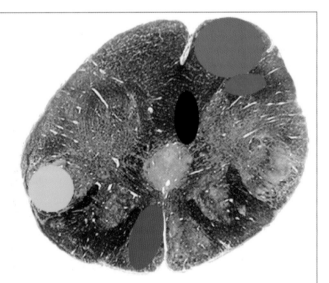

Figure 11.22 Describe the symptoms that would be present in a patient with each of the colored lesions indicated in this myelin-stained caudal medulla oblongata cross section.

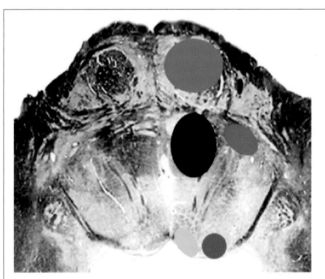

Figure 11.24 Describe the symptoms that would be present in a patient with each of the colored lesions indicated in this myelin-stained mid-pons cross section.

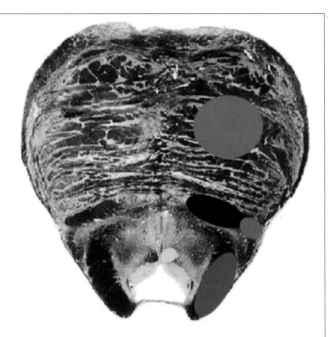

Figure 11.25 Describe the symptoms that would be present in a patient with each of the colored lesions indicated in this myelin-stained rostral pons cross section.

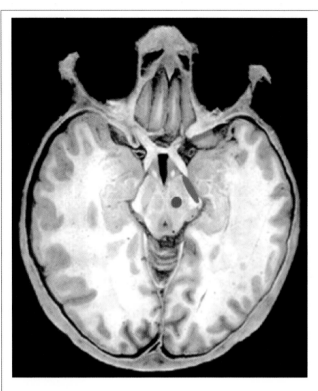

Figure 11.27 Describe the symptoms that would be present in a patient with each of the colored lesions indicated in this fresh tissue midbrain cross section.

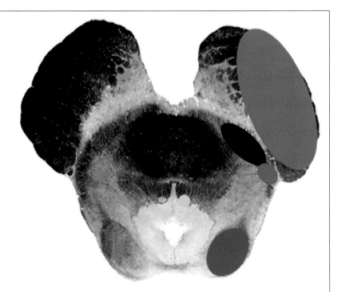

Figure 11.26 Describe the symptoms that would be present in a patient with each of the colored lesions indicated in this myelin-stained midbrain cross section.

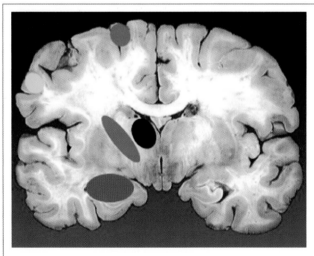

Figure 11.28 Describe the symptoms that would be present in a patient with each of the colored lesions indicated in this fresh tissue frontal (coronal) section at the level of the postcentral gyrus.

Figure 11.29 Describe the symptoms that would be present in a patient with each of the colored lesions indicated in this fresh tissue cortical horizontal section.

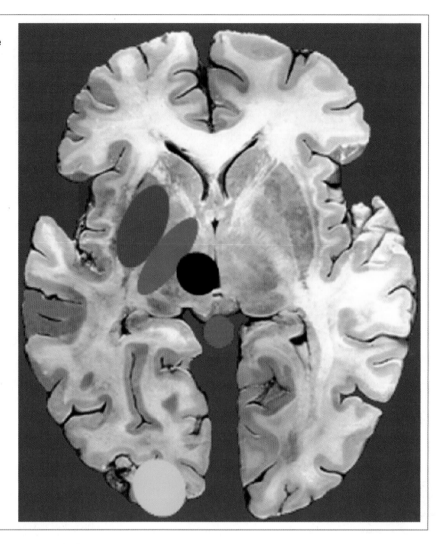

Case 1

A 35-year-old waitress, Ms Kimberly Carson, is involved in a car accident in which she suffers major trauma to her vertebral column. In the emergency room, along with treating her other injuries, her neural status is assessed. The tests reveal that she has lost fine touch sensation and skeletal motor control on the left side of her body below the T12 dermatome, with a loss of pain and temperature from the right side of her body below the L1 dermatome. The on-call neurologist, Dr Tim Lancaster, realizes that she has a loss of function of her spinal cord on the left side at the T12 level (**Brown-Séquard syndrome**) (Figure 11.30) (Dlouhy, *et al.*, 2013).

An MRI of her vertebral column indicates that she has a fractured vertebral body and a hematoma at the T12 spinal level. Surgical removal of the hematoma and stabilization of the broken vertebra takes place quickly.

Ms Carson receives excellent treatment, with the aim to prevent further loss or degeneration of neurons due to inflammation or scar formation. She also has good physical rehabilitation to maintain the muscle tone and function of her lower motor neurons. Within six months of the injury, she has regained a majority of her neural function, although she still has muscle weakness in her left lower limb.

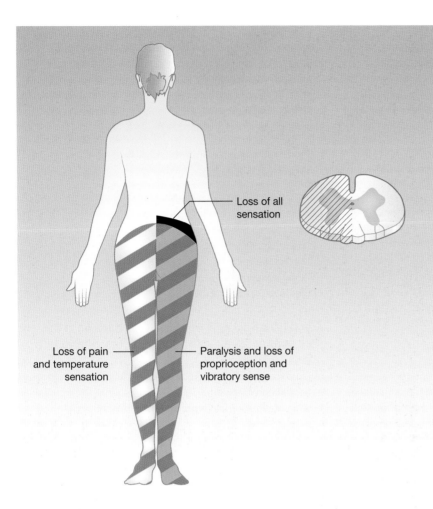

Loss of all sensation

Loss of pain and temperature sensation

Paralysis and loss of proprioception and vibratory sense

Figure 11.30 Symptoms of a spinal cord hemisection on the right side at spinal cord level T12 (Brown-Séquard lesion). Note the loss of pain and temperature on the contralateral side, with a loss of fine touch, proprioception, and skeletal motor control on the ipsilateral side.

Case 2

A 46-year-old homeless man, Mr Richard Jameson, comes to the emergency room of the local county hospital complaining of sporadic, sharp pains. A fourth-year medical student on rotation in the emergency room, Mr Luke Wilson, sees Mr Jameson and, by practicing his history and physical skills, obtains a detailed history and physical. Mr Jameson tells him that these pains have been recurring over the past few years and that other physicians have given him pain medications in the past. Mr Wilson notices that Mr Jameson has a wide stance gait and appears uncoordinated in simple motor tasks. He assumes this is due to excess alcohol consumption, but Mr Jameson denies any use of alcohol or other drugs of abuse. For completeness, Mr Wilson conducts a mini mental status exam and some basic neurologic tests. He notes that Mr Jameson has some reduced mental status, has decreased reflexes, has a decreased pupillary response to light, and fails a Romberg test.

In reviewing the detailed history and physical, Mr Wilson suggests to the resident on-call in the emergency room that Mr Jameson receive further tests

for neuropathies. He suggests that Mr Jameson may have **syphilitic myelopathy** (**tabes dorsalis**) (Berger and Dean, 2014), a degeneration/demyelination of the sensory neurons in the posterior (dorsal) columns. This would explain the majority of Mr Jameson's symptoms.

The on-call resident is dubious of the diagnosis, but because it is a slow night in the emergency room and, for further training for Mr Wilson, decides that a few more tests could be conducted. A complete blood work up, including a specific blood test for syphilis, is ordered. Mr Jameson is given some pain medication for the sharp pains and is asked to return to the emergency room in one week when Mr Wilson will be back.

One week later, with the test results in hand, Mr Wilson, along with a new on-call resident, discuss with Mr Jameson the outcome of the tests. Mr Jameson does have syphilitic myelopathy, probably due to a syphilis infection many years ago. The resident suggests that Mr Jameson has intravenous injections of penicillin to combat the infection. This will prevent any further loss of function, but will probably not help with the already established functional losses. With the treatment, Mr Jameson experiences some relief from the symptoms, although his coordination and gait difficulties continue.

Mr Wilson keeps in touch with Mr Jameson and meets him six months later to follow up on the treatment. In this time frame, Mr Jameson has been able to obtain a low paying labor job which is enough to rent a modest room and to pay for living expenses. He still suffers from some of the complications from the syphilis infection, but has an overall improvement in his health. He expresses his thanks to Mr Wilson for all of his help.

Study questions

1. A 34-year-old female patient presents with a loss of fine touch sensation on the left side of her body below the level of the umbilicus, without the loss of pain or temperature sensation or motor control. The structure lesioned in the spinal cord is the:
a) lateral corticospinal tract
b) anterior corticospinal tract
c) rubrospinal tract
d) fasciculus cuneatus
e) fasciculus gracilis

2. A 27-year-old male patient presents with a loss of pain and temperature sensation on the left side of his body below the level of the nipple without the loss of fine touch sensation. The structure lesioned in the spinal cord is the:
a) right spinothalamic tract
b) left spinothalamic tract
c) right posterior (dorsal) columns
d) left posterior (dorsal) columns
e) anterior commissure

3. A 32-year-old male patient presents with a loss of lower extremity motor control on the left side. He exhibits a Babinski sign and has increased deep tendon reflexes in the left lower extremity. He has no loss of sensation. The structure lesioned in the spinal cord is the:
a) left lateral corticospinal tract
b) right lateral corticospinal tract
c) left sciatic nerve
d) right sciatic nerve
e) right fasciculus gracilis

4. A 44-year-old female patient has a lesion in the right cerebral peduncle in the midbrain. She would present with a loss of:
a) fine touch and pain sensation from the entire left side of the body
b) fine touch and pain sensation from the entire right side of the body
c) skeletal motor control to the entire left side of the body
d) skeletal motor control to the entire right side of the body
e) skeletal motor control to both sides of the body

5. A 56-year-old male patient has a lesion in the right medial lemniscus in the pons. He would present with a loss of:
a) fine touch sensation from the left side of the body
b) fine touch sensation from the right side of the body
c) pain sensation from the left side of the body
d) pain sensation from the right side of the body
e) skeletal motor control to the left side of the body
f) skeletal motor control to the right side of the body

 For more self-assessment questions, visit the companion website at
www.wileyessential.com/neuroanatomy

FURTHER READING

For additional information on the ascending and descending spinal tracts, the following textbooks and review articles may be helpful:

Bader MS. 2013. Herpes zoster: diagnostic, therapeutic, and preventive approaches. *Postgrad Med*, 125(5): 78–91.

Berger JR, Dean D. 2014. Neurosyphilis. *Handb Clin Neurol*, 121: 1461–1472.

Bican O, Minagar A, Pruitt AA. 2013. The spinal cord: a review of functional neuroanatomy. *Neurol Clin*, 31(1): 1–18.

Blumenfeld H. 2002. *Neuroanatomy Through Clinical Cases*. Sinauer Associates, Sunderland, Massachusetts.

Dlouhy BJ, Dahdaleh NS, Howard MA. 2013. Radiographic and intraoperative imaging of a hemisection of the spinal cord resulting in a pure Brown-Séquard syndrome: case report and review of the literature. *J Neurosurg Sci*, 57(1): 81–86.

Felten DL, Shetty A. 2009. *Netter's Atlas of Neuroscience*, 2nd edition. Saunders Elsevier, Philadelphia, Pennsylvania.

Haines DE. 2012. *Neuroanatomy: An Atlas of Structures, Sections and Systems*, 8th edition. Lippincott Williams & Wilkin, Baltimore, Maryland.

Moore KL, Dalley AF, Agur AMR. 2014. *Moore Clinically Oriented Anatomy*, 7th edition. Lippincott, Williams & Wilkins, Philadelphia, Pennsylvania.

Nathanson N, Kew OM. 2010. From emergence to eradication: the epidemiology of poliomyelitis deconstructed. *Am J Epidemiol*, 172(11): 1213–1229.

Patestas MA, Gartner LP. 2006. *A Textbook of Neuroanatomy*. Blackwell Publishing, Malden, Massachusetts.

Robberecht W, Philips T. 2013. The changing scene of amyotrophic lateral sclerosis. *Nat Rev Neurosci*, 14(4): 248–264.

Roy AK, Slimack NP, Ganju A. 2011. Idiopathic syringomyelia: retrospective case series, comprehensive review, and update on management. *Neurosurg Focus*, 31(6): E15 (1–9).

Woolsey TA, Hanaway J, Gado MH. 2008. *The Brain Atlas: A visual guide to the human central nervous system*, 3rd edition. Wiley-Liss, Hoboken, New Jersey.

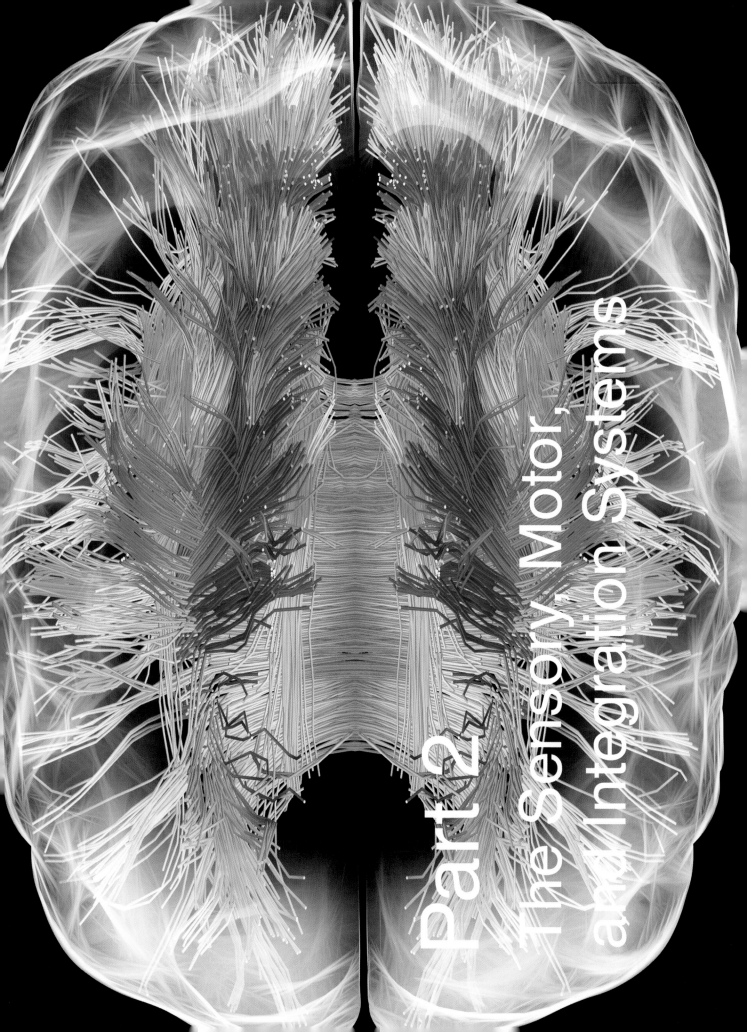

Part 2
The Sensory, Motor, and Integration Systems

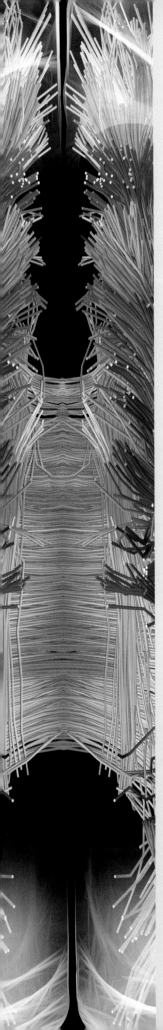

CHAPTER 12
Visual system

Learning objectives

1. Describe and identify the anatomy of the eye.
2. Describe and identify the layered components of the retina.
3. Describe and identify the central components of the visual pathways.
4. Diagnose and discuss clinical problems regarding pupillary light reflexes.
5. Describe visual field defects produced by lesions within the visual pathways.

Development of the eye   177

Optic vesicle – neural tissue from diencephalon

Lens placode – ectoderm

Optic cup

Lens vesicle

Anatomy of the eye   177

Fibrous tunic
1. Sclera – type I collagen, elastic fibers – dura mater extension
2. Cornea – avascular
   a) Corneal epithelium – stratified squamous, non-keratinized
   b) Bowman's membrane – type I collagen, fibrillar lamina
   c) Stroma – thickest layer (90%), parallel type I collagen fibers
   d) Descemet's membrane – thick basement membrane
   e) Corneal endothelium – simple squamous, dehydrate stroma

Vascular tunic
1. Choroid
   a) Posteriorly placed, highly vascularized
   b) Highly pigmented (numerous melanocytes) – light absorption
   c) Bruch's membrane
2. Ciliary body
   a) Ciliary processes – suspensory ligaments of the lens
   b) Aqueous humor production – drainage into canal of Schlemm
   c) Ciliary muscle – smooth muscle, accommodation, oculomotor nerve (III)
3. Iris
   a) Heavily pigmented cells, forms pupil
   b) Muscles: dilator pupillae (sympathetic),constrictor pupillae (parasympathetic)
   c) Melanocyte density determines color

Essential Clinical Neuroanatomy, First Edition. Thomas H. Champney.
© 2016 John Wiley & Sons, Ltd. Published 2016 by John Wiley & Sons, Ltd.
Companion website: www.wileyessential.com/neuroanatomy

4. Lens – biconvex disc
   a) Lens capsule – type IV collagen, glycoproteins, 10–20 µM
   b) subcapsular epithelium – simple cuboidal
   c) lens fibers – long fibers with crystallins
5. Vitreous body – refractile gel (mainly water)
6. Spaces
   a) Anterior chamber
   b) Posterior chamber
   c) Pupil
   d) Vitreous space

Neural tunic (retina)
1. Ten distinct layers (superficial to deep)
   a) Inner limiting membrane
   b) Optic nerve fiber layer
   c) Ganglion cell layer – ganglion cell nuclei
   d) Inner plexiform layer
   e) Inner nuclear layer – bipolar, horizontal, amacrine nuclei
   f) Outer plexiform layer
   g) Outer nuclear layer – rod (120×10^6) and cone (6×10^6) nuclei
   h) Outer limiting membrane
   i) Layer of rods and cones
   j) Pigment epithelium – melanin granules, phagocytosis, nutrition (vitamin A)
2. Optic disc
3. Macula lutea – fovea centralis
4. Neuroglial supporting cells (Müller cells)

Visual system 180

Retina – ganglion cells

Optic nerve (II) – ipsilateral

Optic chiasm
1. Left visual field moves to right optic tract
   a) Left eye – nasal (medial)
   b) Right eye – temporal (lateral)
2. Right visual field moves to left optic tract
   a) Left eye – temporal (lateral)
   b) Right eye – nasal (medial)

Optic tract – contains axons from contralateral visual field

Lateral geniculate nucleus (synapse)

Six layers of neuronal cell bodies

Optic radiations (geniculo-calcarine radiations)

Occipital cortex
1. Synapse above calcarine fissure (area 17) – lower visual field
2. Synapse below calcarine fissure (area 17) – upper visual field

3. Meyer's loop
4. Macular vision projects to caudal occipital cortex

Direct and consensual pupillary light reflexes 182

Retina – ganglion cells

Optic nerve (II) – ipsilateral

Optic chiasm

Optic tract – contains axons from contralateral visual field

Superior colliculus/pretectal area (synapse)

Nucleus of Edinger-Westphal (synapse)

Oculomotor nerve (III) – preganglionic parasympathetic

Ciliary ganglion (synapse)

Sphincter pupillae muscle (constricts)

Accommodation 182

Same pathway as pupillary light reflexes

Except ciliary muscle constricts – lens thickens ("rounds up") naturally

Also, pupillary constriction and eyes converge (medial rectus)

Clinical considerations 182

Glaucoma – increased intraocular pressure

Cataracts – "clouding" of the lens

Retinal detachment – pigment epithelial layer

Lesions in visual system
1. Optic nerve (II) lesion – loss of vision in ipsilateral eye
2. Optic chiasm lesion – bitemporal (heteronymous) hemianopsia
3. Optic tract lesion – homonymous hemianopsia
4. Optic radiation lesion – quandrantanopsia
5. Occipital cortex lesion – homonymous hemianopsia (macular sparing)

Pupillary light reflex lesions
1. Optic nerve (II) lesion
2. Oculomotor nerve (III) lesion

Case studies 188

Pituitary adenoma

Posterior cerebral artery stroke

Study questions 190

Introduction

The next three chapters will focus on the special sensory systems (vision, hearing, balance, taste, and smell). This chapter will examine the visual system: its development, its anatomy, and its distribution through the brain.

Development of the eye

The eye develops as an outgrowth from the diencephalon at approximately 30 days after conception. This outgrowth is referred to as the **optic vesicle**. The lens of the eye is derived from overlying ectoderm which grows into the developing optic cup. The lens is contained within the center of the optic cup and develops independently. As the optic cup develops, the neural tissue folds back on itself, such that there are two layers of tissue contacting each other. These two layers produce a potential space for separation and this can lead to **retinal detachment** (Figure 12.1). As the neural portion of the eye develops, the photoreceptive sensory elements (the rods and cones) are found deep within the layers of the retina. This can

be counter intuitive; the photoreceptors are not on the surface of the retina (closest to the light source), but are actually deep within the neural retina.

Anatomy of the eye

The anatomy of the eye can be divided into three layers or tunics. The first layer is referred to as the **fibrous tunic** and is made of the **cornea** and the **sclera**. The cornea is an avascular transparent structure that allows light to enter the eye and slightly refracts that light. The sclera is made of type I collagen and is an extension of the dura mater of the brain. The typical "white of the eye" is the sclera that is observed through the overlying conjunctiva (Figures 12.2, 12.3).

The cornea is made of five layers, with the outer layer termed the corneal epithelium. The thickest layer of the cornea is the stroma. The stroma is made of parallel type I collagen fibrils and makes up approximately 90% of the thickness of the cornea. The corneal endothelium is found adjacent to the anterior chamber of the eye and it has an important role in removal of water from the stromal layer (Figure 12.4). LASIK surgery for visual acuity

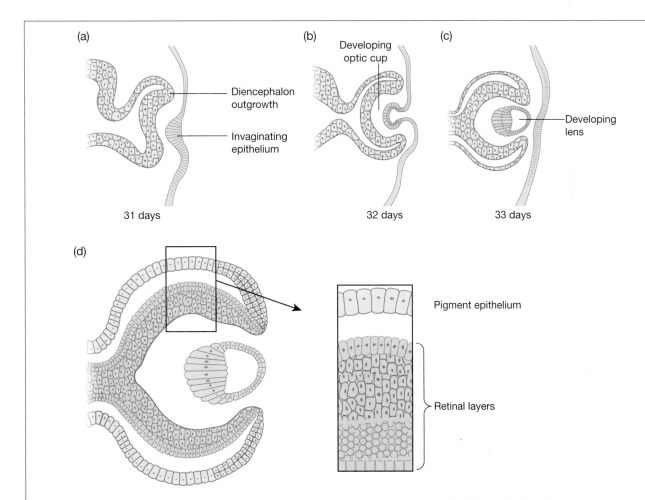

Figure 12.1 Development of the eye. Note the outgrowth of the diencephalon (a), the ingrowth of the epithelium (b) to form the lens (d) and the formation of the optic cup (c). The optic cup folds back on itself and merges with the pigment epithelium leaving a potential space for future retinal detachment.

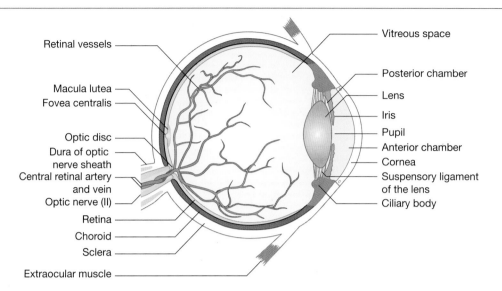

Figure 12.2 A drawing of the anatomy of the eye. Note the outer fibrous layer (the cornea and the sclera), the middle vascular layer (the choroid, ciliary body, iris, and lens) and the inner neural layer (the retina). Note also the optic disc (where the axons exit the globe and the blood vessels enter) as well as the macula lutea and the fovea centralis.

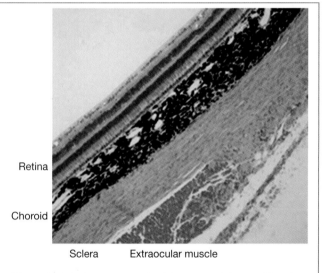

Figure 12.3 A photomicrograph of the layers of the eye. Note the inner retinal layer, the middle choroid layer, and the outer fibrous (scleral) layer.

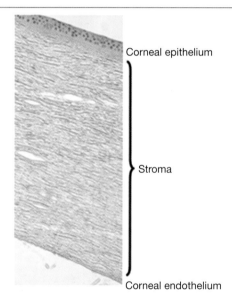

Figure 12.4 A photomicrograph of the cornea. Note the outer cellular, corneal epithelium; the thick middle portion, the stroma; and the inner single cell layer, the corneal endothelium.

involves the removal of a small portion of the stroma, reducing its thickness and altering the refractory nature of the cornea.

The second layer of the eye is referred to as the **vascular tunic** and contains the **choroid**, the **iris**, the **lens**, and the **ciliary body** (Figure 12.2). The choroid is a highly vascular layer that contains many blood vessels, as well as numerous melanocytes for light absorption (Figure 12.3). This layer provides nourishment for the inner neural layer, as well as absorbing any scattered light rays, thus preventing light from producing multiple events on the retina.

The iris, lens, and ciliary body make up an anterior group of vascular tunic structures that modify the amount and quality

of light that enters the eye. The iris acts as a circular curtain to regulate the amount of light that enters the eye. There are two muscles associated with this function. The **dilator pupillae muscle** is made of bands of smooth muscle that radiate from the inner edge of the iris (near the pupil) to the outer edge of the iris. As they contract, they pull the inner edge of the iris towards the outer edge and increase the pupil size (letting more light enter the eye). The other muscle of the iris is the **sphincter pupillae muscle**, which is a circular ring of smooth muscle at the inner edge of the iris. When contracted, this muscle acts

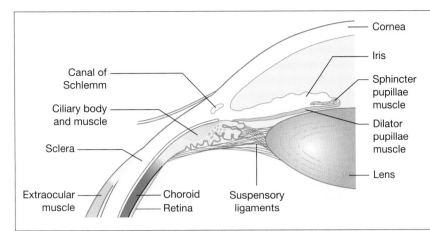

Figure 12.5 A drawing of the anterior aspect of the eye. Note the ciliary body, which produces aqueous humor and the ciliary muscle which relaxes the suspensory ligaments allowing the lens to "round up". Also note the iris with its two integral smooth muscles: the circular sphincter pupillae muscle on the outer edge of the iris and the radial dilator pupillae muscle extending through the iris from inner to outer edge.

like the string of a sack and reduces the pupillary space (decreasing the amount of light that enters the eye). The iris contains a large number of melanocytes to block the incoming light. The melanocyte density determines the iris color, with light-eyed (blue-eyed) individuals having a lower density than dark-eyed (brown-eyed) individuals (Figure 12.5).

The lens is a biconvex disc with specifically oriented crystallin fibers that is responsible for modifying and directing the light image to the appropriate part of the retina. This occurs by the contraction or relaxation of the circular **ciliary muscle** that is found around the outside of the lens. When the circular ciliary smooth muscle contracts, the inner diameter of space that contains the lens is reduced and the lens is then able to round up naturally. As the muscle relaxes, the space around the lens increases, the ligaments holding the lens in place are tightened and the lens is flattened (Figure 12.5). The rounding or flattening of the lens changes the angle of the incoming light and modifies the focal plane of the image (allowing close-up or long-distance viewing). As individuals age, the natural rounding of the lens is diminished, so that the lens remains in a more flattened state, even with ciliary muscle contraction. This leads to older individuals needing reading glasses for near vision.

The ciliary body is responsible for the production of **aqueous humor**, which circulates through the anterior chamber of the eye providing a fluid medium between the cornea, the iris, and the lens. The aqueous humor is produced in the ciliary body, circulates in the posterior chamber, through the pupillary space and into the anterior chamber, where it is drained at the lateral margins of the corneo-scleral junction in the **Canal of Schlemm** (Figure 12.5). If the aqueous humor is not drained adequately (or if too much is produced), then an increase in intraocular pressure in the anterior chamber can occur. This is **glaucoma** and can have serious consequences on vision if left untreated.

The **vitreous body** is not part of the three tunics, but is a refractile gel made up of water and hyaluronic acid that helps hold the lens anteriorly and keeps even pressure on the retina. It also helps to maintain the rounded shape of the eye.

The third layer of the eye is the **neural tunic** and is made of the **retina**. The retina is composed of distinct layers, some

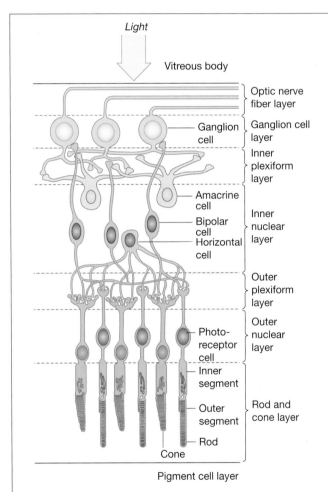

Figure 12.6 A drawing of the layers of the retina. Note that light enters at the top of the drawing and has to pass through many layers to interact at the rod and cones.

with neural cell bodies and others with neural projections (dendrites and axons). The retina can be described as having three cell body layers, with intervening neural projection layers. The layers are described from the superficial (or vitreal) side to the deep (or choroid) side of the retina (Figure 12.6). The first neural projection layer is the **optic nerve fiber layer** that is made of the

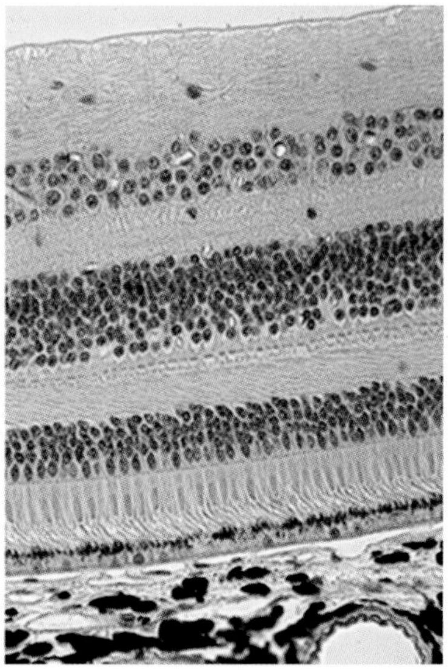

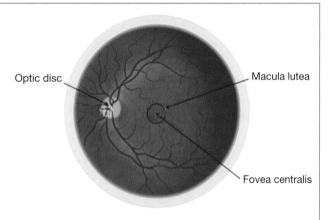

Optic nerve fiber layer

Ganglion cell layer

Inner plexiform layer

Inner nuclear layer

Outer plexiform layer

Outer nuclear layer

Layer of rods and cones

Pigment cell layer

Choroid

Figure 12.7 A photomicrograph of the layers of the retina. Note that light enters at the top of the field and has to pass through many layers to interact at the rod and cones.

Optic disc

Macula lutea

Fovea centralis

Figure 12.8 A drawing of the back of the eye with the optic disc, macula lutea, and fovea centralis identified. Note that the fovea centralis is the region of highest visual acuity and has the highest concentration of cones. Source: Science Photo Library/ Stanford Eye Clinic.

axons that project from the **ganglion cells** of the retina to the brain. These axons course along this outer layer of the retina to leave the orbit via the optic disc and the **optic nerve (II)**. The first cell body layer of the retina is the **ganglion cell layer**, containing the large ganglion cells whose axons project into the optic nerve fiber layer. The next neural projection layer (the **inner plexiform layer**) is made up of axons from the deeper cell body layer (the inner nuclear layer). The **inner nuclear layer** contains the cell bodies of **bipolar**, **horizontal**, and **amacrine cells**. Generally, the horizontal and amacrine cells interact in the inner nuclear layer to

modify the output of the bipolar cells. The bipolar cells have two projections: one which projects through the inner plexiform layer to the ganglion cells and another which projects through the **outer plexiform layer** to the cell bodies for the photoreceptors. Therefore, the next neural projection layer is made of projections from the bipolar cells, while the deeper cell body layer is composed of the **photoreceptor cell bodies** (outer nuclear layer). The photoreceptor cell bodies are either rod or cone cells. The rods are responsible for determining movement and vision in low light conditions, while the cones are responsible for color vision. This is the layer in which the actual photoreception takes place. There are many more rod cells in the eye (approximately 120 million) compared with cone cells (approximately 6 million). They are also not equally distributed in the retina with rod cells more peripherally located and cone cells more centrally located. The final layer of the retina is the **pigment epithelium**, a layer that is responsible for physical and nutritional support of the rods and cones, for stray light absorption, and for phagocytosis of photoreceptor cell elements (Figure 12.7).

When examining the layers of the retina, it is important to realize that light must pass through multiple layers of the retina prior to interacting with the photoreceptive elements of the rods and cones. Once the rods or cones are activated, the neural signal is propagated through the bipolar cells and onto the ganglion cells. The axons from the ganglion cells then project into the brain via the optic nerve (II). Because of this multicellular interaction, the ability to interpret visual signals is already processed within the retina by interactions between the bipolar cells, horizontal cells, amacrine cells, and the ganglion cells.

The retina is not a uniformly thick layer within the eye. There is a region in which photoreception does not occur due to the congregation of the ganglion cell axons as they pass into the optic nerve. This region is referred to as the **optic disc** and is the "blind spot" within the eye. Interestingly, the brain is able to reconstruct the visual portion of the blind spot so that individuals do not "see" a deficit in the visual field. There is also a portion of the retina which is highly sensitive to visual cues and contains a large quantity of cone cells. This area of the retina is thinner and is referred to as the **macula lutea,** with a highly sensitive center region referred to as the **fovea centralis** (Figure 12.8). This is the region in which the eyes will focus when especially high sensitivity is necessary.

Visual pathway

The visual sensory pathway begins with the photoreceptor cells, the rods and cones, within the deep layers of the retina. The activated photoreceptor cells stimulate one limb of the bipolar cell which then passes this signal through its second limb onto the ganglion cells of the retina. The signal from the ganglion cells is then transmitted to the brain via the optic nerve (II). As mentioned previously, this signal is modified prior to the ganglion cells by the amacrine and horizontal cells.

Clinical box 12.1

Physicians routinely examine the internal aspect of the eye utilizing an ophthalmoscope. It is important to understand the normal structures seen in an opthalmoscopic view so that abnormal features can be identified. When examining the retina; the optic disc, the fovea, and macula, as well as branches of the central retinal artery, should be observed (Figure 12.8). In cases of hypertension or diabetic retinopathy, there will be noticeable differences in the size of the blood vessels and the optic disc.

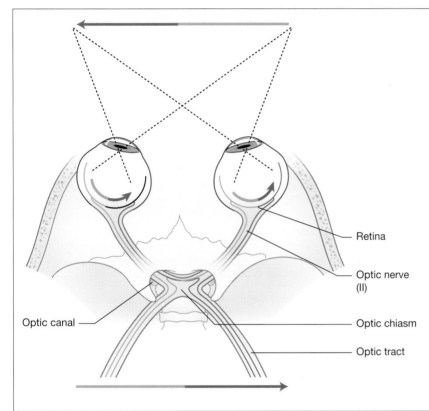

Figure 12.9 A drawing of the optic nerves, optic chiasm, and the optic tracts. Note that each optic nerve carries the visual information from one eye, while in the optic tracts the visual information from the opposite visual field is transmitted. This rearrangement occurs in the optic chiasm.

Retina

Optic nerve (II)

Optic canal

Optic chiasm

Optic tract

The axons from the retinal ganglion cells project through the optic nerve and meet at the **optic chiasm**. Within the optic chiasm, the axons from the right side of the visual field project into the left optic tract, while the axons from the left side of the visual field project into the right optic tract. Therefore, the **optic tract** contains the axons from the contralateral visual field. Another way of interpreting this distribution is that the nasal (medial) portion of the retina from the left eye is in the right optic tract, while the temporal (lateral) portion of the right eye is also in the right optic tract. This is because these two portions of the retina sense visual stimuli in the left visual field, so that they both project to the right optic tract. From

this point onward in the visual pathway, the two visual fields are separate and are in contralateral portions of the brain (Figure 12.9).

The majority of axons within the optic tracts synapse at the **lateral geniculate nuclei**, the thalamic relay nuclei for vision. The lateral geniculate nuclei are highly organized, with six layers of neuronal cell bodies. Recall that all of the sensory input from the spinal cord synapsed within thalamic relay nuclei and this is no different for visual sensory inputs. The axons from the lateral geniculate nucleus project posteriorly through **optic radiations** (geniculo-calcarine radiations) to synapse in the **occipital cortex**. The superior portion of the optic radiations contains the lower visual field from the contralateral side, while the inferior portion of the optic radiations contains the upper visual field from the contralateral side. These inferior optic radiations progress through the temporal lobe in a specialized band, referred to as Meyer's loop. The visual fibers synapse in area 17 of the occipital cortex, with the lower visual field above the calcarine fissure and the upper visual field below the calcarine fissure. The level of highest visual acuity from the macula of the retina is projected to the most caudal region of the occipital cortex (Figures 12.10, 12.11).

Once the visual cortex has received incoming visual information about an object, the details of the object are then processed by other areas of the cortex to provide meaning. This can involve motion and spatial analysis ("where" the object is being seen) as well as form and color of the object ("what" the object is). The dorsal "where" pathways project from the visual cortex to the posterior parietal cortex, while the ventral "what" pathways project from the visual cortex to the lateral temporal cortex. This region of cortex can specifically identify faces, letters, and other common objects. Lesions of these pathways or cortical regions will not affect the actual ability to see, but will impact on the ability to interpret visual information.

When discussing lesions of the visual pathway, it is important to realize that the loss of vision from one eye (or the optic nerve (II)) produces quite different symptoms than the loss of vision produced by a lesion of the optic tract, optic radiations, or occipital cortex. This will be discussed in more detail in the clinical considerations portion of this chapter.

Direct and consensual light reflexes

While the previous paragraphs referred to the visual pathway, there are also light reflex pathways that are clinically significant. When a bright light is shone into a patient's eyes, both pupils should contract equally (using the sphincter pupillae muscles). If a bright light is shone into one eye and the pupil of that eye contracts, this is referred to as a **direct pupillary light reflex**. On the other hand, if a bright light is shone into one eye and the contralateral pupil contracts, this is referred to as a **consensual pupillary light reflex**. These reflexes are mediated by a pathway that is separate from the visual pathway (Figure 12.12).

The light reflex pathway begins at the retina, with the ganglion cell projections through the optic nerve (II) and into the optic chiasm. These ganglion cell axons continue through the optic tract and synapse in the pretectal area of the **superior colliculus**. From the pretectal area, the axons project bilaterally to the **nucleus of Edinger-Westphal**. From the nucleus of Edinger-Westphal, the preganglionic parasympathetic axons travel through the **oculomotor nerve** (III) to synapse in the

ciliary ganglion. The postganglionic parasympathetic fibers from the ciliary ganglion project to the **sphincter pupillae muscle** of the iris to decrease the size of the pupil. Since the projection from the pretectal area is bilateral, the light stimulation in one eye will normally produce pupillary constriction in both eyes (Figures 12.13, 12.14).

Clinically, this can help localize lesions within the visual system. For example, if the optic nerve (II) on the right side were lesioned, then light shone in the right eye would have no effect on either side (no direct or consensual reflex). If, however, light was shone in the left eye, then the pupils in both eyes would constrict (a direct and consensual reflex). As another example, if a lesion occurred in the right oculomotor nerve (III), then light shone in the right eye would produce constriction in the left pupil but not in the right pupil (a consensual, but no direct reflex). If light was shone in the left eye of this patient, then constriction in the left pupil would occur but not in the right pupil (a direct, but no consensual reflex).

This same parasympathetic pathway is used to produce accommodation of the lens when near focus is required. The parasympathetic pathway from the nucleus of Edinger-Westphal controls both pupillary constriction as well as ciliary smooth muscle contraction. In accommodation, the ciliary smooth muscle contracts allowing the lens to naturally round up while the medial rectus muscle turns the eye inward to move the point of focus closer to the eyes.

Clinical considerations

The development of increased intraocular pressure by either overproduction of aqueous humor or blocked drainage of this fluid can produce a clinical condition referred to as **glaucoma**. Glaucoma can cause serious visual complications because of the increased pressure in the anterior chamber of the eye. There are a number of treatments for glaucoma, including surgically increasing the ability to drain the excess aqueous humor. This usually occurs in the region of the canal of Schlemm (Figure 12.5).

With increasing age, the lens of the eye can become opaque (**cataracts**) and produce decreased visual acuity. This can be surgically corrected by removing the lens and replacing it with a fixed man-made material. One complication of the surgery is the loss of accommodation due to the inability of this artificial lens to naturally round up.

If an individual suffers blunt trauma to the eye, a portion of the retina can detach and produce visual disturbances. This detachment usually takes place at the level of the pigment epithelium, which does not interrupt the neural connections of the retina but does impact on the physiological regulation of the retina.

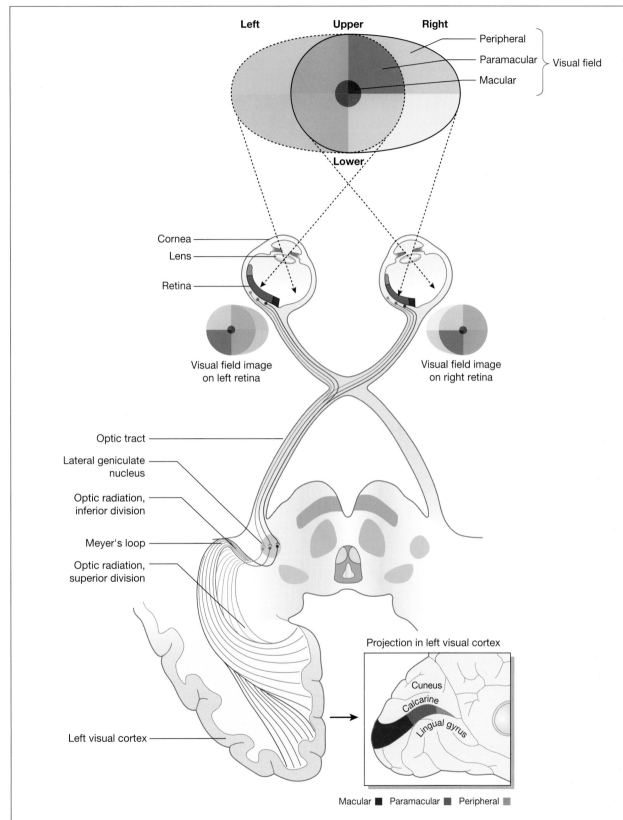

Left **Upper** **Right**

Peripheral
Paramacular ⎫ Visual field
Macular ⎭

Cornea
Lens
Retina

Lower

Visual field image
on left retina

Visual field image
on right retina

Optic tract

Lateral geniculate
nucleus

Optic radiation,
inferior division

Meyer's loop

Optic radiation,
superior division

Projection in left visual cortex

Cuneus
Calcarine
Lingual gyrus

Left visual cortex

Macular ■ Paramacular ■ Peripheral ■

Figure 12.10 A drawing of the visual pathways from the eye to the occipital cortex. Note the visual field distribution in each optic tract, the synapse in the lateral geniculate ganglion, and the optic radiations to the cortex.

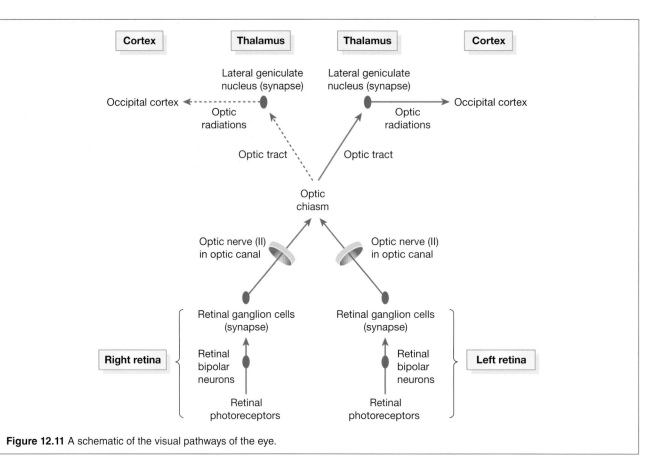

Figure 12.11 A schematic of the visual pathways of the eye.

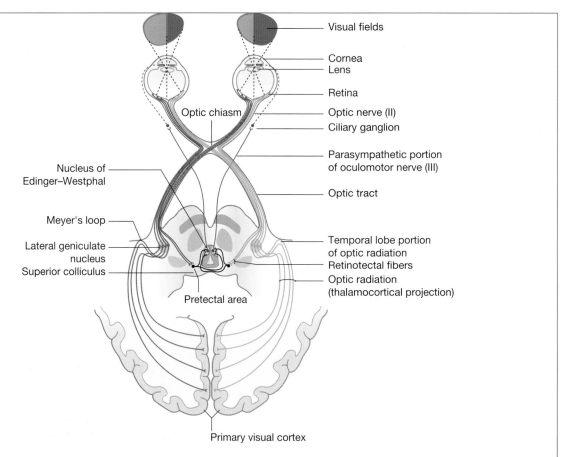

Figure 12.12 A drawing of the visual pathways, as well as the light reflex pathways of the eye. Note the reflex pathway bypasses the geniculate ganglion, synapses in the pretectal area, and projects bilaterally to both parasympathetic motor nuclei.

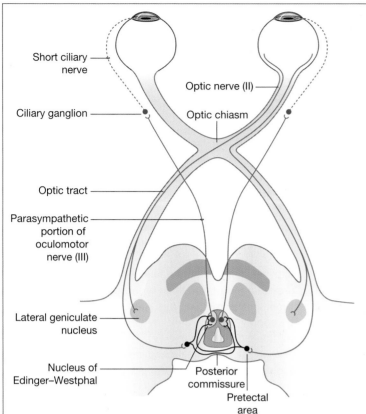

Short ciliary nerve

Ciliary ganglion

Optic nerve (II)

Optic chiasm

Optic tract

Parasympathetic portion of oculomotor nerve (III)

Lateral geniculate nucleus

Nucleus of Edinger–Westphal

Posterior commissure

Pretectal area

Figure 12.13 A drawing of the pupillary light reflex pathways of the eye. Note the pathway bypasses the lateral geniculate nucleus, synapses in the pretectal area, and projects bilaterally to both parasympathetic motor nuclei. Consider what happens when a light is shone into each eye separately and what would happen with lesions of the optic nerve (II) or the oculomotor nerve (III).

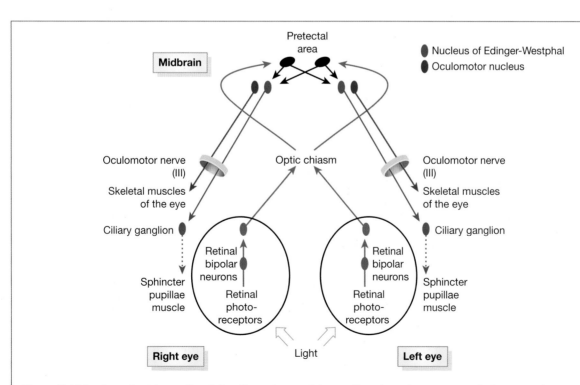

Figure 12.14 A schematic of the pupillary light reflex pathways of the eye. Note the pathway synapses in the pretectal area and projects bilaterally to both parasympathetic motor nuclei. Consider what happens when a light is shone into each eye separately and what would happen with lesions of the optic nerve (II) or the oculomotor nerve (III).

Clinical box 12.2

Recall that the second cranial nerve (optic nerve II) brings the visual information from the retina to the brain, while the oculomotor (III), trochlear (IV), and abducens (VI) nerves control the skeletal muscles that move the eye. Therefore, if one of these motor nerves is damaged, an individual will be able to see the entire visual field, but may have double vision due to misalignment of the eyes. This can be quite problematic for patients and they will alter their behavior to prevent the diplopia (e.g. align their head to limit the visual disturbance or close the affected eye). These extraocular motor deficits are covered in more detail in the chapters that describe the individual cranial nerves (Chapter 7 for the oculomotor (III) and trochlear (IV) cranial nerves; Chapter 6 for the abducens (VI) cranial nerve).

A lesion of the oculomotor nerve (III) would also damage the preganglionic parasympathetic nerves that close the pupil (sphincter pupillae muscle), so an affected patient would have a dilated pupil. On the other hand, the loss of sympathetic innervation to the eye (from the upper thoracic spinal cord, through the ascending sympathetic trunk, superior cervical ganglia, internal carotid arterial plexus onto the ophthalmic artery, and through the ciliary nerves to the dilator pupillae muscle) will produce a constricted pupil and, depending on the site of the lesion, may also produce other autonomic loses (e.g. Horner's syndrome).

A lesion of the trigeminal nerve (V) or the facial nerve (VII) can also impact on the function of the eye. These two nerves are involved in the corneal blink reflex as well as regulating the production of tears (lacrimation), both vital for proper eye function. Blinking helps move the lacrimal fluid across the eye keeping the cornea moist, as well as preventing damage to the eye. The blink reflex begins with the sensory nerve fibers in the cornea that relay their activity through the ophthalmic branch of the trigeminal nerve (V). These first order sensory nerves are pseudounipolar neurons with their cell bodies in the trigeminal ganglion. The central processes of these neurons project to the main sensory nucleus of the trigeminal in the pons, where they synapse. Interneurons from the main sensory nucleus project bilaterally to both facial nuclei. They synapse on motor cell bodies that project through the facial nerve (VII) and drive the contraction of the orbicularis oculi muscles, causing both eyelids and the surrounding skin to contract. Therefore, a stimulus on one cornea causes both eyelids to close. There is also a visual blink reflex that utilizes the visual stimulus of something approaching the eye (through the optic nerve (II)) to activate the facial nucleus and nerve, causing the eyelids to close quickly. Consider how a patient would present with a lesion in the ophthalmic division of the trigeminal nerve (V) or with a lesion in the facial nerve (VII).

One of the important messages from this chapter is to identify the location of lesions based on the presentation of the patient. For example, if a patient has a loss of vision in one eye, that would be due to a lesion in the optic nerve (II). However, if the patient has a loss of vision in the temporal (lateral) portions of both visual fields, then an optic chiasm lesion would be considered. This is referred to as **bitemporal (heteronymous) hemianopsia**. If the patient were to present with a loss of vision in the temporal field of one eye and the nasal field of the other eye (a one-sided visual field deficit), the patient would have an optic tract lesion on the side of the nasal deficit. This is referred to as **homonymous hemianopsia**. If only one quarter of the visual field is lost, this is referred to as **quadrantanopia** and occurs with an optic radiation lesion (recall that the superior optic radiation carries the inferior portion of the contralateral visual field, while the inferior radiation carries the superior portion of the contralateral visual field). Finally, if a patient presents with homonymous hemianopsia but retains macular vision, this is usually due to a lesion within the contralateral occipital cortex. It is important to be able to identify the location of lesions based on patient presentations and, likewise, it is important to be able to identify the symptoms that would occur if a particular lesion is identified (Figures 12.15, 12.16).

As mentioned previously, it is also valuable to determine the deficits that would occur in the pupillary light reflex when a patient has an optic nerve (II) lesion or an oculomotor nerve (III) lesion.

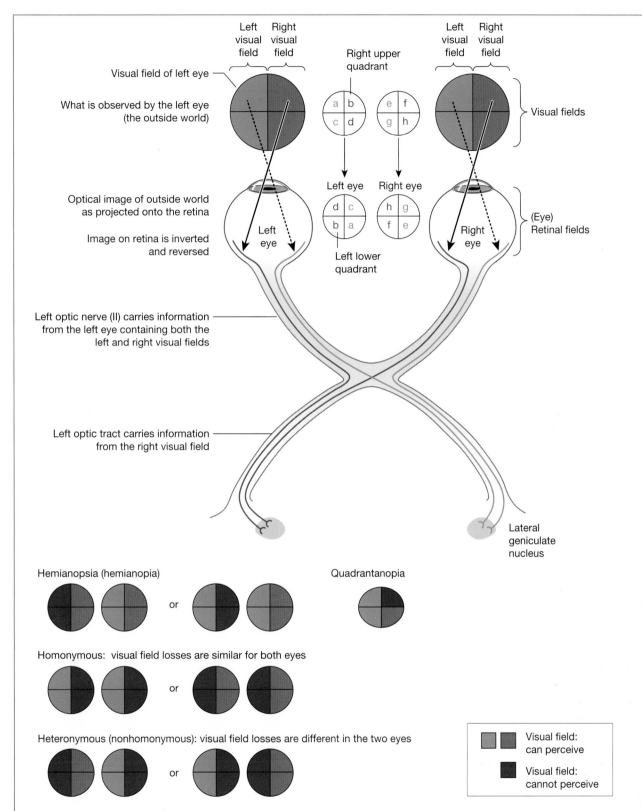

Figure 12.15 A drawing of the visual fields and retinal fields of the eye. Note the difference between the visual fields, the retinal fields, and the visual information carried by the optic nerves (II) and optic tracts. Note also the different names that are used to denote losses in visual fields.

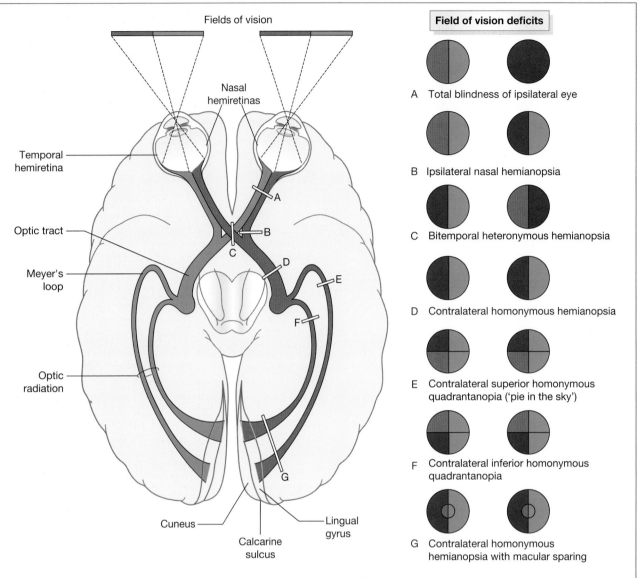

Fields of vision

Nasal
hemiretinas

Temporal
hemiretina

Optic tract

Meyer's
loop

Optic
radiation

Cuneus

Calcarine
sulcus

Lingual
gyrus

Field of vision deficits

A Total blindness of ipsilateral eye

B Ipsilateral nasal hemianopsia

C Bitemporal heteronymous hemianopsia

D Contralateral homonymous hemianopsia

E Contralateral superior homonymous
quadrantanopia ('pie in the sky')

F Contralateral inferior homonymous
quadrantanopia

G Contralateral homonymous
hemianopsia with macular sparing

Figure 12.16 A drawing of the visual pathways of the eye, with lesions in the pathway indicated. Note the different visual field losses that occur with lesions in different parts of the pathway.

Case 1

Audrey Masters, a 56-year-old law enforcement officer, had been experiencing some metabolic disturbances for the past few months. She did not seek clinical help, because she thought this was a natural part of her aging process. However, she began experiencing headaches, occasional diplopia, and a transient loss of peripheral vision. This was a cause for concern, so she visited her local emergency room after a particularly long episode. The physician in the emergency room, Dr Janice Nations, took a detailed history and physical.

She found that Ms Masters had visual disturbances (both in peripheral vision and in extraocular muscles). She took blood to have it tested for hormonal changes and scheduled Ms Masters to have an MRI of the pituitary region, since she thought that a pituitary adenoma could be causing the symptoms.

Once the blood tests and MRI results were obtained, Ms Masters met with a neurologist, Dr Jack Waters. He confirmed that Ms Masters had a space occupying structure in the region of the pituitary that was placing pressure on the chiasm of the optic nerve (II) and on the oculomotor nerve (III) (Figure 12.17). This could account for the peripheral visual deficits, since the mass was compressing the axons crossing in the optic chiasm – the nasal retinal ganglion fibers that carry visual information from the peripheral

(temporal) field of vision (Figures 12.9, 12.10). Ms Masters was also hyperthyroid and this could be due to the cells in the mass. Ms Masters was provided with a number of alternatives, but opted to have neurosurgery to remove the mass. Once the mass was removed, it was biopsied to reveal a **pituitary adenoma**. The removal of this benign tumor eliminated the visual symptoms and, luckily, the neurosurgery did not damage the optic nerve (II) or the oculomotor nerve (III), so their function was fully restored. Ms Masters did continue to have hormonal disturbances, so she had multiple follow-up sessions with an endocrinologist.

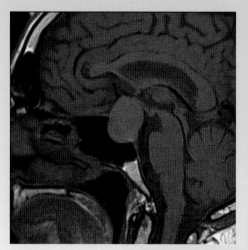
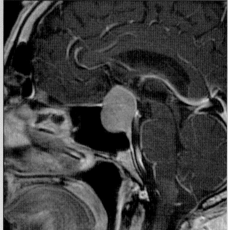
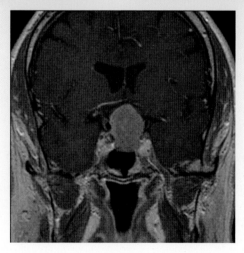

Figure 12.17 Two sagittal magnetic resonance images of a patient with a pituitary adenoma (without and with contrast) as well as a frontal magnetic resonance image of the adenoma. Note the large size of the adenoma and how it places pressure on the optic (II) nerve and the contents of the cavernous sinuses.

Case 2

A 62-year-old attorney, Mr Dave Harrison, had a high stress job with concomitant high blood pressure. He was too busy for doctor's appointments and, although feeling unwell at times, he continued to work. One evening at 7.30 pm, while still working at the office, he experienced a sudden headache and collapsed. His long-suffering secretary called an ambulance and Mr Harrison was taken to the emergency room of the local hospital.

Upon awakening, Mr Harrison realized there was something different about his vision. At the hospital, the neurologist on call, Dr Tom Simpson, took a history and did a neurological exam. He found the only deficit that Mr Harrison exhibited was a loss of vision in the right visual field with some macular sparing. Mr Harrison had an MRI that indicated a **stroke** in the **left posterior cerebral artery** as it supplies the left occipital cortex (Figure 12.18). Mr. Harrison received immediate treatments to prevent further neuronal loss from the stroke.

In the ensuing months, Mr Harrison had difficulty getting around, because he would bump into things that he would have seen in his right visual field. He returned

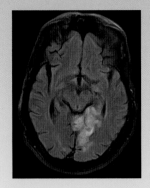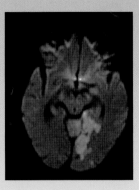

Figure 12.18 Two axial magnetic resonance images of a patient with a left posterior cerebral stroke (infarct). Note the extent of the occipital cortex that is damaged due to the infarct.

to work part time, took medication for his blood pressure, and did try to limit his stress. Over time, he had some restoration of his vision in the right visual field, but he had difficulties with naming objects or explaining scenes in that field of vision even though he could see them.

Study questions

1. A patient presents with a loss of vision. Upon testing, it is determined that the patient has lost vision in the left temporal visual field and the right nasal visual field. Therefore, the patient would have a lesion in the:
a) left optic tract, producing homonymous hemianopsia
b) right optic tract, producing homonymous hemianopsia
c) left optic nerve, producing heteronymous hemianopsia
d) right optic nerve, producing heteronymous hemianospia
e) left optic tract, producing heteronymous hemianopsia
f) right optic nerve, producing homonymous hemianopsia

2. If a patient had a lesion in the right nucleus of Edinger-Westphal, then a light shone in the right pupil would produce:
a) no direct effect on right pupil size, but a consensual effect on left pupil size
b) a direct effect on right pupil size, but no consensual effect on left pupil size
c) no direct effect on left pupil size, but a consensual effect on right pupil size
d) a direct effect on left pupil size, but no consensual effect on right pupil size
e) a direct effect on right pupil size and a consensual effect on left pupil size
f) a direct effect on left pupil size and a consensual effect on right pupil size

3. If a patient has a lesion in the left occipital cortex, they would present with:
a) loss of pupillary reflexes in the right eye and vision from the right visual field
b) loss of pupillary reflexes in the left eye and vision from the left visual field
c) intact pupillary reflexes in the right eye, but loss of vision from the right visual field
d) intact pupillary reflexes in the left eye, but loss of vision from the left visual field

4. Glaucoma can be due to an increase in aqueous humor production from the:

a) corneo-scleral junction
b) vitreous body
c) ciliary body
d) pigment epithelium
e) choroid

5. The signal from the retinal photoreceptors propagates through the _____ to reach the ganglion cells.

a) amacrine cells
b) horizontal cells
c) basket cells
d) bipolar cells
e) stellate cells

For more self-assessment questions, visit the companion website at
www.wileyessential.com/neuroanatomy

FURTHER READING

For additional information on the visual system, the following textbooks and review articles may be helpful:

Bae YJ, Kim JH, Choi BS, Jung C, Kim E. 2103. Brainstem pathways for horizontal eye movement: pathologic correlation with MR imaging. *Radiographics*, 33(1): 47–59.

Blumenfeld H. 2002. *Neuroanatomy Through Clinical Cases*. Sinauer Associates, Sunderland, Massachusetts.

Duong DK, Leo MM, Mitchell EL. 2008. Neuro-ophthalmology. *Emerg Med Clin North Am*, 26(1): 137–180.

Felten DL, Shetty A. 2009. *Netter's Atlas of Neuroscience*, 2nd edition. Saunders Elsevier, Philadelphia, Pennsylvania.

Haines DE. 2012. *Neuroanatomy: An Atlas of Structures, Sections and Systems*, 8th edition. Lippincott Williams & Wilkin, Baltimore, Maryland.

Moore KL, Dalley AF, Agur AMR. 2014. *Moore Clinically Oriented Anatomy*, 7th edition. Lippincott, Williams & Wilkins, Philadelphia, Pennsylvania.

Patestas MA, Gartner LP. 2006. *A Textbook of Neuroanatomy*. Blackwell Publishing, Malden, Massachusetts.

Wilhelm H. 2011. Disorders of the pupil. *Handb Clin Neurol*, 102: 427–466.

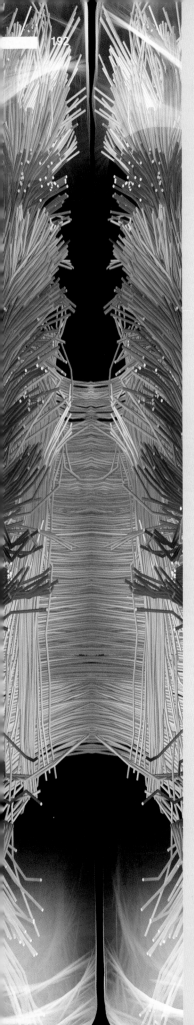

CHAPTER 13
Auditory and vestibular system

Essential Clinical Neuroanatomy, First Edition. Thomas H. Champney.
© 2016 John Wiley & Sons, Ltd. Published 2016 by John Wiley & Sons, Ltd.
Companion website: www.wileyessential.com/neuroanatomy

Auditory ossicles
1. Malleus – tensor tympani muscle (trigeminal nerve V$_3$)
2. Incus
3. Stapes – stapedius muscle (facial nerve VII)

Structure
1. Osseous (bony) labyrinth – filled with perilymph
2. Membranous labyrinth – filled with endolymph
3. Round window and oval window

Cochlea
1. Scala vestibuli
2. Scala tympani
3. Cochlear duct (scala media)
4. Tectorial membrane
5. Basilar membrane
6. Neuroepithelial (hair) cells

Cochlear nerve (of vesitbulocochlear VIII)
1. Bipolar neurons
2. Spiral ganglion
3. Tonotopically organized

Cochlear nuclei (pontomedullary junction) – second order cell bodies
1. Posterior cochlear nucleus – lateral lemniscus – inferior colliculus
2. Anterior cochlear nucleus – superior olive – lateral lemniscus – inferior colliculus
3. Bilateral projections through brain stem

Inferior colliculus (of midbrain)

Medial geniculate (of thalamus)

Auditory cortex
1. Auditory radiations
2. Primary auditory cortex (area 41, Heschl's gyrus)

Semicircular canals (anterior, posterior, lateral) – angular acceleration
1. Ampullae – crista ampullaris – cupula
2. Neuroepithelial (hair) cells

Utricle and saccule – linear acceleration, gravity (head tilt)
1. Maculae – otoliths
2. Neuroepithelial (hair) cells

Vestibular ganglia – superior and inferior
1. Bipolar neurons
2. Vestibular nerve (of vestibulocochlear VIII)

Vestibular nuclei (pons/rostral medulla) – second order cell bodies
1. Lateral vestibular nucleus – lateral vestibulospinal tract (body balance)
2. Medial vestibular nucleus – medial vestibulospinal tract (head and neck)
3. Inferior vestibular nucleus – medial vestibulospinal tract (head and neck)
4. Superior vestibular nucleus – medial longitudinal fasciculus

Medial longitudinal fasciculus (MLF)
1. Interconnects eye muscle nuclei (oculomotor, trochlear, and abducens) with the vestibular nuclei (vestibulo-ocular reflex)
2. Primarily with superior and medial vestibular nuclei

Cerebellum
1. Direct axons from vestibular ganglia as well as from vestibular nuclei
2. Project to the flocculonodular lobe and vermis
3. Provide information on balance during complex motor functions

Cerebrum – ascending fibers to the thalamus and cortex

Mechanical hearing defects – tympanic membrane or ossicles

Neural hearing defects
1. Unilateral deafness occurs proximal to the cochlear nuclei
2. Central lesions produce bilateral effects
3. Acoustic neuroma, tinnitus

Vestibular defects – balance/equilibrium
1. Vertigo
2. Nystagmus

Ménière's disease

Inferior colliculus lesion

Introduction

The auditory and vestibular systems are interrelated because they use similar sensory neurons within the inner ear and transmit that information to the central nervous system via the same cranial nerve, the **vestibulocochlear nerve (VIII)**. Interestingly, both the auditory and vestibular systems use the same type of receptor cells to perceive the sensory information. These are **neuroepithelial (hair) cells**.

Development

The development of the ear can be divided into three sections: the external ear, the middle ear, and the inner ear. The external ear develops from the first and second pharyngeal arches along the rudimentary neck, with the external auditory canal formed by the first pharyngeal cleft. An outgrowth of endoderm from the primitive pharynx forms the first pharyngeal pouch and this becomes the auditory tube and middle ear. The bones of the middle ear are formed from the first and second pharyngeal arches. The inner ear is formed from ectodermal derivatives termed **otic placodes** and these eventually develop into the cochlea and vestibular systems.

External ear

The external ear is composed of the auricle (pinna), the external auditory meatus, and the tympanic membrane (Figure 13.1). The external ear is a relatively simple structure which helps direct the sound waves to the tympanic membrane. As the sound waves hit the **tympanic membrane**, it vibrates, producing the first mechanical transduction of sound waves in the auditory system. The vibration of the tympanic membrane causes the vibration of three small bones within the middle ear, which further conduct the sound waves to the inner ear.

Middle ear

The middle ear is an air-filled space (the **tympanic cavity**) and it has the same external air pressure because of the **auditory tube** (a tube between the middle ear and the pharynx). When working properly, the middle ear should have the same air pressure as the external environment, keeping the pressure on both sides of the tympanic membrane equal. During a change in altitude or when underwater, an individual may feel pressure in their middle ear due to the difference in pressures on either side of the tympanic membrane. To relieve this pressure, individuals yawn or exert a positive Valsalva maneuver to open the auditory tube and equalize the pressure.

The **malleus** (the first middle ear ossicle) is attached to the tympanic membrane and also to the **incus** (the second middle ear ossicle). The incus is further attached to the **stapes** (the third middle ear ossicle). The stapes sits in an oval shaped window that connects to the inner ear (Figures 13.1, 13.2). Therefore, when the tympanic membrane vibrates, the malleus moves, causing the incus to move and the stapes is pushed into the inner ear, setting up a concomitant vibration

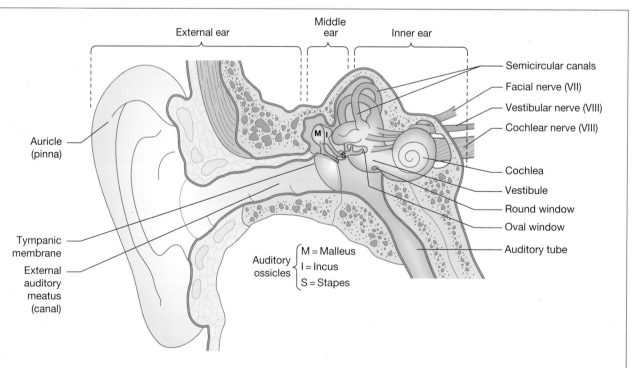

Figure 13.1 A drawing of the anatomy of the ear. Note the external ear consists of the auricle, the external auditory meatus, and the tympanic membrane. The air-filled middle ear contains the three ear ossicles: the malleus, the incus, and the stapes. The fluid-filled inner ear consists of the cochlea (for hearing) and the semicircular canals (for balance).

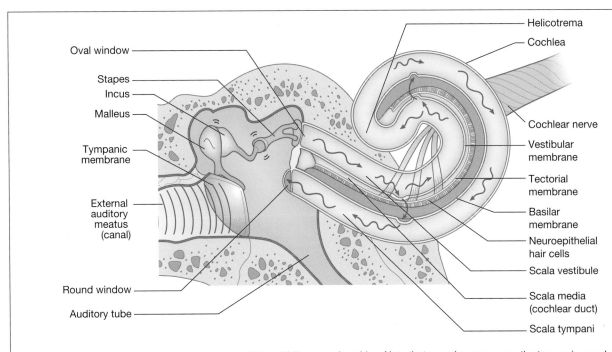

Figure 13.2 A schematic drawing of the anatomy of the middle ear and cochlea. Note that sound waves cause the tympanic membrane to vibrate, which moves the malleus, incus, and stapes. The foot plate of the stapes pushes into the oval window, setting up a concomitant vibration in the perilymphatic fluid of the cochlea. This fluid vibration produces a shearing force along specific parts of the tectorial membrane depending on the frequency of the vibration, with high pitches near the oval window and low pitches towards the end of the cochlea (helicotrema).

within the inner ear. At this point, the sound waves in the air have been transduced across the tympanic membrane and through the malleus, incus, and stapes to reach the fluid-filled inner ear.

This mechanical transduction of sound waves is important for hearing since it allows for the intensity of the sound waves to be modified before reaching the inner ear. Two muscles attach to the bony ossicles, providing a mechanism to dampen the amount of vibration transduced from the tympanic membrane to the inner ear. These two muscles are the **tensor tympani muscle**, which attaches to the malleus, and the **stapedius muscle**, which attaches to the stapes. Interestingly, the tensor tympani muscle is innervated by the trigeminal nerve (V), while the stapedius muscle is innervated by the facial nerve (VII). When contracted, these two muscles stabilize the ossicles and prevent them from vibrating as robustly as normal (Figure 13.2). For example, when attending a loud event such as a rock concert, these two muscles contract and the loud music is dampened so as not to damage the inner ear. After the concert, when it is quiet, the muscles remain contracted in anticipation of a loud sound and, therefore, most normal sounds appear reduced and friends may have to speak loudly in order to be heard. This reaction can, however, only take place when sounds increase over time and the muscles have a chance to respond to these changes. Therefore, a gunshot, which produces a very loud sound in a very short time frame, does not allow enough time for the muscles to respond and damage to the inner ear can occur.

Inner ear

The inner ear is a hollowed out space within the petrous portion of the temporal bone. This is referred to as the **osseous labyrinth** and it is filled with a fluid called **perilymph**. Within the osseous labyrinth is a membranous sack, the **membranous labyrinth**, filled with **endolymph** (Figures 13.1, 13.3). The inner ear communicates with the middle ear by way of two small windows: an **oval window** (filled by the stapes) and a **round window** (filled with a membrane). As the stapes pushes into the oval window, the fluid in the inner ear is compressed and passes through the cochlea, and eventually displaces the membrane of the round window. Therefore, the round window can act as a pressure relief valve within the inner ear. The inner ear has two components, the **cochlea** for hearing and the **vestibular apparatus** for balance and positional sense.

Auditory system

The **cochlea** is the portion of the inner ear responsible for hearing and looks like a snail shell, with 2½ turns to its body. This rolled up tube is subdivided internally into three compartments: the **scala vestibuli**, the **scala tympani**, and the **scala media** (cochlear duct). The scala vestibuli and scala tympani are filled with perilymph and are separated from the scala media (filled with endolymph) by two membranes: the **vestibular membrane** and the **basilar membrane**. Within the basilar membrane, specialized neuroepithelial receptor cells have

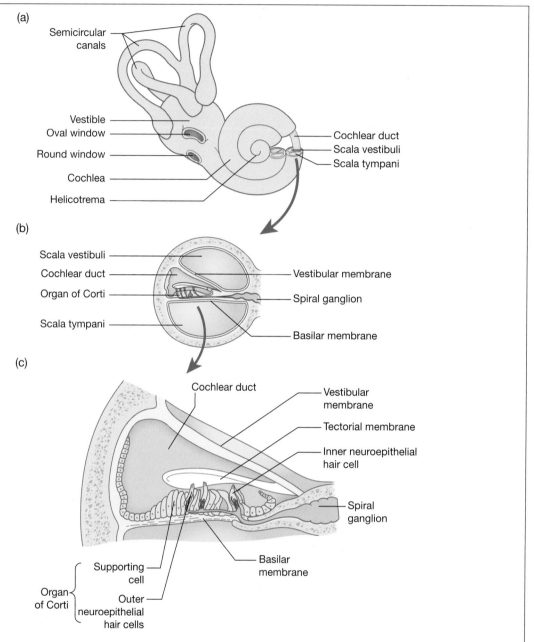

(a)

Semicircular canals

Vestible
Oval window
Round window
Cochlea
Helicotrema

Cochlear duct
Scala vestibuli
Scala tympani

(b)

Scala vestibuli
Cochlear duct
Organ of Corti
Scala tympani

Vestibular membrane
Spiral ganglion
Basilar membrane

(c)

Cochlear duct

Vestibular membrane
Tectorial membrane
Inner neuroepithelial hair cell
Spiral ganglion
Basilar membrane

Supporting cell
Organ of Corti
Outer neuroepithelial hair cells

Figure 13.3 A drawing of the bony labyrinth of the inner ear (a) with a cross section of the cochlear duct (b and c). Note within the cochlear duct, the firm tectorial membrane resting on the tips of the hair cells. As the basilar membrane is moved, due to the pressure wave in the perilymph of the scala tympani, this produces a shearing force of the hair cells against the tectorial membrane – deflecting the stereocilia and producing an ionic change.

projections from their apical surface (sterocilia and kinocilia) that rest against a firm **tectorial membrane** (Figure 13.3c).

When sound waves produce a vibration of the stapes which compresses the perilymph in the oval window, this wave of fluid is transferred through the scala tympani and the scala vestibuli. As the wave of fluid displaces the basilar membrane, the stereocilia (kinocilia) of the neuroepithelial cells are deflected because of their resistance against the tectorial membrane. This deflection produces a change in ionic conductance which stimulates the firing of **bipolar neurons** that project into the central nervous system. The

cell bodies for these bipolar neurons are found in the central portion of the spiraled duct and are referred to as **spiral ganglia**. Note that the movement of specific sections of the basilar membrane and its associated neuroepithelial hair cells occurs for specific wavelengths of fluid (Figures 13.2, 13.3). Therefore, different pitches of sound deflect different portions of the basilar membrane and specific bipolar neurons fire for specific pitches. This is known as a **tonotopic** arrangement and this means that sound is already subdivided into pitches at the time of the first neuronal activity. Likewise, the intensity of the sound can be determined by the "height" of the wavelength, so that both intensity and pitch are determined prior to neuronal signaling. If the spiral tube were unrolled and the specific wavelengths of hearing mapped on the tube, it would be observed that high pitches (~15,000 Hz) would deflect the basilar membrane near the oval window, while lower pitches (~50 Hz) would deflect the membrane near the end of the tube (the **helicotrema**) (Figure 13.2).

The bipolar neurons that originate in the cochlea and have their cell bodies in the spiral ganglia continue through the cochlear portion of the vestibulocochlear nerve (VIII) into the brain stem to synapse on the **cochlear nuclei** (Figure 13.4). The posterior (dorsal) and anterior (ventral) cochlear nuclei are found near the pontomedullary junction of the brain stem. The second order cell bodies that are found in the posterior cochlear nucleus send their axons through the

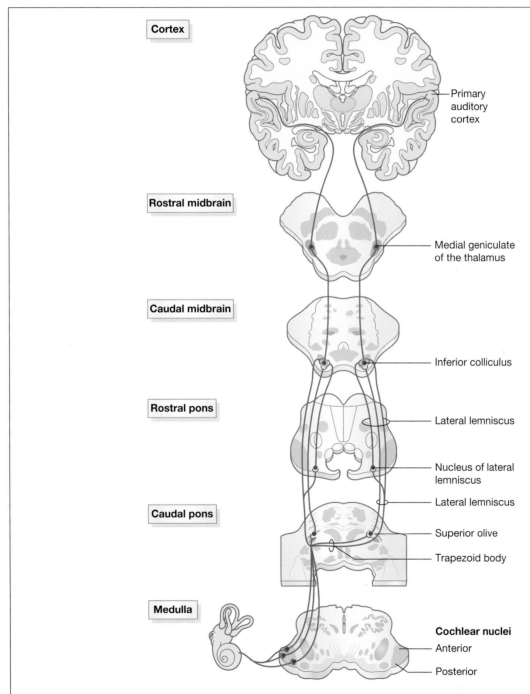

Figure 13.4 A drawing of the central pathways from the cochlear nuclei to the cortex. Note that the projections from the cochlear nuclei are bilateral, passing to the opposite side through the trapezoid body to ascend in the lateral lemniscus. Some fibers synapse in the superior olive, while others continue to the inferior colliculus. From the inferior colliculus, axons project to the medial geniculate nucleus, with subsequent axons projecting to the primary auditory cortex of the temporal lobe.

lateral lemniscus to the contralateral **inferior colliculus** in the midbrain. The second order cell bodies that are found in the anterior cochlear nucleus send some of their axons to the ipsilateral **superior olive** and then to the lateral lemniscus and inferior colliculus. Other axons from the anterior cochlear nucleus decussate to the contralateral lateral lemniscus and project to the contralateral inferior colliculus (Figures 13.4, 13.5). Therefore, the second order axons from the cochlear nuclei project bilaterally through the brain stem, so that each inferior colliculus receives input from both sets of cochlear nuclei.

The axons from the inferior colliculus project to the **medial geniculate** of the thalamus, where they synapse. These axons leave the medial geniculate by way of the auditory radiations to synapse in the **primary auditory cortex** (area 41, Heschl's gyrus) in the temporal lobe. All of the projections from the cochlear nuclei through the inferior colliculus and medial geniculate to the auditory cortex retain the tonotopic arrangement observed in the cochlea. Therefore, there are specific regions of the auditory cortex for recognition of specific pitches of sound (Figure 13.6).

Clinically, since the projections from the cochlear nuclei to the inferior colliculus are bilateral, it is less likely for a patient to have unilateral hearing deficits due to a central neural lesion. If a unilateral hearing deficit is observed, the lesion would generally be found in the inner ear, the cochlear nerve, or the cochlear nuclei.

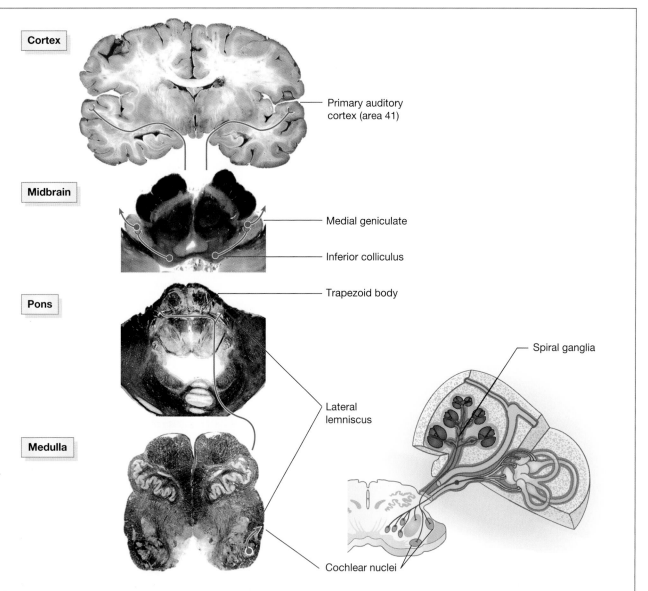

Figure 13.5 A composite of myelin stained cross sections and a fresh tissue section showing the central pathways from the cochlear nuclei to the cortex. Note that the projections from the cochlear nuclei are bilateral, passing to the opposite side through the trapezoid body to ascend in the lateral lemniscus to the inferior colliculus. From the inferior colliculus, axons project to the medial geniculate nucleus, with subsequent axons projecting to the primary auditory cortex of the temporal lobe.

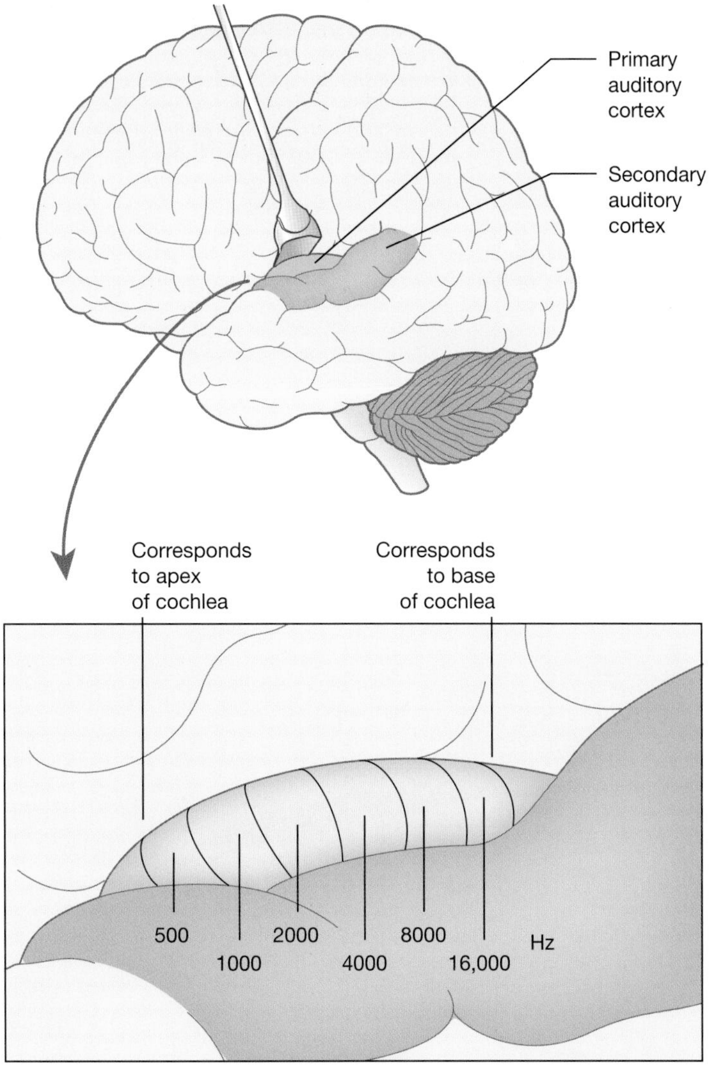

Primary
auditory
cortex

Secondary
auditory
cortex

Corresponds
to apex
of cochlea

Corresponds
to base
of cochlea

500   2000   8000   Hz
   1000   4000   16,000

Figure 13.6 A drawing of the primary and secondary auditory cortices in the temporal lobe. Note the tonotopic arrangement of pitches in the primary auditory cortex.

Vestibular system

The other part of the inner ear contains the **semicircular canals**, the **utricle**, and the **saccule** that comprise the vestibular system. The semicircular canals are three half-moon shaped tubes oriented in the three primary planes. They are the **anterior**, **posterior**, and **lateral** semicircular canals (Figure 13.8). At one end of each tube is a dilated portion (the **ampulla**), which contains neuroepithelial receptor cells embedded in a gelatinous matrix (Figure 13.9). When an individual rotates their head in a specific direction, the fluid flows past the ampulla, deflecting the stereocilia of the neuroepithelial receptor cells and producing an ionic change which stimulates **bipolar cell** dendrites located adjacent to the receptor cells. This means that the semicircular canals sense angular acceleration in each of the three primary planes.

The **utricle** and **saccule** are regions in the inner ear that contain specific **macula** (neuroepithelial hair cells in a gelatinous matrix with crystalline material on the upper surface of the matrix). These crystals (**otoliths**) provide a slight downward force produced by gravity, so that there is a continuous slight deflection of the associated stereocilia of the neuroepithelial hair cells (Figure 13.10). This provides individuals with a generalized sense of gravitational pull, leading to the ability to distinguish "up" and "down". The macula in the utricle is oriented horizontally (for horizontal acceleration), while the macula in the saccule is oriented vertically (for vertical acceleration). During acceleration, the otoliths do not move as readily as the body and therefore cause a rearward deflection of the neuroepithelial hair cells. Once a standard speed is reached, the otoliths return to their normal position and no further acceleration is experienced.

Clinical box 13.1

The second order axons from the cochlear nuclei interact at the superior olivary complex to determine sound localization. This is based on the difference in the amount of time it takes signals from the right and left ear to reach the superior olive. If the signal from the right ear arrives more quickly, then the sound should be closer to the right ear.

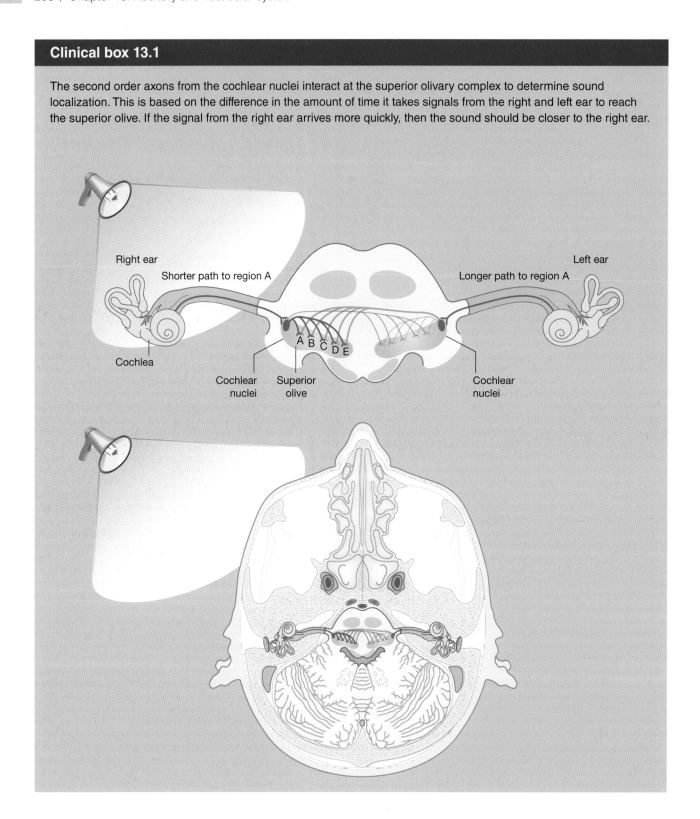

During braking, the opposite phenomenon takes place, in which the otoliths continue in the forward direction and cause a forward deflection of the neuroepithelial hair cells. In this way, the utricle and saccule provide the sensation of linear acceleration as well as gravity. When the stereocilia of the neuroepithelial hair cells are deflected, they produce an ionic change which again causes the firing of adjacent **bipolar cell** dendrites.

The bipolar cell nuclei for the semicircular canals and the utricle/saccule are found in the superior and inferior **vestibular ganglia**. The central processes of these bipolar cells project through the vestibular portion of the

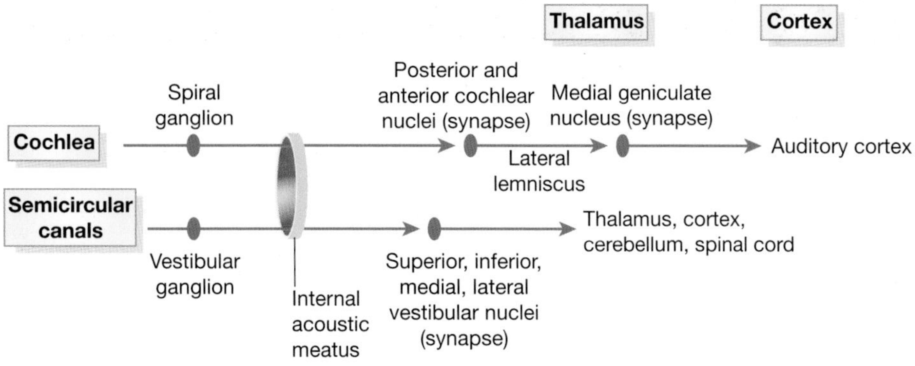

Figure 13.7 A schematic of the vestibulocochlear nerve (VIII) and the distribution of its fibers into the central nervous system.

Clinical box 13.2

There are simple tests that can be used to determine whether there is a conductive hearing loss (external or middle ear defects) compared to a sensorineural hearing loss (cochlea or vestibulocochlear nerve (VIII)). The **Rinne test** asks patients to listen to a tuning fork just outside each ear (air conduction) as well as a tuning fork placed against the mastoid process (bone conduction). Normally, a patient will hear better with air conduction, but, if there is conductive hearing loss, he will hear better with bone conduction (since it bypasses the external and middle ear). With the **Weber test**, a tuning fork is put on the top of the head in the center (vertex) and the patient is asked in which side the sound is louder. In a normal individual, the intensity of the sound should be the same on both sides. With a conductive, mechanical hearing loss, the sound is louder on the affected side, while, with a sensorineural hearing loss, the sound is louder on the unaffected side.

The bilateral nature of the auditory signal from the cochlear nuclei to the cortex can make it difficult diagnostically to localize lesions in the central auditory pathway. Generally, central auditory lesions produce a loss of hearing acuity that cannot be localized to a specific side of the body. Without other symptoms to help localize the lesion, it can be quite difficult to determine where in the central pathway the lesion has occurred. However, with the advent of increased resolution in neuroimaging, especially magnetic resonance imaging, it is now more commonplace to localize the lesions by direct observation of neural tissue damage.

---

vestibulocochlear nerve (VIII) (Figure 13.4). These axons enter the brain stem and the majority synapse on vestibular nuclei located in the pons and rostral medulla (a few axons continue directly into the cerebellum). There are four **vestibular nuclei**: the lateral, medial, inferior, and superior vestibular nuclei. The second order cell bodies in the lateral vestibular nuclei send their axons inferiorly in the lateral **vestibulospinal tract** to the spinal cord to provide balance information to the spinal cord motor axons. The medial and inferior vestibular nuclei send their axons into the medial **vestibulospinal tract** to the upper spinal cord to help maintain balance in the head and neck. The superior vestibular nuclei send their axons into the **medial longitudinal fasciculus** (Figure 13.11). The medial longitudinal fasciculus is important in connecting the vestibular system with the eye muscle nuclei (oculomotor, trochlear, and abducens). This allows for the vestibulo-ocular reflex: the ability of the eyes to track an object while the head is moving.

Some central processes from the vestibular ganglia, as well as axons from the vestibular nuclei, project to the cerebellum, primarily to the **flocculonodular lobes** and the **vermis**, to provide information on balance and positional sense during complex motor functions. In addition, the vestibular nuclei send fibers to the **thalamus** (ventral posterior nucleus) and from there axons project to the **cortex** (Figure 13.12). These two pathways allow for vestibular information to be continuously processed during motor functions, as well as providing awareness of the body's motion and position (Khan and Chang, 2013).

Clinical considerations

Clinically, auditory deficits are divided into two components: **mechanical hearing defects** and **neural hearing defects**. Mechanical hearing defects include loss of the tympanic membrane or the middle ear ossicles. Neural hearing

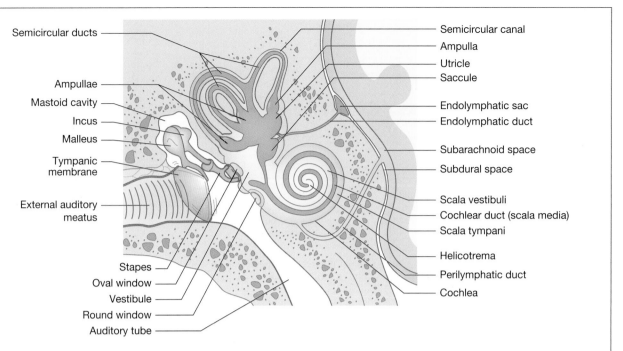

Figure 13.8 A drawing of the anatomy of the middle and inner ear, with the portions of the vestibular system (semicircular canals, utricle, and saccule) highlighted. Note the endolymphatic duct and sac that project to the subdural space of the cranial cavity.

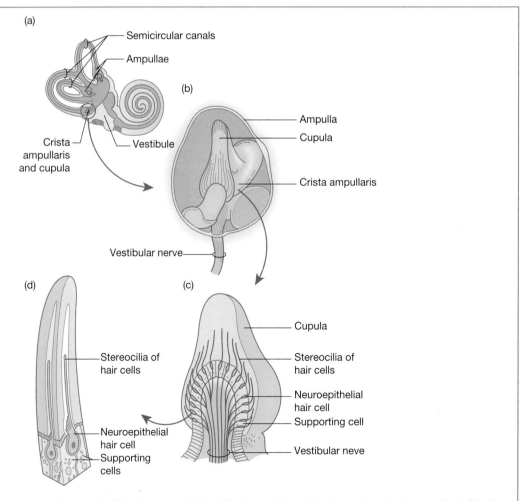

Figure 13.9 A drawing of the semicircular canals of the inner ear with the dilated ampullae and their associated crista ampullaris (a). Note the gelatinous cupula with the stereocilia of the hair cells inside (b–d). As the fluid in the semicircular canals is moved (due to twisting or turning of the head), the cupula is bent and the hair cell responds by releasing ions onto the nearby bipolar nerve fiber of the vestibular nerve, creating an action potential.

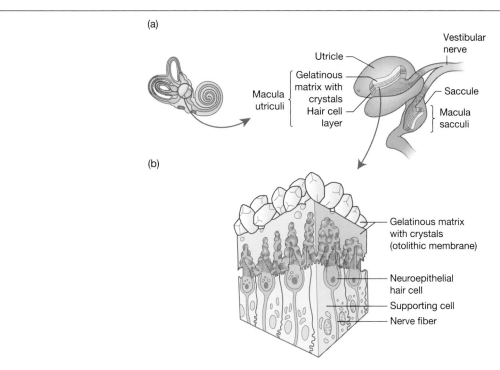

(a)

Utricle

Vestibular nerve

Macula utriculi { Gelatinous matrix with crystals / Hair cell layer

Saccule

Macula sacculi

(b)

Gelatinous matrix with crystals (otolithic membrane)

Neuroepithelial hair cell

Supporting cell

Nerve fiber

Figure 13.10 A drawing of the utricle and saccule of the inner ear (a). Note the gelatinous matrix with the stereocilia of the hair cells inside and the crystalline otoliths on the surface (b). As the fluid in the utricle and saccule is moved (due to gravity or acceleration), the gelatinous matrix is shifted and the hair cells respond by releasing ions onto the nearby bipolar nerve fibers of the vestibular nerve, creating an action potential.

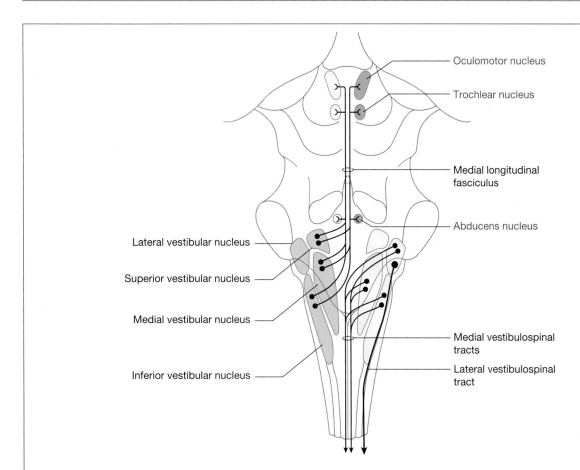

Oculomotor nucleus

Trochlear nucleus

Medial longitudinal fasciculus

Abducens nucleus

Lateral vestibular nucleus

Superior vestibular nucleus

Medial vestibular nucleus

Inferior vestibular nucleus

Medial vestibulospinal tracts

Lateral vestibulospinal tract

Figure 13.11 A drawing of a superior view of the brain stem with the projections of the second order neurons from the vestibular nuclei. Note the lateral vestibular nuclei contribute to the lateral vestibulospinal tract, while the inferior and medial vestibular nuclei contribute to the medial vestibulospinal tract and the medial longitudinal fasciculus. The superior vestibular nuclei contribute to the medial longitudinal fasciculus to help coordinate eye, head, and neck musculature.

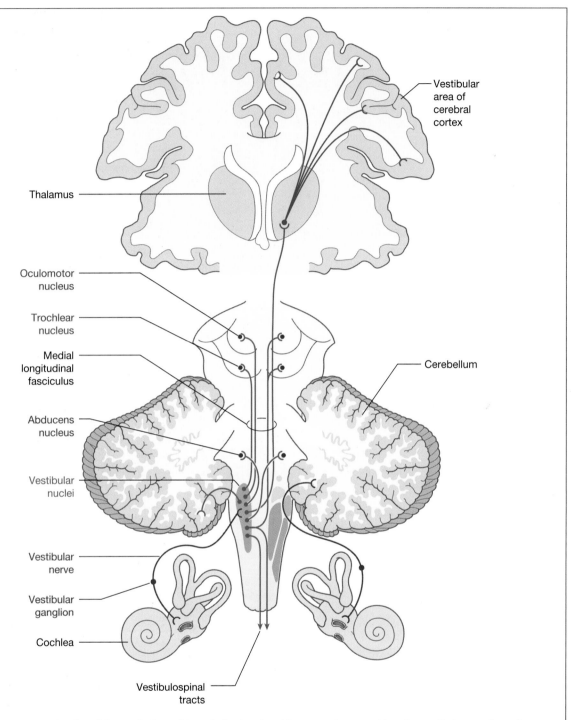

Thalamus

Oculomotor
nucleus

Trochlear
nucleus

Medial
longitudinal
fasciculus

Abducens
nucleus

Vestibular
nuclei

Vestibular
nerve

Vestibular
ganglion

Cochlea

Vestibulospinal
tracts

Vestibular
area of
cerebral
cortex

Cerebellum

Figure 13.12 A schematic drawing of the vestibular pathways indicating the wide range of outputs. Note the vestibular ganglia project to the vestibular nuclei or to the cerebellum directly. The vestibular nuclei project to the cerebellum, spinal cord (vestibulospinal tracts), brain stem motor nuclei (medial longitudinal fasciculus), and thalamus, with subsequent axonal projections to the cortex.

Clinical box 13.3

Testing vestibular function may not be helpful in determining the actual site of a lesion – only determining that the vestibular system is dysfunctional. The current use of neuroimaging is much more helpful in localizing region-specific abnormalities. Historically, three different tests can be used to examine vestibular function. The **rotation test** involves a patient sitting on a rotating stool with his head tilted forward approximately 30 degrees. The clinician spins the patient on the stool in one direction for approximately 30 seconds at a constant acceleration. Then the rotation is stopped. The clinician examines the eyes of the patient throughout the procedure. During the spinning, a normal patient's eyes will slowly move in the opposite direction of the rotation (slow phase) and will then rapidly swing back in the same direction of rotation (fast phase). This is referred to as **nystagmus** (Figure 13.14). Once the spinning stops, the patient's eyes will display the opposite nystagmus with the fast phase in the opposite direction of the spinning. This may last about a minute. At the same time, if the patient attempts to stand (with support), he will lean towards the direction of rotation and may experience vertigo in the opposite direction. A patient with vestibular defects will not exhibit these normal behaviors and may have exaggerated responses.

Positional testing (Dix-Hallpike maneuver) involves a patient sitting up with her eyes open. The clinician (supporting the patient's head) then briskly brings her to a lying down position with her head rotated 90 degrees (so that one ear is facing downward) over the end of the bed. The clinician then examines the patient's eyes for nystagmus. If nystagmus is delayed for a few seconds, is in the opposite direction upon sitting upright, and is less noticeable after a few repetitions of the test (habituation/fatigable), then this is a positive outcome of the test and indicates a peripheral or inner ear condition. If, however, the nystagmus occurs without any delay, there is no habituation on repeat testing and there is nystagmus without vertigo, then this is considered a negative outcome and may indicate a more central lesion.

Caloric testing involves placing cold or warm water into the external auditory meatus of a patient and determining if nystagmus occurs. A patient is usually in the sitting position with the head tilted backwards about 60 degrees. Cold water is introduced into the external auditory meatus and any nystagmus produced is recorded. After a time period for equalization, warm water is introduced and the determination of nystagmus is re-examined. In normal individuals, the cold water should produce an opposite direction (fast phase) nystagmus, while the warm water should produce same direction (fast phase) nystagmus. The mnemonic COWS (cold opposite, warm same) is used to remember this relationship. This test indicates an intact vestibulo-ocular pathway.

defects involve the loss of the neuroepithelial hair cells within the cochlea, lesions to the cochlear portion of the vestibulo-cochlear nerve (VIII), or central neural lesions. Unilateral deafness can be produced by mechanical hearing defects on the ipsilateral side or by neural lesions proximal to the cochlear nuclei on the ipsilateral side. Lesions distal to the cochlear nuclei will not produce unilateral deficits due to the bilateral projections that leave the nuclei (Gokhale, *et al.*, 2013).

The facial nerve (VII) and the vestibulocochlear nerve (VIII) pass through the **internal acoustic meatus** in the temporal bone. Any space filling object found in the meatus can compress the nerves and produce a loss in facial nerve (VII) or vestibulocochlear nerve (VIII) function. For example, a cancer in the glial support cells for these nerves (Schwanoma, referred to as an **acoustic neuroma**) can compromise the function of both of these nerves (Figure 13.13).

Damage to the inner ear or the vestibulocochlear nerve (VIII) will quite often produce hearing loss (or tinnitus) and vestibular disturbances. Vestibular symptoms without any hearing deficit usually point to central lesions (vestibular nuclei, cerebellar, or cerebral damage).

Recall that all of the vestibular sensory components are in the inner ear (semicircular canals and utricle/saccule), so defects in the external and middle ear affect hearing and not the vestibular system. Because the vestibular system projects widely throughout the central nervous system and its sensory components are not localizable (like touch, vision, or sound), determining specific lesions in the vestibular system can be difficult. Patients with vestibular defects will often mention "dizziness", vertigo, and unsteadiness as symptoms. These symptoms can be due to many disorders, not just vestibular defects, so a careful and complete neurological exam is required (Smouha, 2013).

Vestibular defects generally occur in the inner ear, with disruptions in the semicircular canals or the utricle/saccule. These can produce alterations in balance and equilibrium, leading patients to complain of dizziness or **vertigo**. A common vertigo/vestibular disorder (benign paroxysmal positional vertigo) occurs when an individual changes position and experiences vertigo. This is believed to be due to debris in the semicircular canals that causes abnormal bending of the hair cells and an increased firing of the associated neurons. The unique interrelationship between the vestibular nuclei and the motor nuclei of the eye can lead to alterations in eye motion, referred to as **nystagmus** (Figure 13.14). Identifying nystagmus in patients can be indicative of vestibular or cerebellar defects.

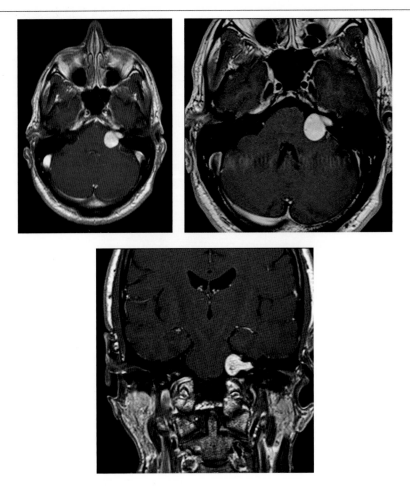

Figure 13.13 Two axial and one frontal magnetic resonance image of a patient with an acoustic neuroma. Note that the space-filling mass has compressed the facial nerve (VII) and the vestibulocochlear nerve (VIII) in the internal acoustic meatus.

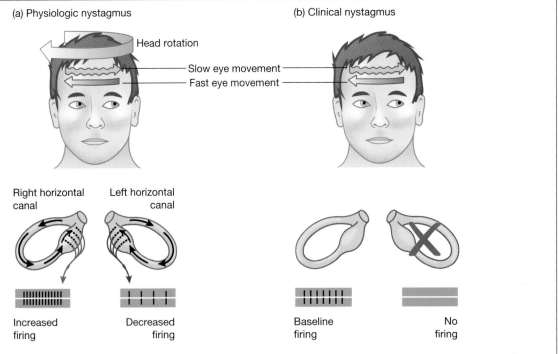

Figure 13.14 A drawing of the production of physiologic and clinical nystagmus. Note that the eyes have two separate motions: a slow phase and a rapid (saccadic) phase. In physiologic nystagmus, an imbalance in firing from each horizontal canal produces the characteristic eye movements, with the fast phase in the same direction as the initial head movement (a). In clinical nystagmus, an imbalance in firing from each horizontal canal (or a central processing defect) can produce the same characteristic eye movements (b).

Certain drugs can be toxic to the otoliths (ototoxic) (e.g. gentamicin) and can produce vestibular symptoms, due to the loss of the otoliths. Other drugs (alcohol, anticonvulsants) can produce vestibular symptoms (dizziness, vertigo, unsteadiness) by interfering with neurotransmission. Some of the drug treatments can be reversible, while others can cause permanent damage. In addition, medical conditions (e.g. anemia, thyroid disease) can produce vestibular symptoms. With vestibular symptoms produced by a wide range of conditions and treatments, clinicians need to carefully examine patients who present with dizziness, vertigo, or unsteadiness.

Case 1

A 35-year-old auto mechanic, Mr Randy Thomas, began noticing short periods of disorientation, along with a ringing in his ears, and diminished hearing. The first few instances he didn't do anything, since he regained his hearing and balance after a short period of time. A prolonged period of disorientation while he was driving convinces him to see his physician.

His physician, Dr Mark Jackson, collects a detailed history and physical. After a number of tests and referral to a neurologist and audiologist, the team of physicians concludes that Mr Thomas has **Ménière's disease**. Dr Jackson explains to Mr Thomas that this disease appears to be due to an increase in production of endolymphatic fluid in the inner ear, causing disturbances in balance (vestibular function) and hearing. Dr Jackson suggests a number of alternatives (corticosteroid injections, surgical approaches, pharmacologic and/or physiotherapy). Mr Thomas decides on a less aggressive treatment regimen, so opts for physiotherapy, with some pharmacologic treatments.

These treatments help prevent the occurrence of other episodes, but Mr Thomas still has small bouts of disorientation and hearing loss. He eventually opts for a surgical decompression of the endolymphatic sac, which removes all of the symptoms for approximately nine months (Pullens, et al., 2013). The bouts begin to return and he decides he wants a more permanent solution. After much more discussion with Dr Jackson and his neurologist, Mr Thomas chooses to have the vestibular portion of his vestibulocochlear nerve cut on the affected side. The surgery is successful and Mr Thomas has no vestibular function and some reduced hearing after recovery. He has some disorientation from loss of vestibular input, but physiotherapy is helpful in retraining his brain to adapt to unilateral vestibular input. He remains symptom free (but with reduced hearing) five years after the surgery.

Case 2

A 40-year-old accountant, Mrs Jasmine Brown, was being treated for metastases from breast cancer when the nurses administering her treatment recognized that Mrs Brown was having difficulty understanding them during normal conversation. They could see that she responded to sounds, but that she was having difficulty following the conversation. They suggested that she meet with a neurologist and audiologist.

Mrs Brown met with a neurologist, Dr Joan Thompson, who performed a complete neural examination and found no loss in hearing sensitivity, but did find a decrease in word recognition. After an MRI, Dr Thompson located small lesions in the **inferior colliculi** of Mrs Brown's midbrain (Figure 13.15) (Champoux, et al., 2007). Dr Thompson encouraged Mrs Brown to continue her chemotherapy and explained that they would monitor her auditory deficits. Mrs Brown also met with an auditory therapist to help her with word understanding.

With remission of her cancer and cessation of her chemotherapy, Mrs Brown did not have any immediate change in her word recognition deficit. However, six months later, she had a noticeable increase in word recognition ability, although she did not have a full recovery.

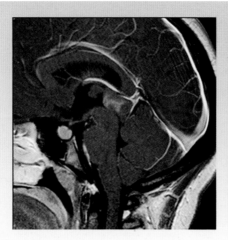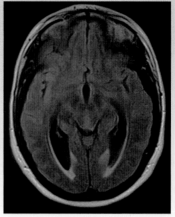

Figure 13.15 A sagittal and axial magnetic resonance image of a patient with a tectal glioma. Note the hyperintense region of the tectum in the sagittal view.

Study questions

1. If a 63-year-old male patient has facial nerve (VII) paralysis along with hearing deficits, his physician could suspect a space occupying mass in the:
a) external acoustic meatus
b) internal acoustic meatus
c) facial canal
d) tegmentum of the midbrain
e) tectum of the midbrain

2. If a 57-year-old female patient has a cortical stroke that produces a hearing loss, which region of her cortex would be expected to be damaged?
a) frontal
b) parietal
c) temporal
d) occipital
e) insular

3. If a 62-year-old male patient has a lesion in the pons that produces a hearing loss, which of the following structures could be involved?
a) pontocerebellar fibers
b) inferior cerebellar peduncle

c) spinothalamic tract
d) medial lemniscus
e) lateral lemniscus

4. Otoliths in the vestibular system are associated with:
a) angular acceleration in the semicircular canals
b) linear acceleration in the semicircular canals
c) angular acceleration in the utricle/saccule
d) linear acceleration in the utricle/saccule
e) gravity determination in the semicircular canals

5. The neural tract involved in the production of nystagmus during a vestibular disorder is the:
a) lateral lemniscus
b) medial lemniscus
c) spinothalamic tract
d) solitary tract
e) medial longitudinal fasciculus

For more self-assessment questions, visit the companion website at
www.wileyessential.com/neuroanatomy

FURTHER READING

For additional information on the auditory and vestibular systems, the following textbooks and review articles may be helpful:

Bizley JK, Cohen YE. 2013. The what, where and how of auditory-object perception. *Nat Rev Neurosci*, 14(10): 693–707.

Blumenfeld H. 2002. *Neuroanatomy Through Clinical Cases*. Sinauer Associates, Sunderland, Massachusetts.

Champoux F, Paiement P, Mercier C, Lepore F, Lassonde M, Gagné JP. 2007. Auditory processing in a patient with a unilateral lesion of the inferior colliculus. *Eur J Neurosci*, 25(1): 291–297.

Felten DL, Shetty A. 2009. *Netter's Atlas of Neuroscience*, 2nd edition. Saunders Elsevier, Philadelphia, Pennsylvania.

Gokhale S, Lahoti S, Caplan LR. 2013. The neglected neglect: auditory neglect. *JAMA Neurol*, 70(8): 1065–1069.

Haines DE. 2012. *Neuroanatomy: An Atlas of Structures, Sections and Systems*, 8th edition. Lippincott Williams & Wilkin, Baltimore, Maryland.

Khan S, Chang R. 2013. Anatomy of the vestibular system: a review. *NeuroRehabilitation*, 32(3): 437–443.

Moore KL, Dalley AF, Agur AMR. 2014. *Moore Clinically Oriented Anatomy*, 7th edition. Lippincott, Williams & Wilkins, Philadelphia, Pennsylvania.

Patestas MA, Gartner LP. 2006. *A Textbook of Neuroanatomy*. Blackwell Publishing, Malden, Massachusetts.

Pullens B, Verschuur HP, van Benthem PP. 2013. Surgery for Ménière's disease. *Cochrane Database Syst Rev*. 28 (1–21).

Smouha E. 2013. Inner ear disorders. *NeuroRehabilitation*, 32(3): 455–462.

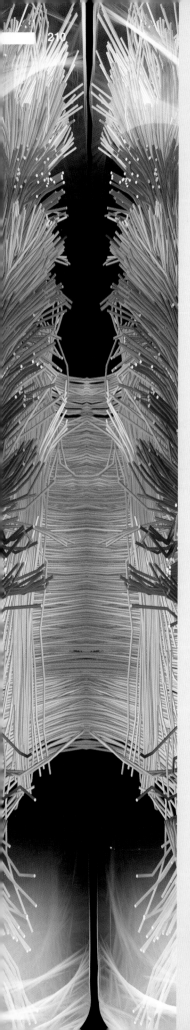

CHAPTER 14
Olfaction and taste

Learning objectives

1. Describe and identify the anatomy of the olfactory system.
2. Describe and identify the central components of the olfactory pathways.
3. Describe and identify the anatomy of the taste system.
4. Describe and identify the central components of the taste pathway.
5. Diagnose and discuss clinical problems regarding taste and olfaction.

Essential Clinical Neuroanatomy, First Edition. Thomas H. Champney.
© 2016 John Wiley & Sons, Ltd. Published 2016 by John Wiley & Sons, Ltd.
Companion website: www.wileyessential.com/neuroanatomy

2. First order, pseudounipolar neurons in:
   a) Anterior ⅔ tongue: lingual nerve (V_3), chorda tympani (VII), facial nerve (VII), geniculate ganglion (cell bodies), facial nerve (VII), solitary tract, solitary nucleus (gustatory)
   b) Posterior ⅓ tongue: glossopharyngeal nerve (IX), inferior (petrosal) ganglion, glossopharyngeal nerve (IX), solitary tract, solitary nucleus (vagus nerve (X) may also contribute)

Central connections of taste system

1. Solitary nucleus (rostral, gustatory) – second order cell bodies
2. Second order fibers via central tegmental tract (bilaterally) to the
3. Thalamus (VPM)
4. Third order neurons project to the taste cortex (postcentral gyrus/ insula) and orbitofrontal cortex (interaction with smell sensation)

5. Projections to hypothalamus and amygdala (taste aversion)

Introduction

The special senses of olfaction and taste are similar in their ability to detect chemical signals in the air or in the saliva. These signals are then transmitted to the brain as neural activity, where they are interpreted as smell or taste. The special sensation of smell is highly diverse, resulting in the ability to distinguish thousands of different chemical compounds. The special sensation of taste is, however, much more restricted and is only able to distinguish about five different modalities. Combined, these two systems produce an individual's ability to distinguish fine wines, good food, or toxic compounds.

Olfactory system

The olfactory system begins in the superior portion of the nasal cavity with specialized olfactory neurons that are embedded in the mucosal epithelium. The dendritic portions of these bipolar neurons (**olfactory nerves (I)**) have specialized chemoreceptors that can distinguish thousands of different compounds. These neurons are unique in that they die off and regenerate many times. They are one of only a few neural cells that have a regenerative capacity. These bipolar neurons send their central processes through foramina in the cribriform plate of the ethmoid bone to synapse in the **olfactory bulbs**.

The olfactory bulbs are found on the inferior surface of the frontal cortex and are located in close contact with the ethmoid bone (Figure 14.1). The bulbs contain second order neurons that receive input from the bipolar olfactory neurons. There are two types of second order neurons: tufted cells and mitral cells.

These neurons interact with other interneurons in the olfactory bulbs (periglomerular cells and granule cells). The olfactory bulbs are highly organized and, when viewed histologically, contain a layer of spherical collections of nuclei referred to as glomeruli. Interestingly, there are afferent fibers to the olfactory bulbs from the contralateral olfactory bulb and other brain regions that can modulate the function of the olfactory bulb. This allows processing of the olfactory information within the olfactory bulb (Figure 14.2). The second order axons from the olfactory bulbs project through the olfactory tracts towards the brain. Some of these axons synapse in the **anterior olfactory nucleus** located within the olfactory tracts. This nucleus sends axons to the contralateral olfactory bulb, providing intercommunication between the two olfactory bulbs.

The second order axons in the olfactory tracts divide into two smaller tracts: a medial tract (striae) and a lateral tract (striae). The medial tract primarily provides communication with the contralateral olfactory bulb. The lateral tract contains projections to the cortex and amygdala. The lateral tract projects directly to the **primary olfactory cortex** (piriform and periamygdaloid cortex) and does not synapse in the thalamus (Figure 14.3). This is unique for sensory input to the brain; all other sensory input is relayed to the cortex via the thalamus.

From the primary olfactory cortex, neural projections of olfactory information are distributed to the limbic system, the thalamus, and frontal cortex for an individual's conscious perception of smell. Specific areas of the cortex process smell and taste information together to produce the perceptions of flavor and food identification.

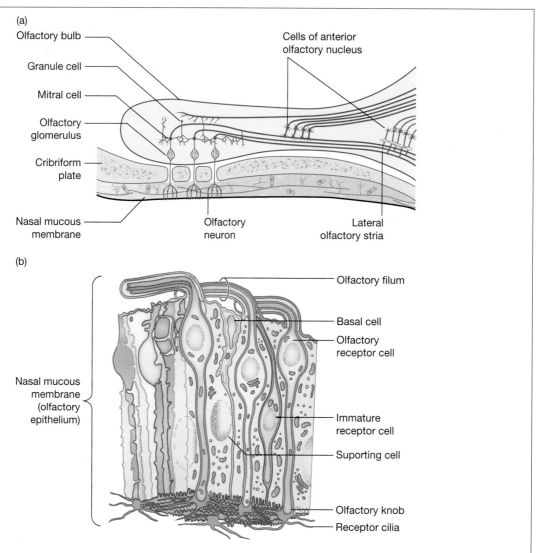

(a)

Olfactory bulb

Granule cell

Mitral cell

Olfactory glomerulus

Cribriform plate

Nasal mucous membrane

Cells of anterior olfactory nucleus

Olfactory neuron

Lateral olfactory stria

(b)

Nasal mucous membrane (olfactory epithelium)

Olfactory filum

Basal cell

Olfactory receptor cell

Immature receptor cell

Suporting cell

Olfactory knob

Receptor cilia

Figure 14.1 A drawing of the olfactory anatomy. Note the olfactory nerves located in the nasal mucosa (b) that have processes that pass through the cribriform plate and synapse in the olfactory bulb (a).

Some projections from the lateral olfactory tracts proceed directly to the amygdala and olfactory tubercle, providing olfactory information to deep-seated limbic structures which can produce smell memories and emotional responses. This may be why smells can be so evocative of memories and emotions.

Taste system

The taste system begins in the taste buds located on the fungiform and circumvallate papillae of the tongue. The **taste buds** are specialized chemoreceptor cells found within the epithelium of the tongue and respond to one of five different tastes. These five tastes are bitter, salty, sweet, sour, and a specialized "savory taste" referred to as umami. These tastes are a relatively primitive means to detect chemical compounds that could be toxic to the individual.

When the taste buds are activated, they produce an ionic change in the peripheral process of the first order, pseudounipolar neuron adjacent to the taste bud. These neurons have different pathways to enter the central nervous system dependent on their location on the tongue. Those neurons in the anterior two-thirds of the tongue course on the lingual nerve, the chorda tympani nerve, and the facial nerve (VII), to enter the brain stem, where they course in the **solitary tract** to synapse in the gustatory portion of the **solitary nucleus**. These neurons have their cell bodies located in the geniculate ganglion of the facial nerve (VII). Those pseudounipolar neurons in the posterior one-third of the tongue course on the glossopharyngeal nerve (IX) to enter the brain stem and then enter the solitary tract to synapse in the gustatory portion of the solitary nucleus. These neurons have their cell bodies in the inferior (petrosal) ganglion of the glossopharyngeal nerve (IX). Additionally, some taste buds

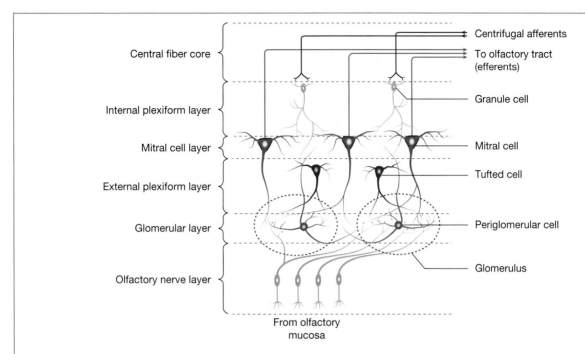

Figure 14.2 A drawing of the anatomy of the olfactory bulb. Note that the olfactory neurons synapse in a glomerulus with periglomerular cells, and processes from tufted cells and mitral cells. The mitral cells provide the main second order neuronal output pathways from the olfactory bulb. Interestingly, there are centrifugal afferents from the other olfactory bulb and from specific brain regions that can impact on processing within the olfactory bulb.

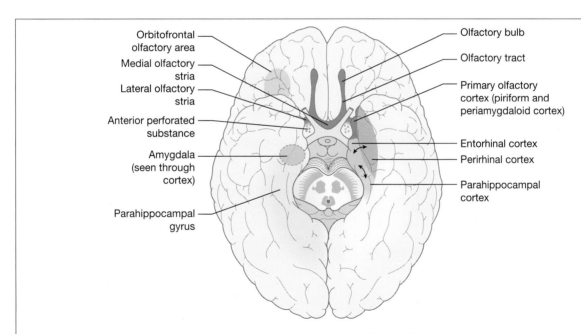

Figure 14.3 A drawing of the base of the brain with the olfactory system highlighted. Note the olfactory bulbs and the olfactory tracts contain second order sensory neurons. The majority of these neurons project to the primary olfactory cortex on the medial side of the temporal lobe (without synapsing in the thalamus). There are also neurons that directly project to limbic structures.

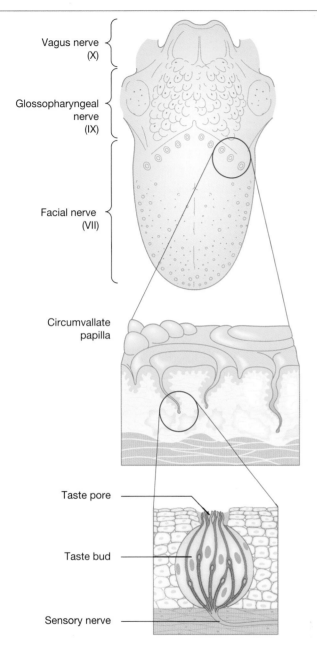

Vagus nerve
(X)

Glossopharyngeal
nerve
(IX)

Facial nerve
(VII)

Circumvallate
papilla

Taste pore

Taste bud

Sensory nerve

Figure 14.4 A drawing of a taste bud on a circumvallate papilla of the tongue. Note that taste from the anterior two-thirds of the tongue is carried by the facial nerve (VII) while taste from the posterior one-third of the tongue is carried by the glossopharyngeal nerve (IX). Sensation from scattered taste buds on the epiglottis is carried by the vagus nerve (X).

These projections are bilateral, so that taste sensation from one side of the tongue is projected to both the right and left thalamus and cortex. From the thalamus, the third order neurons project to the taste cortex, that part of the postcentral gyrus of the parietal lobe that is adjacent to the insula (Figures 14.4, 14.5). Third order neurons also project to other parts of the **insular cortex** to interact with olfactory sensation, leading to an individual's ability to identify and catalog specific flavors. In addition, third order neurons project to the **orbitofrontal cortex** to add emotional and decision-making aspects to flavors. Likewise, there are direct projections from the solitary nucleus to the hypothalamus and amygdala, providing taste sensory information for food intake regulation, taste memories, and taste aversion (Figures 14.6, 14.7).

Clinical box 14.1

Testing for smell and taste deficiencies is relatively straightforward. Smell tests generally provide a small piece of paper with a distinctive smell (coffee) that an individual can identify (e.g. the University of Pennsylvania Smell Identification Test). When conducting the tests, it is important not to use substances that irritate the nasal mucosa (such as ammonia), which may be sensed by pain fibers. Since smell is distributed bilaterally from the olfactory bulbs to the cortex, the inability to smell unilaterally indicates a peripheral loss at the bipolar neurons. Bilateral losses or diminished sense of smell can be peripheral (loss of both sets of bipolar neurons) or central (lesions of the olfactory bulbs, olfactory tracts, or cortical lesions).

Testing for taste deficiencies involves the use of sugar, salt, or lemons applied in small swabs to the tongue. This can indicate losses over the surface of the tongue, both unilaterally and bilaterally. Note that a loss of taste sensation bilaterally on the tongue (without any significant bilateral face trauma) can be indicative of a central deficit, since taste is projected from the tongue ipsilaterally until the central tegmental tract (Figure 14.5).

While these tests are not usually used during neurological exams, smell tests can be helpful in the diagnosis of a number of neural disorders (e.g. Alzheimer's and Parkinson's). Some clinicians suggest the use of a baseline smell test during middle age which can then be used to compare with results of future smell tests.

---

are scattered over the epiglottis and upper larynx and these cells interact with branches from the vagus nerve (X) which also project to the solitary tract and solitary nucleus (Figure 14.4, 14.5).

The second order cell bodies located in the solitary nucleus send their projections via the **central tegmental tract** to the **thalamus** (ventroposterior medial portion).

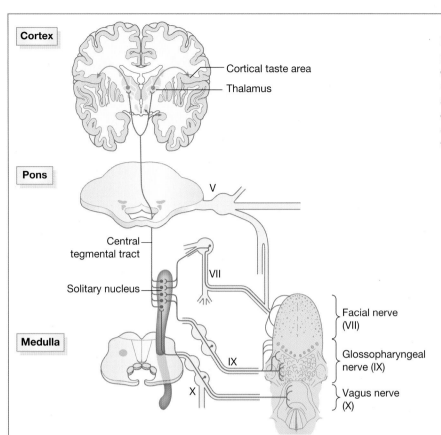

| Cortex |

Cortical taste area
Thalamus

| Pons |

V

Central tegmental tract

VII

Solitary nucleus

| Medulla |

IX

X

Facial nerve (VII)

Glossopharyngeal nerve (IX)

Vagus nerve (X)

Figure 14.5 A drawing of the central taste pathways. Note that taste from all three cranial nerves converges on the gustatory (rostral) portion of the solitary nucleus. The second order neurons project through the central tegmental tract bilaterally to reach each thalamus. Third order neurons from the thalamus project to the cortical taste area.

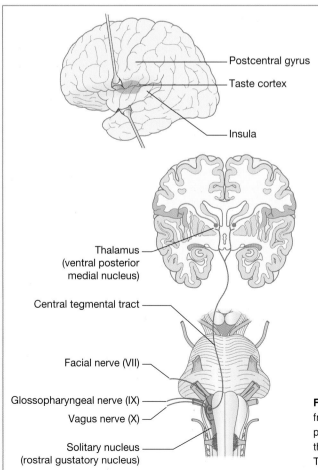

Postcentral gyrus
Taste cortex
Insula

Thalamus (ventral posterior medial nucleus)

Central tegmental tract

Facial nerve (VII)

Glossopharyngeal nerve (IX)

Vagus nerve (X)

Solitary nucleus (rostral gustatory nucleus)

Figure 14.6 A drawing of the central taste pathways. Note that taste from all three cranial nerves converges on the gustatory (rostral) portion of the solitary nucleus. The second order neurons project through the central tegmental tract bilaterally to reach each thalamus. Third order neurons from the thalamus project to the cortical taste area.

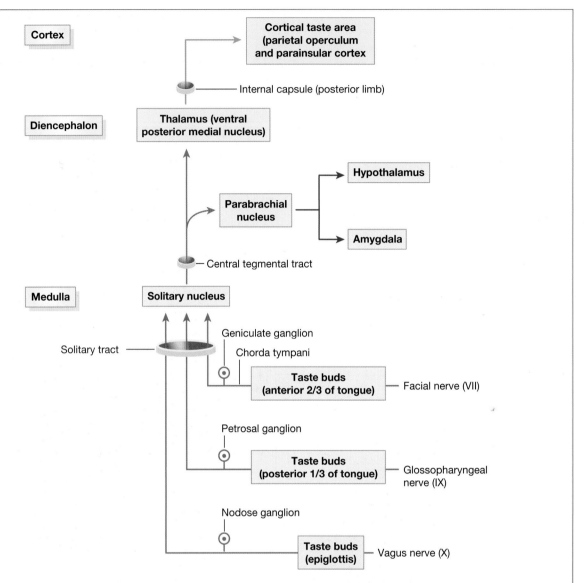

Figure 14.7 A schematic drawing of the central taste pathways. Note that taste from all three cranial nerves converges on the gustatory (rostral) portion of the solitary nucleus. The second order neurons project through the central tegmental tract bilaterally to reach each thalamus. Third order neurons from the thalamus project to the cortical taste area. Note that there are also collateral branches from the central tegmental tract that project to the hypothalamus and amygdala for regulation of feeding behavior and taste aversion.

Clinical considerations

Anosmia is the term for a patient's inability to distinguish smells. This can be indicative of more global neural deficits. For example, patients with early-onset **Alzheimer's disease** or **Parkinson's disease** frequently complain of a lack of smell and taste prior to the more debilitating aspects of the disease. It has been found that over 50% of individuals over the age of 65 have a diminished sense of smell, indicating that a loss of smell occurs naturally in an aging population (Doty and Kamath, 2014).

Lesions that produce a loss of smell can occur peripherally or centrally. Peripheral lesions generally occur where the olfactory neurons (I) pass through the **cribriform plate**. A fracture of the plate or any trauma in that region may damage the olfactory

neurons. A lesion of this type may be self-healing because of the regenerative ability of the olfactory neurons (although a complete recovery is rare). A central lesion in the olfactory tracts or the cortex is generally more permanent since these neurons are unable to regenerate. Smell sensations are sent to both olfactory bulbs and from there to the cortex bilaterally; therefore, it is difficult to localize central lesions based on smell deficits.

Lesions that produce a loss of taste can also occur peripherally or centrally. Peripheral lesions can involve a number of cranial nerves due to the distributional differences of taste from the tongue. If a patient has a loss of taste sensation from the anterior two-thirds of the tongue, then the lingual branch of the trigeminal nerve (V), the chorda tympani nerve, or the **facial nerve (VII)** could be involved. To discriminate which nerve is affected, other sensory or motor deficits need to be assessed. If the patient loses taste sensation from the posterior one-third of the tongue, then the **glossopharyngeal nerve (IX)** can be involved. A central lesion that produces a loss of taste sensation will generally involve taste from the whole surface of the tongue and can be due to a lesion in the **solitary tract**, **solitary nucleus**, central tegmental tract, or lesions in the thalamus or cortex. These lesions invariably involve wider areas of the brain stem or cortex and therefore produce additional symptoms besides a loss of taste.

Case study

A 28-year-old, third-year medical student, Mr Frank Burns, is involved in a car accident in which he suffers head trauma. After regaining consciousness, Mr Burns notices that clear fluid is running out of his nose. After transport to the hospital and treatment for his other injuries, Mr Burns realizes that the clear fluid was cerebrospinal fluid that was leaking through a fracture in the **cribriform plate** of the ethmoid bone (Figure 14.8). The leak is controlled with a nasal pack of gauze, but

Mr Burns recalls that his sense of smell may be affected due to a loss of his olfactory neurons.

Luckily, six weeks after the accident, Mr Burns realizes his sense of smell is returning when he notices that his morning toast smells burnt. He remembers that the olfactory neurons are one of a few sets of neurons that can regenerate. Six months after the accident, Mr Burns has recovered a portion of his sense of smell, but has not had a complete recovery. He has been delayed in completing his third year of medical school, but will complete his requirements and is on schedule to graduate with his class.

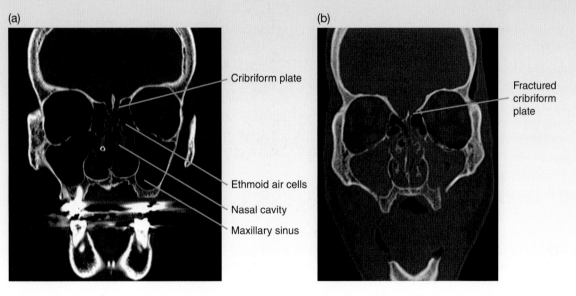

(a)

Cribriform plate

Ethmoid air cells

Nasal cavity

Maxillary sinus

(b)

Fractured cribriform plate

Figure 14.8 (a) Frontal magnetic resonance images of a normal and (b) a fractured cribriform plate. Note, in the image on the right, the discontinuity of the cribriform plate as well as the fluid-filled maxillary sinuses and nasal cavity.

Study questions

1. A 27-year-old male suffers a fracture of the cribriform plate of the ethmoid bone in an automobile accident. The nerves damaged include the:
a) olfactory nerves (I)
b) medial olfactory tract (second order axons)
c) lateral olfactory tract (second order axons)
d) chorda tympani nerve
e) lingual nerve (V)
f) facial nerve (VII)

2. A 25-year-old male suffers a fracture of the mandible during a fight in a bar. It is later found that he has lost taste and general sensation over the anterior portion of his tongue on the side of the fracture. The nerve that is damaged is the:
a) maxillary nerve
b) buccal nerve
c) glossopharyngeal nerve (IX)
d) vagus nerve (X)
e) lingual nerve

3. Taste fibers (first order sensory fibers) can be carried by a variety of cranial nerves, yet they all synapse in the:
a) geniculate ganglion
b) inferior (petrosal) ganglion
c) superior (jugular) ganglion
d) solitary nucleus
e) dorsal nucleus

4. The cortical region that processes olfactory and taste sensations to provide an emotional and decision-making component to flavors is the:
a) superior temporal gyrus
b) lateral portion of the precentral gyrus
c) lateral portion of the postcentral gyrus
d) medial portion of the precentral gyrus
e) medial portion of the postcentral gyrus
f) orbitofrontal cortex

5. The medial olfactory tract is responsible for projection of olfactory fibers to the:
a) amygdala
b) piriform cortex
c) periamygdaloid cortex
d) contralateral olfactory bulb
e) thalamus

For more self-assessment questions, visit the companion website at
www.wileyessential.com/neuroanatomy

FURTHER READING

For additional information on taste and olfaction, the following textbooks and review articles may be helpful:

Blumenfeld H. 2002. *Neuroanatomy Through Clinical Cases*. Sinauer Associates, Sunderland, Massachusetts.

Breslin PA, Huang L. 2006. Human taste: peripheral anatomy, taste transduction, and coding. *Adv Otorhinolaryngol*, 63: 152–190.

Dipatrizio NV. 2014. Is fat taste ready for primetime? *Physiol Behav*, 136:145–154.

Doty RL, Kamath V. 2014. The influences of age on olfaction: a review. *Front Psychol*, 5: 20 (1–20).

Felten DL, Shetty A. 2009. *Netter's Atlas of Neuroscience*, 2nd edition. Saunders Elsevier, Philadelphia, Pennsylvania.

Giessel AJ, Datta SR. 2014. Olfactory maps, circuits and computations. *Curr Opin Neurobiol*, 24(1): 120–132.

Haines DE. 2012. *Neuroanatomy: An Atlas of Structures, Sections and Systems*, 8th edition. Lippincott Williams & Wilkin, Baltimore, Maryland.

Malaty J, Malaty IA. 2013. Smell and taste disorders in primary care. *Am Fam Physician*, 88(12): 852–859.

Moore KL, Dalley AF, Agur AMR. 2014. *Moore Clinically Oriented Anatomy*, 7th edition. Lippincott, Williams & Wilkins, Philadelphia, Pennsylvania.

Patestas MA, Gartner LP. 2006. *A Textbook of Neuroanatomy*. Blackwell Publishing, Malden, Massachusetts.

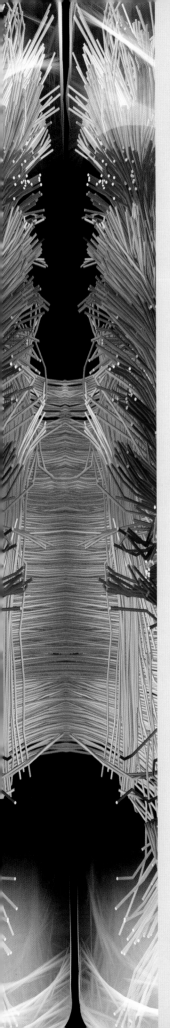

CHAPTER 15
Central motor control

Learning objectives

1. Describe the functions of each level of the motor system hierarchy.
2. Describe the nervous system structures involved in the motor system hierarchy.
3. Describe the connections and functions of the corticospinal, reticulospinal, rubrospinal, tectospinal, and vestibulospinal tracts.
4. Discuss the function of the basal ganglia, cerebellum, and motor cortex.
5. List the anatomy and components of the basal ganglia.
6. Describe the direct and indirect basal ganglia pathways and their relation to movement disorders.

Levels of motor control 221

Highest level – strategy
1. Why move? Goals to be achieved
2. Structures
   a) Neocortical association areas (sensations, memories)
   b) Basal ganglia

Middle level – tactics
1. How, what, and when to move? Sequence of muscles used, timing
2. Structures
   a) Motor cortex (areas 4 and 6)
   b) Cerebellum

Lowest level – execution
1. Move! Activation of motor neurons
2. Structures
   a) Brain stem
   b) Spinal cord

Essential Clinical Neuroanatomy, First Edition. Thomas H. Champney.
© 2016 John Wiley & Sons, Ltd. Published 2016 by John Wiley & Sons, Ltd.
Companion website: www.wileyessential.com/neuroanatomy

Motor pathways 221

Motor cortex
1. Precentral gyrus (area 4)
2. Premotor area and supplementary motor area (area 6)
3. Posterior parietal cortex (areas 5 and 7) – sensory input
4. Motor homunculus

Lateral pathways – voluntary movement
1. Corticospinal tract (pyramidal)
   a) Longest tract
   b) Largest tract (one million axons)
   c) Primary motor cortex ($\frac{2}{3}$) and somatosensory cortex ($\frac{1}{3}$)
   d) Descends through internal capsule, cerebral peduncle (midbrain), and pyramid (medulla – decussates) to lateral corticospinal tract (spinal cord)
   e) Synapses in anterior (ventral) horn
2. Rubrospinal tract
   a) Arises in red nucleus; input from ipsilateral cortex and contralateral cerebellum
   b) Decussates and descends through lateral medulla
   c) Synapses in anterior (ventral) horn

Anteromedial pathways – posture and locomotion
1. Anterior corticospinal tract
   a) Primary motor cortex ($\frac{2}{3}$) and somatosensory cortex ($\frac{1}{3}$)
   b) Descends through internal capsule, cerebral peduncle (midbrain), and pyramid (medulla)
   c) Does not decussate (ipsilateral) into anterior corticospinal tract (in anterior column of spinal cord)
   d) Synapses bilaterally in anterior (ventral) horn to control trunk musculature
2. Reticulospinal tracts
   a) Pontine (medial) – enhances antigravity reflexes
   b) Medullary (lateral) – relaxes antigravity reflexes
   c) Arise in the reticular formation of the pons or the medulla; input from cerebral cortex
   d) Descends ipsilaterally through medulla and spinal cord
   e) Synapse in anterior (ventral) horn
3. Vestibulospinal tract
   a) Orientation of head to objects in space; balance and posture
   b) Arises in vestibular nuclei; input from cerebellum and motor cortex
   c) Descends through medial medulla
   d) Bilateral projection: stabilizes head, keeps eyes stable

e) Ipsilateral projection: upright and balanced posture
f) Both synapse in anterior (ventral) horn
4. Tectospinal tract
   a) Orientation of head and eyes for fovea placement
   b) Arises from superior colliculus; input from retina, visual cortex, auditory cortex, and somatosensory areas
   c) Decussates and descends in medial midbrain and medulla
   d) Synapses in anterior (ventral) horn

Cortical regulation of movement 225

Parietal cortex (areas 5 and 7)
1. Sensory input
2. Output to premotor area (area 6)

Prefrontal cortex (dorsolateral region)
1. Decision making, consequential input
2. Output to premotor area (area 6)

Cerebellar regulation of movement 225

Planned execution of voluntary, multi-joint movements

Directs the motor cortex for proper direction, timing, and force

Based on predictions of previous outcomes (learned)

Coordinated execution of continuing motion – error correction

Basal ganglia regulation of movement 225

Anatomy
1. Caudate nucleus
2. Putamen (caudate + putamen = striatum)
3. Globus pallidus (putamen + globus pallidus = lentiform nucleus)
   a) External globus pallidus
   b) Internal globus pallidus
4. Subthalamic nucleus (related, not strictly part of basal ganglia)
5. Substantia nigra (related, not strictly part of basal ganglia)

Pathway
1. Input from prefrontal, parietal and motor cortex
   a) Excitatory
   b) Glutaminergic fibers
2. Striatum (caudate and putamen)
3. Globus pallidus
   a) Majority of neurons are inhibitory
   b) GABAergic
4. Output to ventral lateral thalamic nucleus then to cortex

Function

1. Globus pallidus to cortex
   a) Internal globus pallidus neurons are spontaneously active
   b) Inhibit the excitatory ventral thalamic nucleus
   c) Motor cortex is continually not excited ("quiet")
2. Cortex to putamen to cortex
   a) Direct pathway – excitatory
      i. Cortical input (excitatory)
      ii. Substantia nigra input (excitatory)
      iii. Excites putamen (inhibitory output)
      iv. Inhibits internal globus pallidus
      v. Inhibited internal globus pallidus excites motor cortex
   b) Indirect pathway – inhibitory
      i. Cortical input (excitatory)
      ii. Excites putamen (inhibitory output)
      iii. Inhibits external globus pallidus (inhibitory output)
      iv. Inhibits subthalamic nucleus (excitatory output)
      v. Excites internal globus pallidus
      vi. Excited internal globus pallidus inhibits motor cortex

Basal ganglia disorders

1. Hyperkinetic disorders – Huntington's disease (chorea)
   a) Chorea – jerky movements, dance-like
   b) Dementia
   c) Psychiatric disorders
2. Hypokinetic disorders – Parkinson's disease
   a) Resting tremor (pill rolling)
   b) Rigidity
   c) Lack of expression
   d) Difficulty starting and stopping movements
3. Athetosis – slow, writhing motions
4. Ballismus
   a) Flailing, flinging motions of the extremities
   b) Hemiballismus – unilateral, due to contralateral lesion in subthalamic nucleus

Cerebellar disorders – ataxia

Cortical disorders – spasticity

Introduction

After receiving sensory information, the brain of an individual decides what response should be undertaken. If a motor output is determined to be appropriate, the central nervous system must then put into play specific pathways to ensure a proper motor response. The first level to be addressed is **strategic**. For example, what are the goals to be achieved by initiating motion? The cortical association areas and the basal ganglia are involved in developing this motor strategy. The second level of motor control is **tactical**. This utilizes the motor cortex and the cerebellum to develop the sequence and timing of muscles to produce the specific motion required. Finally, the third level of motor control is the **execution** of the motor output: the actual activation of the motor neurons to the spinal cord and then out to the specific muscles involved.

As a good example of this hierarchy of motor control, consider a professional tennis player. The player has numerous sensory inputs in the form of visual cues from the opposing player, visual information about the conditions (temperature, wind speed), auditory information, as well as internal sensations about the status of his body and his ability to perform. All of this information is processed and the tennis player then strategically decides which hit he will make with his racket. As the ball approaches the racket, he utilizes both sensory memories (the feel of the racket) and motor memories (many hours of hitting tennis balls in the past) to develop the tactics he will use to hit the ball into a specific trajectory. He is continually processing incoming sensory information, while developing the specific tactical motor output. Then, utilizing his proprioceptive input, he directs the muscles of his upper extremity (as well as the rest of his body) to initiate the hitting motion with the ball directed to a specific target. Notice how all three levels of motor control are utilized in this example (Figure 15.1).

Motor pathways

Beginning with the third level of motor control, **execution**, the neural cell bodies for direct motor control are found in the precentral gyrus (Brodmann's area 4) of the cortex. Anterior to the precentral gyrus are motor planning areas that provide input to the precentral gyrus. These are the premotor area and supplementary motor area (Brodmann's area 6). Likewise, there is sensory input to the precentral gyrus from the posterior parietal cortex (Brodmann's areas 5 and 7).

The precentral gyrus has a specific distribution for motor control that is anatomically distinct. This is the **motor homunculus**, which begins within the sagittal suture and extends laterally along the cortex to the insular region. Therefore, a small lesion or stroke can have precise impact on specific motor output based on the homuncular location of the lesion (Figure 15.2).

The cell bodies in the precentral gyrus project inferiorly through the brain and brain stem to form the **corticospinal**

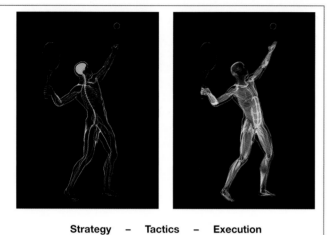

Strategy – Tactics – Execution

Figure 15.1 A drawing of a tennis player utilizing sensory input to calculate the strategic hit to make, then developing the specific tactics to make the hit, followed by the actual activation (execution) of the muscles for the hit to be effective. Note how strategy, tactics, and execution are involved in complex motor activity. Source: Science Photo Library/Sciepro.

tract. This is the longest tract in the brain and contains the largest number of axons, over one million. The axons descend through the internal capsule into the cerebral peduncle in the midbrain and pass through the pyramid in the medulla. In the caudal medulla, the axons decussate to enter the contralateral lateral corticospinal tract, where they descend through the spinal cord to synapse on alpha motor neurons and interneurons in the anterior (ventral) horn. Recall that the cell bodies of the lower motor neurons in the anterior horn project through the anterior (ventral) root into the spinal nerve, eventually to synapse on the skeletal muscle of interest. Notice that the motor execution pathway is a two neuron pathway: **upper motor neurons** from the cortex to the anterior horn and **lower motor neurons** from the anterior horn to the skeletal muscle (Chapter 11 and Figure 15.3).

This same type of pathway exists for the motor nuclei in the brain stem (**corticobulbar tract**). Upper motor neurons in the precentral gyrus have descending axons in the internal capsule and the cerebral peduncle, which synapse on the motor nuclei for cranial nerves (such as the trigeminal or facial motor nuclei). These drive lower motor neurons for the jaw muscles and facial muscles (Figure 15.4).

While the corticospinal tract is the most important of the descending motor tracts, there are other descending tracts as well. The **rubrospinal tract**, for example, arises in the red nucleus of the midbrain (receiving information from the ipsilateral cortex and contralateral cerebellum), decussates and descends through the medulla and spinal cord to synapse in the

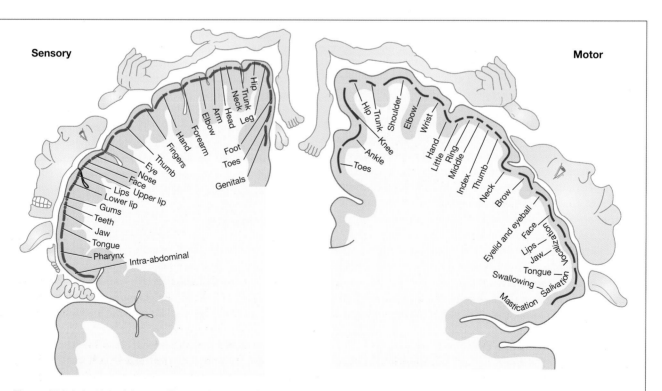

Figure 15.2 A drawing of the specific somatosensory and motor distribution on the postcentral and precentral gyri, respectively. This distribution is termed a homunculus. Note that specific lesions in either of the gyri will produce specific sensory or motor losses.

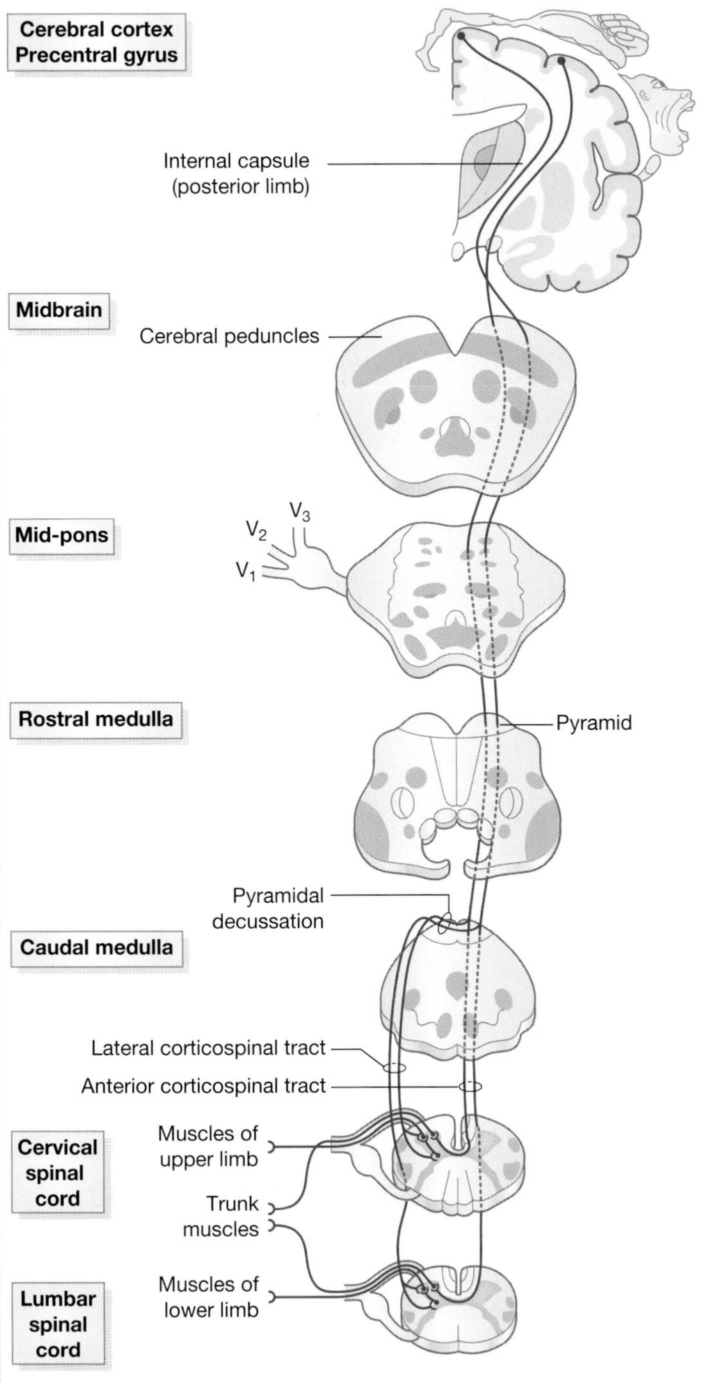

Figure 15.3 A view of the descending voluntary motor pathways (corticospinal tracts) from the cortex through the brain stem to the spinal cord. Note the decussation of the upper motor neurons in the caudal medulla oblongata.

anterior horn. Recall that the rubrospinal tract runs in close proximity to the lateral corticospinal tract in the lateral column of the spinal cord. The overall importance of the rubrospinal tract in humans is still being debated, with some individuals suggesting that it is of limited importance.

The **anterior column** of the spinal cord is mainly involved with postural and reflex motor activities and contains four descending pathways: the reticulospinal, the vestibulospinal, the tectospinal, and the anterior corticospinal tract. For details about each of these tracts, Chapter 11 can be reviewed. The **anterior corticospinal tract** is a small tract that branches from the lateral corticospinal tract in the medulla prior to its decussating. The anterior corticospinal tract descends ipsilaterally and provides motor innervation to the trunk musculature bilaterally (on both the ipsilateral and contralateral side) to help maintain balance and posture during other large voluntary motor activities (such as playing tennis).

The **reticulospinal tract** has numerous roles including the maintenance of antigravity reflexes. It arises in the reticular

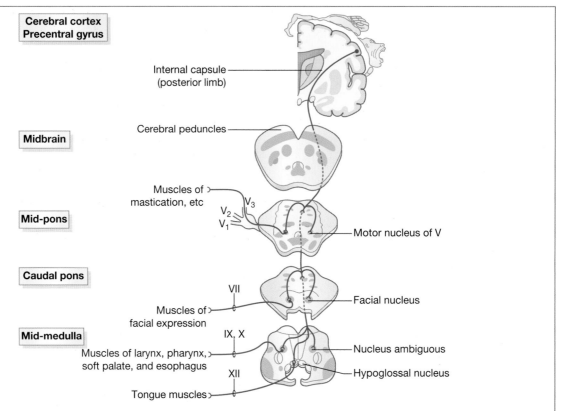

Figure 15.4 Schematic view of the descending motor pathways (corticobulbar tracts) from the cortex through the brain stem to the cranial nerve nuclei, controlling the skeletal muscles of the jaw (trigeminal V), the muscles of the face (facial VII), the muscles of the pharynx and larynx (glossopharyngeal IX and vagus X), and the muscles of the tongue (hypoglossal XII). Note the bilateral projection of the upper motor neurons to the majority of these cranial nerve nuclei. Two notable exceptions exist: the lower portion of the facial nerve (VII) is contralateral, not bilateral, and the hypoglossal nerve (XII) to the tongue is contralateral, not bilateral.

formation of the pons and medulla and descends ipsilaterally through the spinal cord to synapse in the anterior (ventral) horn. This tract receives input from the cerebral cortex and cerebellum and provides this information to the anterior horn cells in the spinal cord. By modifying antigravity reflexes, this tract helps to maintain posture and balance.

The medial and lateral **vestibulospinal tracts** are responsible for the orientation of the head to objects in space as well as helping to maintain balance and posture (see Chapter 13). The tracts arise from the vestibular nuclei in the brain stem and descend through the medulla into the spinal cord, where they project to both the ipsilateral and contralateral anterior horn cells. The vestibular nuclei receive direct sensory input from the inner ear, as well as input from the cortex and cerebellum. This information is then projected to the anterior horn cells of the spinal cord to help maintain balance and posture, as well as stabilizing the head and eyes during motor activity.

The **tectospinal tract** is responsible for the orientation of the head and eyes in space. The tract arises from the **superior colliculus** in the midbrain, decussates and descends through the brain stem to synapse in the anterior horn cells of the

cervical spinal cord. This allows for fine motor control of the neck muscles to orient the head and eyes towards a specific object of interest. The superior colliculus receives input from the retina, the visual cortex, the auditory cortex, and other somatosensory areas. The tectospinal tract is only found in the cervical spinal cord and does not descend further into the thoracic or lumbar portions of the spinal cord.

With the preceding information, it can be concluded that the lateral column of the spinal cord directs voluntary motor activity, while the anterior column of the spinal cord is primarily engaged in balance, posture, and reflex motor activity. Also, it is important to realize that much of this descending information is congregated at the anterior horn cells to produce the final motor activity via the lower motor neurons. Therefore, while the corticospinal tract directs the voluntary motor activity to the anterior horn cells, the horn cells also receive input from the tracts within the anterior column which can modify the final anterior horn cell activity. As an example, think back to the tennis player previously discussed. As the player sees the tennis ball and prepares to return the ball (utilizing the sensory system and corticospinal tract), he may feel his foot slip, causing a change in the vestibular system which can relay this information to the anterior horn cells, modifying the final output and slightly altering the swing of the racket.

Central control of movement

There are three primary regions of the central nervous system that deal with the control of movement. These are the **motor cortex**, the **basal ganglia**, and the **cerebellum** (Figure 15.5). The motor cortex is involved in the planning and direction of voluntary motor output. The basal ganglia act to initiate and maintain the proper speed and smoothness of motor activity. The cerebellum is responsible for integrating balance and other sensory components to produce complex motor activity. By utilizing all three of these regions, motor output from the central nervous system can be coordinated with sensory input, can be maintained and propagated appropriately, and can produce extremely fine motor activity.

As mentioned previously, the **motor cortex** is composed of the precentral gyrus (area 4), which is the final motor output pathway from the cortex. The firing from this area is modified by input from the parietal cortex (areas 5 & 7) and the premotor area of the frontal cortex (area 6). These are the cortical areas that regulate the planning and initiation of motor activity. In addition, the prefrontal cortex provides decision making to the premotor area for volitional motor control.

Recall from Chapter 10, that the **cerebellum** is involved in the sensory/motor coordination of complex motor activity. The cerebellum receives sensory input from the vestibular nuclei as well as from numerous areas of the cortex. It sends its outputs back to the cortex as well as into the brain stem.

This provides for a continuous **error correction loop** in motor execution so that the proper motor activities occur. The cerebellum is also involved in learned motor activity (such as riding a bicycle), as well as directing the motor cortex for the proper direction, timing, and force of the motor output.

The third component of central nervous system control of movement is the **basal ganglia**. The basal ganglia are located deep within the cortical regions of the brain lateral to the thalamus. The basal ganglia provide a **continuous feedback loop** to the cortex for proper initiation and maintenance of motor activity. This is especially apparent in patients with basal ganglia disorders.

The basal ganglia are composed of specific anatomical subsets: the **caudate nucleus**, the **putamen**, and the **globus pallidus**. The globus pallidus can be further subdivided into two components, the external and internal globus pallidus. Combining the caudate nucleus and the putamen into one structure produces the **striatum**. Likewise, combining the putamen and the globus pallidus into one structure produces the **lenticular (lentiform) nuclei**.

Understanding the three-dimensional structure of the basal ganglia within the telencephalon can be difficult (Figure 15.6). The putamen is lateral to the globus pallidus and these two structures are found between the external and internal capsules. The internal capsule separates the thalamus from these structures (Figure 15.7). The caudate arises from the anterior portion of the putamen and extends superiorly and then postero-laterally to project into the temporal lobe, where it ends at the amygdala. Therefore, the head of the caudate can be found anteriorly and superiorly to the putamen, while the tail of the caudate can be found inferiorly and laterally to the putamen within

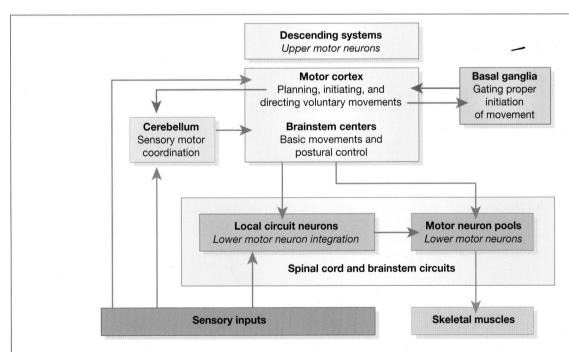

Figure 15.5 Schematic view of the interrelationship between the motor cortex, the basal ganglia, and the cerebellum, on central control of movement. Note that sensory input occurs at the cortex, the cerebellum and in the spinal cord.

Figure 15.6 A drawing of the relationship of the basal ganglia with the other deep cortical structures. Note that the internal capsule separates the thalamus medially from the basal ganglia laterally. Also, the head of the caudate nucleus arises from the anterior aspect of the putamen, the body of the caudate extends superiorly and laterally around the putamen to end as the tail of the caudate in the deep temporal lobe.

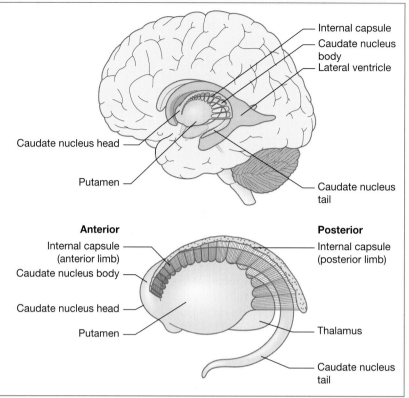

Figure 15.7 A drawing of an axial section of the brain at the level of the basal ganglia. The left hemi-section is a superior view, while the right hemi-section is an inferior view. Note the relationship of the basal ganglia (putamen, caudate nucleus, and globus pallidus) to the external capsule, internal capsule, and thalamus.

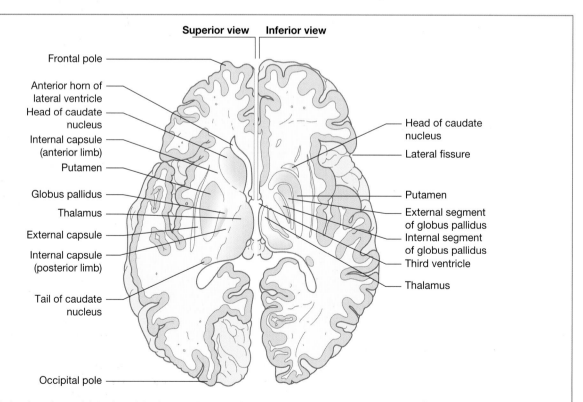

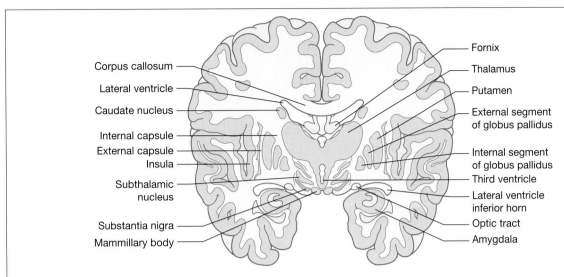

Figure 15.8 A drawing of an oblique section of the brain at the level of the basal ganglia. Note the relationship of the basal ganglia (putamen, caudate nucleus, and globus pallidus) to the external capsule, internal capsule, and thalamus.

the temporal lobe (Figure 15.8). Two other anatomical regions are functionally associated with the basal ganglia, but are not specifically a part of the basal ganglia. These are the **subthalamic nucleus** and the **substantia nigra**. The subthalamic nucleus is located in the region associated with its name, just inferior to the thalamus. The substantia nigra is found in the midbrain, adjacent to the cerebral peduncles and is named based on its black appearance (increased presence of melanin). When examining an oblique section of the brain and brain stem, the proximity of the basal ganglia to the substantia nigra can be easily observed (Figures 15.9, 15.10).

The neural input into the basal ganglia arises from the prefrontal cortex, the parietal cortex, and the motor areas of the frontal cortex (areas 4 and 6). These inputs are **excitatory** (glutaminergic) and enter the basal ganglia by way of the **striatum** (caudate and putamen) (Figure 15.11). These inputs are then relayed by a number of different circuits throughout the basal ganglia to produce a final output from the **internal globus pallidus** to the thalamus (ventral lateral nucleus), which then projects back to the frontal cortex (Figure 15.12). The internal globus pallidus produces a **tonic inhibitory output** to the thalamus which is then relayed as an inhibitory signal to the motor cortex (Figure 15.13). By modifying this tonic inhibition, increased motor activity can occur. As can be seen, this produces a feedback loop from the cortex through the basal ganglia back to the cortex, which can modify ongoing motor activity.

Within the basal ganglia, there are two main circuits. The first circuit is referred to as the **direct pathway** and involves **excitatory** stimulation from the cortex and substantia nigra to the striatum (putamen and caudate). This excitation of the striatum produces an inhibition of the internal globus pallidus which **decreases the tonic inhibition** from the globus pallidus to the thalamus, resulting in an **increase** in firing to the motor cortex. Therefore, in the direct pathway, the excitatory input produces an

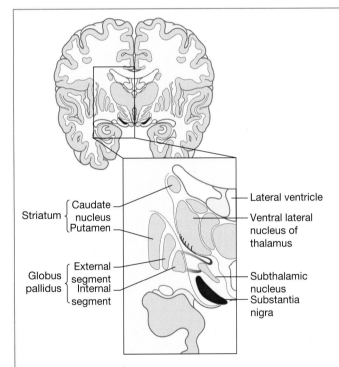

Figure 15.9 A drawing of a detailed oblique, section of the brain at the level of the basal ganglia. Note the relationship of the basal ganglia (putamen, caudate nucleus, and globus pallidus) to the subthalamic nucleus and the substantia nigra.

excitatory output at the cortex (Figure 15.14). The second circuit is referred to as the **indirect pathway** and utilizes the direct pathway with two additional intermediate steps. Again, excitatory input from the cortex stimulates the striatum (putamen and caudate), which then inhibits the **external globus pallidus**. The inhibition of the external globus pallidus leads to less inhibition of the

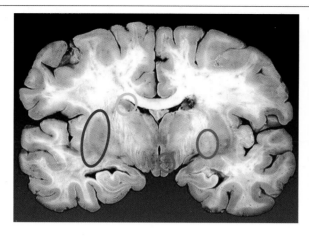
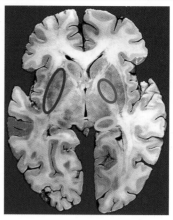

Figure 15.10 Identify the structures associated with the basal ganglia in these coronal and horizontal brain sections.

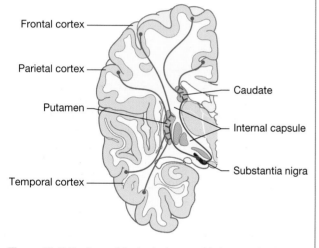

Figure 15.11 Regions of the brain that provide input to the basal ganglia. Note that the majority of inputs enter the caudate or the putamen (the striatum) and that they are excitatory.

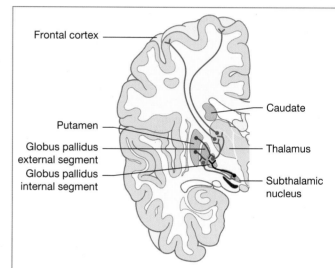

Figure 15.12 The interconnections and main output pathway of the basal ganglia. Note that the main output of the basal ganglia is from the internal globus pallidus to the thalamus and that this is a tonic inhibitory output.

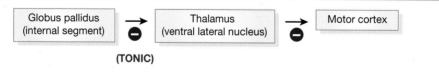

Figure 15.13 The main output of the basal ganglia is from the internal globus pallidus to the thalamus. Note that this is a tonic (continuous) inhibition of the thalamus that then inhibits the motor cortex.

subthalamic nucleus, which produces an excitatory input to the internal globus pallidus. This **excitation** of the tonic inhibition from the internal globus pallidus leads to a decrease in thalamic firing and a **decrease** in firing at the motor cortex (Figure 15.15). Notice that the indirect and direct pathways share the same excitatory input pathways and utilize the same output pathway from the internal globus pallidus. This means that the balance of activity between each pathway dictates the increase or decrease in tonic inhibition from the internal globus pallidus. A reasonable take home message is that the **direct pathway is excitatory** to the motor cortex, while the **indirect pathway is inhibitory** to the motor cortex (Figure 15.16). Imagine if there were a disruption in one pathway, how the other pathway would then dominate the output and produce disorders in motor activity.

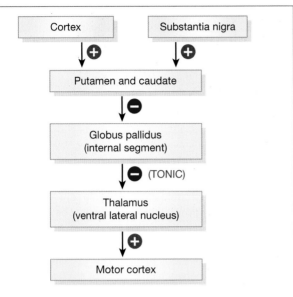

Figure 15.14 The direct pathway of basal ganglia regulation of motor activity begins with excitatory input from the cortex and substantia nigra to the striatum (putamen and caudate). The striatum then inhibits the internal globus pallidus. Note that the inhibition of the internal globus pallidus releases the tonic inhibition of the thalamus, producing an excitation at the cortex.

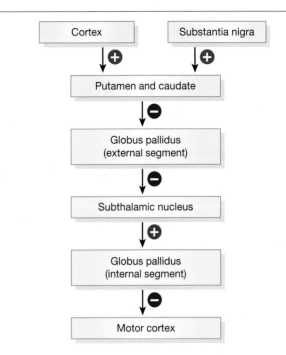

Figure 15.15 The indirect pathway of basal ganglia regulation of motor activity begins with excitatory input from the cortex and substantia nigra to the striatum (putamen and caudate). The striatum then inhibits the external globus pallidus. The external globus pallidus inhibits the subthalamic nucleus. The output from the subthalamic nucleus to the internal globus pallidus is stimulatory, producing an increase in the tonic inhibition of the thalamus. This leads to an inhibition at the cortex.

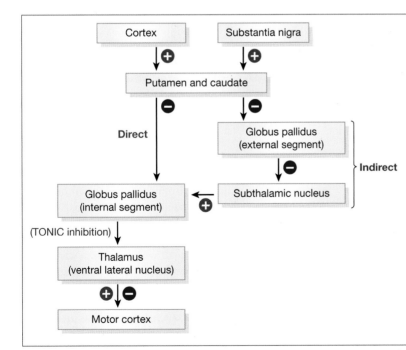

Figure 15.16 The combined direct and indirect pathways of basal ganglia regulation of motor activity. Excitatory input from the cortex and substantia nigra to the striatum (putamen and caudate) inhibits both the internal and external globus pallidus. The external globus pallidus inhibits the subthalamic nucleus. The output from the subthalamic nucleus to the internal globus pallidus is stimulatory. Therefore, there is an inhibitory signal from the striatum (direct pathway) and a stimulatory signal from the subthalamic nucleus (indirect pathway) modulating the tonic inhibition from the internal globus pallidus. This provides balance in the basal ganglia control of motor function. Note that the effect of the direct pathway on the cortex is excitatory, while the effect of the indirect pathway at the cortex is inhibitory.

Clinical box 15.1

Testing for motor disturbances can be difficult because of the numerous pathways involved in regulating motor function. Generally, clinicians begin to test for motor losses at the periphery (lower motor lesions) and then move centrally (upper motor lesions, cortical lesions, basal ganglia disturbances, or cerebellar problems). A detailed neurological exam is especially important to collect the full complement of symptoms presented by the patient (see Chapter 17). As mentioned in Chapter 11, a patient with a peripheral lower motor neuron lesion will present with muscle atrophy, hypotonia, and decreased deep tendon reflexes. A lower motor neuron loss can involve peripheral nerve compressions, such as a herniated disk in the vertebral column or carpal tunnel syndrome. These will usually have accompanying sensory deficits. The losses may occur over specific spinal cord levels (myotomal distribution).

Upper motor neuron lesions can involve the lateral corticospinal tract in the spinal cord, the corticospinal tract in the brain stem, the cerebral peduncle in the midbrain, or specific portions of the internal capsule. Patients with these lesions present with a Babinski sign, increased deep tendon reflexes, and hypertonia. These losses may be regional, but usually cover multiple myotomes and usually present with other deficits, depending on the location and extent of the lesion. Lesions of the precentral gyrus can produce upper motor neuron symptoms as well, since this is the location of the cell bodies for these neurons. Patients with losses in the premotor areas of the cortex usually present with difficulties in complex motor skills, especially those requiring coordination between both sides of the body (e.g. requiring the right hand to catch a ball thrown by the left hand).

Patients with basal ganglia disorders will usually have involuntary motor disturbances when at rest. These can be quite variable, ranging from smooth, large motions to mild tremors, depending on the disorder. When performing a willful motor activity, the patient's symptoms may be reduced or disappear.

Patients with cerebellar disorders, on the other hand, usually present with symptoms during a motor activity. These can include ataxia, gait disturbances, or difficulties with learned motor skills (e.g. riding a bicycle).

With the advent of excellent neurological imaging techniques (computed tomography and magnetic resonance imaging), the localization of lesions in the motor system has been improved. With the results of a detailed neurologic exam and an understanding of the neuroanatomy involved, the clinician can focus on specific regions of interest when examining these images, for confirmation of a diagnosis.

Clinical considerations

Disorders in the output pathway of motor control can be divided into two components, an **upper motor neuron lesion** or a **lower motor neuron lesion**. Upper motor neuron lesions include deficits in the precentral gyrus of the cortex, the internal capsule, the corticospinal tracts as they descend in the cerebral peduncles or pyramids, and the lateral corticospinal tract in the spinal cord. Lower motor neuron lesions include deficits in the anterior (ventral) horn cells in the spinal cord as well as the peripheral axonal projections to the skeletal muscles. To diagnose which of these two pathways is involved in a patient with a motor deficit, the clinician should collect information on the state of the muscles and the function of the patient's reflexes (Table 11.2 from Chapter 11).

Normally, if a blunt object is run along the sole of the foot from the heel to the toes, the patient's toes will curl down (towards the sole). However, if a patient has an upper motor neuron lesion, the patient's toes will fan upward (away from the sole). This is termed a **Babinski sign**. Newborn children that have not yet learned to walk may also exhibit a Babinski sign, since their upper motor neurons are not fully developed. Other signs associated with **upper motor neuron lesions** include increased muscle tone and increased deep tendon reflexes, without muscle wasting. Signs of **lower motor neuron lesions**, on the other hand, include muscle atrophy, fasciculations and fibrillations, decreased muscle tone, and decreased deep tendon reflexes (Table 11.2 from Chapter 11).

The first basal ganglia disorder to consider is a **hyperkinetic disorder** such as **Huntington's disease (chorea)**. Chorea consists of jerky, dance-like motions and can be found in a number of disorders, including Huntington's disease and dementia. If you recall that a person who designs dance movements is called a choreographer, you can understand where the term chorea originates. In Huntington's disease, there is a **decline in the indirect pathway** in the basal ganglia. This leads to less tonic inhibition from the internal portion of the globus pallidus, causing **increased excitation** to the cortex and leading to hyperkinetic motions (Figure 15.17). Huntington's disease is an autosomal dominant disease that only manifests in middle age; therefore, individuals with the disease can pass it on to their children before they know they have the disease. Genetic tests are available and the basic mechanisms of the disease are understood. There are, however, no treatments available and only the management of symptoms is currently offered.

The second basal ganglia disorder is the opposite of a hyperkinetic disorder – a **hypokinetic disorder**. **Parkinson's disease** is one example of a hypokinetic disorder. Patients

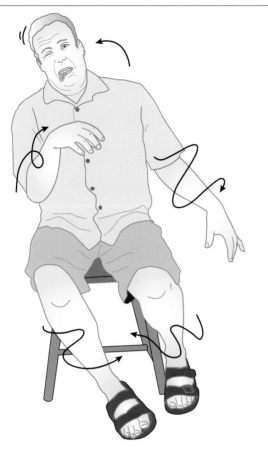

Figure 15.17 A drawing of a patient with Huntington's disease exhibiting chorea-like motions. This individual has a hyperkinetic disorder in his basal ganglia that produces less tonic inhibition of motor cortex activity.

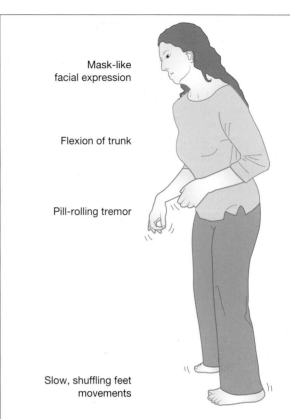

Mask-like facial expression

Flexion of trunk

Pill-rolling tremor

Slow, shuffling feet movements

Figure 15.18 A drawing of a patient with Parkinson's disease exhibiting a pill-rolling tremor and a "mask-like" facial expression. This individual has a hypokinetic disorder in her basal ganglia that produces more tonic inhibition of motor cortex activity.

with this disease exhibit a resting tremor with a characteristic "pill rolling" motion with their fingers. These patients also exhibit a lack of facial expression and have rigidity in the muscles of their extremities. In addition, patients can have difficulty starting and stopping specific motor events (Figure 15.18). The mechanism of Parkinson's disease is well characterized and is due to a degeneration of dopaminergic cells in the **substantia nigra**. Lack of substantia nigra input to the striatum (notably dopamine input) produces an excessive stimulation of the indirect basal ganglia pathway, while diminishing the direct basal ganglia pathway. This produces more tonic inhibition from the internal portion of the globus pallidus, causing **decreased excitation** to the cortex and leading to hypokinetic motor activity. One mechanism for treating Parkinson's disease is to provide the patient with more of the precursor for dopamine synthesis (l-dopa) which can help alleviate the endogenous loss of dopamine from the substantia nigra. This can slow the progressive symptoms of the disease, but it is not a cure. Deep brain stimulation, through surgically-implanted electrodes, can also be used to reverse the symptoms of Parkinson's disease.

Other motor system disorders include **athetosis**, which is a slow, writhing motion, and **ballismus**, which is a flailing and flinging motion of the extremities. When ballismus occurs unilaterally, it is referred to as **hemiballismus** and can be due to a lesion in the contralateral subthalamic nucleus. Recall how a lesion of the subthalamic nucleus would impact on the indirect basal ganglia pathway and produce excessive motor activity.

While the description of these motor system disorders seems straightforward, it should be apparent that there are numerous anatomical regions involved in these disorders and that a range of severity can be seen in patients, based on the involvement of anatomical and neurochemical systems. Recall that the cortex, the cerebellum, and the basal ganglia are all involved in regulation of motor activity. Therefore, a defect in any of these regions can produce motor deficits. In a simplistic manner, descending motor pathway deficits generally produce **spasticity**, while cerebellar disorders generally produce **ataxia**. Basal ganglia disorders, on the other hand, generally produce **hypokinetic** or **hyperkinetic** symptoms. In reality, however, distinguishing the actual site of the deficit by analyzing a patient's clinical symptoms can be quite difficult, due to the complex interrelationships between these pathways.

Case 1

A 32-year-old nurse, Ms Robin Phillips, was driving her car when she was hit by an overly aggressive driver who cut in front of her on the expressway. She sustained a rapid motion head injury in which she was rendered unconscious. She was transported to a regional hospital by the emergency medical technicians that responded to her accident.

After regaining consciousness, while still in the hospital, Ms Phillips becomes aware of her inability to move her right lower limb. A neurologist, Dr Jill Smith, performs a complete neurological exam. After the exam, Ms Phillips is found to have a loss of skeletal motor control in her right thigh, leg, and foot, with no other skeletal motor losses. Luckily, she does not have sensory or cognitive losses.

During the examination, Dr Smith runs the handle of her reflex hammer up the sole of Ms Phillips' right foot and notices that her toes flare out (**Babinski sign**), while doing the same procedure on Ms Phillips' left foot, her toes curl under normally. Dr Smith also notices that Ms Phillips has increased muscle tone and increased deep tendon reflexes in her right lower extremity.

Dr Smith discusses her findings with Ms Phillips, explaining that she appears to have an **upper motor neuron lesion**, perhaps due to a contusion of the cerebral peduncles in her midbrain (Figure 15.19) or at some other point in the descending corticospinal tract. With time and physical therapy, Ms Phillips regains partial function in her lower extremity, but she is unable to regain full motor control.

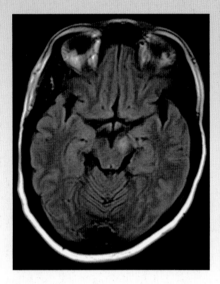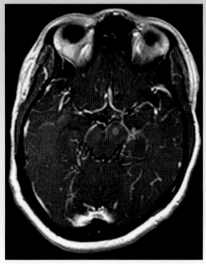

Figure 15.19 Axial magnetic resonance images (without and with contrast) of a patient with a left cerebral peduncle lesion. Note the hyperintense area in the left cerebral peduncle of the midbrain.

Case 2

A 58-year-old faculty member in the philosophy department of the local university, Dr Ron Church, began experiencing tremors in his right hand that were noticeable when he tried to sit in his easy chair and read. The tremors occurred while his hand was at rest, but were not noticeable when he turned the pages of his book. He thought this was a sign of aging and did not discuss the symptoms with his physician. As time passed, the tremor in his right hand worsened and he noticed a slight tremor in his right foot as well.

At his next annual physical exam, he mentioned the tremors to his physician, Dr Randy King, who could observe

the tremors himself. Dr King also noticed that Dr Church had a "flat" expressionless facial appearance. Dr King suggested that Dr Church have a full neurological exam to determine if other subtle neurologic symptoms existed.

After a complete neurologic exam, Dr Church is diagnosed with **Parkinson's disease** due to a decline in dopaminergic neurons in the substantia nigra. Dr King prescribes pharmacologic compounds that can increase dopamine levels to offset the loss that is occurring. This is a stopgap measure and does not treat the underlying cause of the disease; it merely provides an exogenous way to increase central dopamine levels.

The pharmacologic treatments reduce the tremors and provide a better lifestyle for Dr Church, but, over time, the dose needs to be increased to maintain the same level of control. Ten years after the initial diagnosis, Dr Church is having noticeable side effects due to the high dosage of the drugs, with less ability to control the symptoms. In discussion with his neurologist and Dr King, they begin looking at other alternatives to the drug therapy. One alternative is the use of implantable electrodes placed in the subthalamic nucleus, which when activated can reduce Parkinson's symptoms (Figure 15.20). This surgical procedure in conjunction with lower doses of the drugs can provide good control.

Dr Church is assessed to be a good candidate for the procedure and he believes this will help control his symptoms, so he agrees to undergo the surgery. After the surgery with the implants activated, Dr Church has much better motor control and is satisfied with the results.

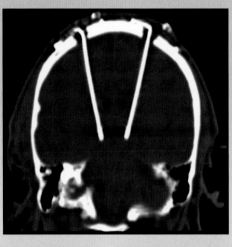

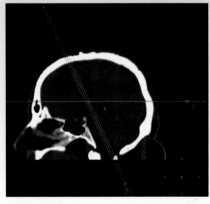
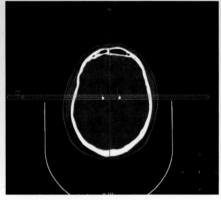

Figure 15.20 Frontal, sagittal, and axial computed tomograph images of a patient with deep brain stimulation electrodes to reduce the symptoms of Parkinsonism.

Study questions

1. Which of the following structures is involved in the indirect pathway of the basal ganglia, but not the direct pathway?
a) putamen
b) substantia nigra
c) subthalamic nucleus
d) internal globus pallidus
e) thalamus

2. A 45-year-old female patient with a hyperkinetic disorder, such as Huntington's chorea, has a(n):
a) decrease in the tonic activity of the internal globus pallidus
b) increase in the tonic activity of the internal globus pallidus
c) decrease in the tonic activity of the external globus pallidus
d) increase in the tonic activity of the external globus pallidus
e) inhibitory activity in the external globus pallidus
f) excitatory activity of the external globus pallidus

3. A 48-year-old male patient presents with muscle atrophy in the muscles of his left hand, with no change in his reflexes. His physician would need to look carefully at the:

a) right precentral gyrus of the cortex
b) right cerebral peduncle
c) pyramids in the medulla
d) left lateral corticospinal tract
e) left anterior (ventral) horn of the cervical spinal cord

4. A 37-year-old female patient has a loss of motor function on the right side of her face below the eye, but not on her right forehead or the left side of her face. Her physician would expect to find a lesion in the:

a) left facial nerve (VII)
b) right facial nerve (VII)
c) face area in the precentral gyrus of the right cortex
d) face area in the precentral gyrus of the left cortex

5. The striatum is composed of the:

a) putamen and caudate nucleus
b) putamen and globus pallidus
c) globus pallidus and caudate nucleus
d) globus pallidus and subthalamic nucleus
e) putamen and subthalamic nucleus

For more self-assessment questions, visit the companion website at
www.wileyessential.com/neuroanatomy

FURTHER READING

For additional information on central motor control, the following textbooks and review articles may be helpful:

Beitz JM. 2014. Parkinson's disease: a review. *Front Biosci (Schol Ed)*, 6: 65–74.

Blumenfeld H. 2002. *Neuroanatomy Through Clinical Cases*. Sinauer Associates, Sunderland, Massachusetts.

Bosch-Bouju C, Hyland BI, Parr-Brownlie LC. 2013. Motor thalamus integration of cortical, cerebellar and basal ganglia information: implications for normal and Parkinsonian conditions. *Front Comput Neurosci*, 7:163 (1–21).

Felten DL, Shetty A. 2009. *Netter's Atlas of Neuroscience*, 2nd edition. Saunders Elsevier, Philadelphia, Pennsylvania.

Fisher SD, Reynolds JN. 2014. The intralaminar thalamus – an expressway linking visual stimuli to circuits determining agency and action selection. *Front Behav Neurosci*, 8: 115 (1–7).

Haines DE. 2012. *Neuroanatomy: An Atlas of Structures, Sections and Systems*, 8th edition. Lippincott Williams & Wilkin, Baltimore, Maryland.

Moore KL, Dalley AF, Agur AMR. 2014. *Moore Clinically Oriented Anatomy*, 7th edition. Lippincott, Williams & Wilkins, Philadelphia, Pennsylvania.

Patestas MA, Gartner LP. 2006. *A Textbook of Neuroanatomy*. Blackwell Publishing, Malden, Massachusetts.

Ward P, Seri S, Cavanna AE. 2013. Functional neuroanatomy and behavioural correlates of the basal ganglia: evidence from lesion studies. *Behav Neurol*, 26(4): 219–223.

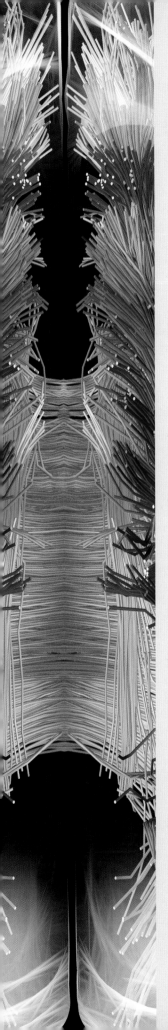

CHAPTER 16
Limbic system

Learning objectives

1. Identify the components of the limbic system.
2. Describe the functions of the amygdala.
3. Describe the functions of the hippocampal formation.
4. Describe the clinical deficits associated with loss of the amygdala or hippocampus.

Essential Clinical Neuroanatomy, First Edition. Thomas H. Champney.
© 2016 John Wiley & Sons, Ltd. Published 2016 by John Wiley & Sons, Ltd.
Companion website: www.wileyessential.com/neuroanatomy

Introduction

The limbic system is a unique part of the nervous system which is responsible for a number of lower-level cognitive functions. These include homeostatic mechanisms, emotions, memory, reward, and olfactory recognition. Many of these functions occur in evolutionarily older regions of the brain. While the basic role of the limbic system is understood, there are still many aspects to the system that are not well described.

Anatomy of the limbic system

The anatomy of the limbic system is comprised of numerous regions of the brain that surround or are in close proximity to the diencephalon. These include the cingulate gyrus and orbito-frontal cortex, the hippocampus, the amygdala, the mammillary bodies and fornix, the hypothalamus, specific thalamic nuclei, the nucleus accumbens (ventral striatum), the insula, and the olfactory system. As can be seen, the majority of these structures are found in the deep central portion of the brain in regions that are believed to be evolutionarily older (Figure 16.1). Evolutionary old cortex (archicortex) is simplistic, with only three cellular layers, compared with more recent cortex (neocortex) that is complex, with six cellular layers. Many of the cortical parts of the limbic system have archicortex, indicating the older evolutionary age of the limbic system.

The **cingulate gyrus** and **orbitofrontal cortex** are located just superior and anterior to the corpus callosum, respectively. This places them in close proximity to the other structures of the limbic system. The **hypothalamus**, the thalamus, the **mammillary bodies**, and the **fornix** are all found in the diencephalon, deep to the corpus callosum (Figure 16.2). Each fornix is a neural tract that extends from the deep temporal lobe posteriorly, superiorly, and medially around the thalamus to project into the mammillary body (Figure 16.3). At the anterior end near the mammillary bodies, each fornix communicates with its opposite member (Figure 16.4). The temporal end of the fornix merges into the **hippocampus** in the medial temporal lobe. The hippocampus, when viewed in cross section, has the appearance of a seahorse lying on its back (Figure 16.5). This is the reason it was named the hippocampus (the scientific name for the seahorse). The substructure of the hippocampus is divided into the **dentate gyrus**, the **subiculum**, and the **parahippocampal gyrus**. Extensive research has been completed on the detailed structure and function of the hippocampus. Anterior to the hippocampus in the temporal lobe is the **amygdala**. The amygdala contains three nuclei, referred to as the central nucleus, medial nucleus, and basolateral nucleus (Figures 16.6, 16.7). These nuclei interact with each other and have neural connections with the other regions of the limbic system. Therefore, the structures of the limbic system are in close proximity and interconnected by specific neural pathways.

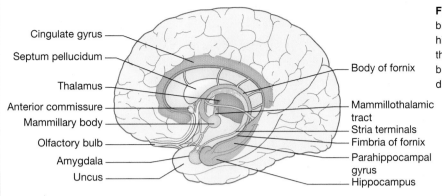

Figure 16.1 A midsagittal drawing of the brain with the brain stem removed to highlight the limbic structures. Note how the limbic structures are found deep in the brain and have a close relationship with the diencephalon.

Cingulate gyrus
Septum pellucidum
Thalamus
Anterior commissure
Mammillary body
Olfactory bulb
Amygdala
Uncus

Body of fornix
Mammillothalamic tract
Stria terminals
Fimbria of fornix
Parahippocampal gyrus
Hippocampus

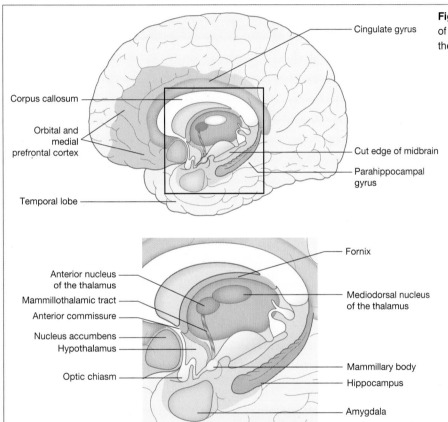

Figure 16.2 A drawing of the components of the limbic system with the area around the diencephalon magnified.

Cingulate gyrus
Corpus callosum
Orbital and medial prefrontal cortex
Temporal lobe
Cut edge of midbrain
Parahippocampal gyrus

Anterior nucleus of the thalamus
Mammillothalamic tract
Anterior commissure
Nucleus accumbens
Hypothalamus
Optic chiasm

Fornix
Mediodorsal nucleus of the thalamus
Mammillary body
Hippocampus
Amygdala

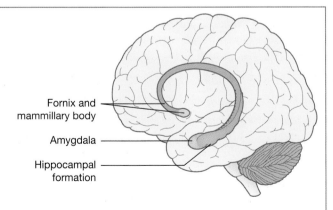

Fornix and mammillary body
Amygdala
Hippocampal formation

Figure 16.3 A drawing of the brain with the relationship between the fornix, the hippocampus, amygdala, and mammillary body.

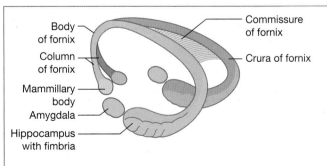

Body of fornix
Column of fornix
Mammillary body
Amygdala
Hippocampus with fimbria

Commissure of fornix
Crura of fornix

Figure 16.4 A schematized drawing of the hippocampus, fornix, and mammillary bodies. Note how each fornix can communicate with the opposite fornix through its commissure.

Figure 16.5 A myelin-stained coronal section of the brain with the hippocampus highlighted.

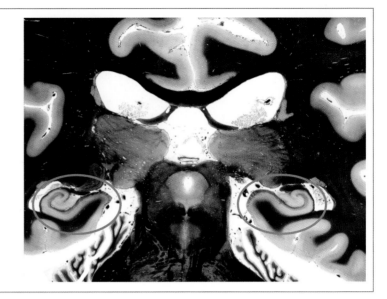

Figure 16.6 A drawing and myelin-stained coronal section of the amygdala with its location in the anterior medial temporal lobe.

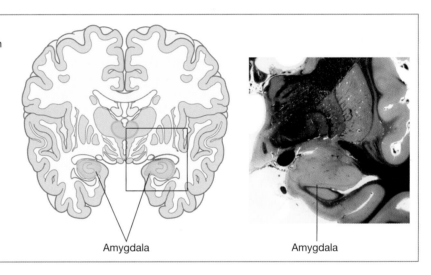

Amygdala   Amygdala

Figure 16.7 A myelin-stained coronal section of the brain with the amygdala highlighted. Note that this coronal section is anterior to Figure 16.5. Also, note the basal ganglia structures: the putamen, caudate nucleus, and the globus pallidus.

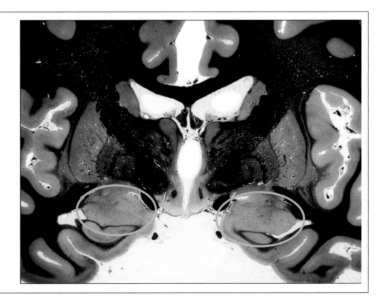

Clinical box 16.1

The microanatomy and neural circuitry of the hippocampus within the medial portion of the temporal lobe has been described in great detail. While this has been valuable in elucidating the function of the hippocampus in relation to memory formation, it is not as clinically relevant. Damage to the hippocampus disrupts the hippocampal microcircuitry and leaves the hippocampus non-functional. Therefore, knowing the type of fibers involved, the neurotransmitters used, or other details cannot, at present, be used clinically to restore hippocampal function.

For those interested in the cellular anatomy of the hippocampal formation, it can be subdivided into six sub-regions: the subiculum laterally, the hippocampus proper with four regions of Ammon's horn (CA1–CA4), and the dentate gyrus, medially. These regions have been "rolled up" like a carpet, so that the subiculum is adjacent to the dentate. Each of these has a unique microarchitecture based on the three layers of the archicortex: a molecular layer, a pyramidal or granule cell layer, and a polymorphic layer. These regions communicate with each other by a microcircuitry that includes the perforant pathway, the alvear pathway, mossy fibers, and Schaffer collaterals. Inputs to the hippocampus are from the association areas of the cortex, as well as from septal areas, and the contralateral hippocampus via commissural fibers. The outputs from the hippocampus project back to the association areas as well as to the diencephalon and septal areas by way of the fornix. A simplistic hypothesis is that the association areas bring the sensory "memory" information into the hippocampus for consolidation with the septal areas, adding emotional or contextual components. The outputs to the association areas are for long-term memory storage, with feedback to the other areas.

A unique aspect of the hippocampus is the ability of the neurons to develop a form of sustained neuronal firing, described as **long-term potentiation**. It is believed that this process aids in the development of memories. Because of the increased sensitivity to neural activity within the hippocampus, it can be one of the focal sites of epilepsy. The hippocampus has also been implicated in the forgetfulness that occurs with age and with the memory disturbances that occur with dementia, such as Alzheimer's disease.

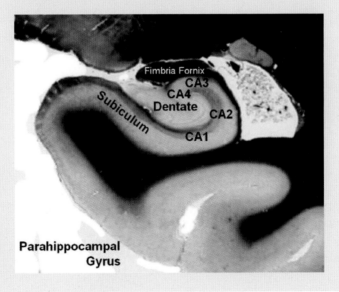

Historically, a pathway was described in the limbic system: the **Papez circuit** (Figure 16.8). This is a reciprocal feedback circuit that connects the hippocampus through the fornix to the mammillary bodies, from the mammillary bodies to the anterior thalamic nucleus, with projections to the cingulate gyrus of the cortex. The cingulate gyrus has connections back to the hippocampus, completing the circuit. While the connections in the circuit undoubtedly exist, it has been shown that each of these limbic structures interacts with numerous other components in a much more complex fashion than the simplistic nature depicted by the Papez circuit.

Another well-described pathway that involves limbic system structures includes the **medial forebrain bundle** which projects from the ventral tegmental area to the amygdala, the nucleus accumbens, the septum, the hypothalamus, and the prefrontal cortex (Figure 16.9). All of these structures interact with each other, as well as with the hypothalamus, to produce a balanced and coordinated response to external stimuli.

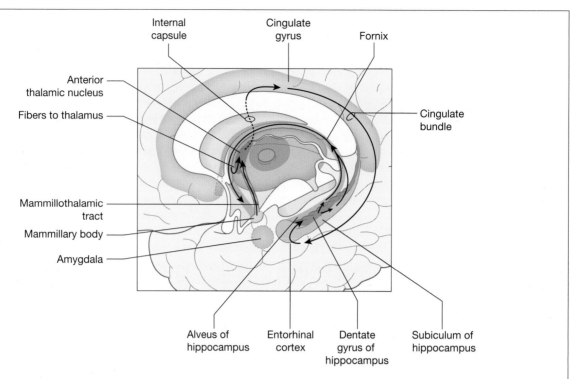

Figure 16.8 A drawing of a medial view of the brain with the brain stem removed, highlighting the Papez circuit within the limbic system.

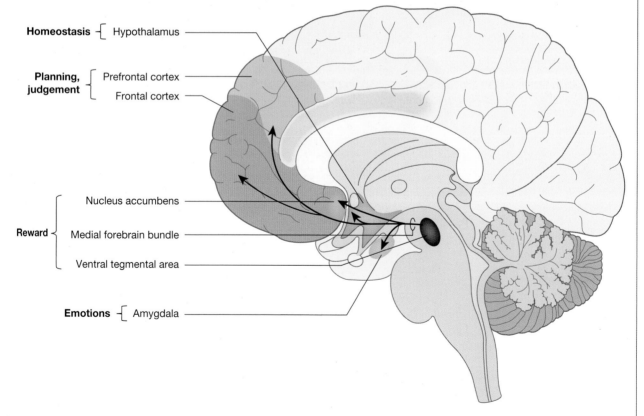

Figure 16.9 A drawing of the medial forebrain bundle and its connections with cortical, hypothalamic, and limbic structures. Note the functions associated with each of these areas and how they can interact via connections with the medial forebrain bundle.

Functions of the limbic system

Memory and learning

The ability to learn new declarative information and to recall that information takes place in the **hippocampus**. The acquisition of verbal memories occurs in the dominant hippocampus (usually the left side), while the acquisition of spatial memories occurs in the non-dominant hippocampus. The long-term storage of information is not as well understood and appears to be disseminated more widely throughout the cortex. The knowledge that the hippocampus is the acquisition site for new memories is due in great part to a specific patient who, in 1953, had bilateral surgical removal of the hippocampus to alleviate seizures. This famous patient, referred to as HM (Henri Molaison), has provided unique insights into the acquisition of memories. HM was unable to acquire any new memories, but retained his previously acquired memories. A more detailed and fascinating description of HM's contribution to neuroscience can be found in his scientific obituary (Squire, 2009).

Emotional experience and expression

The experience and expression of emotions utilizes the **amygdala** as one of the major neural centers. The amygdala regulates mood, aggression, social cues, and other behaviors (Adolphs, 2012; Koelsch, 2014). The amygdala appears to attach social and/or emotional meaning to sensory information. It also acts as the site of recognition of fear, as well as a mediator of emotional memories. In addition, the amygdala provides the source for the startle reflex: the ability to react to a new stimulus in an appropriate manner. For

---

Clinical box 16.2

Our understanding of the role of the hippocampus in learning and memory is substantially due to one man's surgical outcome that was examined for years afterward. Over 60 years ago, this patient, referred to as HM, had the medial aspects of his temporal lobes surgically removed to prevent epileptic seizures. As soon as the surgery was over, it was found that he could no longer acquire new, declarative memories. This is referred to as **anterograde amnesia** as opposed to retrograde amnesia, which occurs when previous memories are lost. HM was studied for decades after his surgery to understand how the **hippocampus** is involved in acquisition of new memories and learning.

It was found, for example, that HM could not remember new names, the current president, or information that he was told the previous day. However, he still remembered his address from his childhood and he remembered who the president was prior to his surgery. Interestingly, his motor memories (e.g. riding a bike) were not affected and he could learn new, non-declarative types of information. If he was given a three-dimensional puzzle to solve, he could complete a few steps in one day. The next day, he would not remember ever seeing the puzzle, but he would be able to complete the first steps quickly and then move onto subsequent steps. Within a few days, he would have solved the puzzle, but could not recall seeing the puzzle before (a "conflict" between his inability to remember declarative memories and his ability to learn new non-declarative memories). For further information on HM and his contribution to neuroscience research, an excellent tribute to him was written after his death (Squire, 2009).

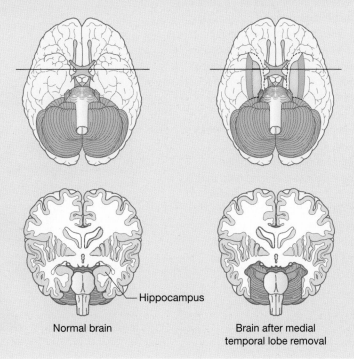

Normal brain

Brain after medial temporal lobe removal

Hippocampus

example, patients with rare bilateral amygdala lesions (**Klüver-Bucy syndrome**) (Kusano, *et al.*, 2012) display flattened emotions and have an inability to recognize fearful objects. These patients also have hyperorality (the need to place things in their mouth) and hypersexuality (the uninhibited acting out of sexual desires).

Homeostasis

One of the main functions of the limbic system is to maintain homeostasis within the body. This primarily falls in the realm of the **hypothalamus**. The hypothalamus contains numerous small tightly packed nuclei that respond to environmental changes with neural activity (Chapter 8). These include water balance (thirst), hunger/satiety, temperature regulation, circadian rhythms, and other functions. While the hypothalamus is the primary site in homeostatic regulation, there are many other inputs to the hypothalamus from the cortex, the brain stem, and other parts of limbic system, which can impact on homeostasis and autonomic function. Further details on hypothalamic function can be found in recent review articles (Buijs, 2013; Buijs *et al.*, 2013; Flouris, 2011; Schneeberger *et al.*, 2014).

Reward

The reward pathway is a pleasure, motivation and reinforcement pathway that provides positive responses to basic drives such as feeding and sexual activity. It is also associated with addictive behaviors and is involved in the pleasure observed with drugs of abuse. It is a dopaminergic pathway (mesolimbic) that involves both limbic and cortical structures, most notably the ventral tegmental area and the nucleus accumbens (Figure 16.9). While the nucleus accumbens appears to be the primary site of the pleasure/reward responses, it interacts with the hypothalamus (for pleasure responses to feeding and sex), the hippocampus (for memories related to pleasure), the amygdala (for emotional aspects of pleasure) and the prefrontal cortex (for cognitive aspects of pleasure). Therefore, there is an interplay with many limbic structures in the expression of pleasure and reward (Arias-Carrion, *et al.*, 2014).

Olfactory sensation and processing

While the olfactory system is sensory for smell, it also has direct connections with components of the limbic system. Specifically, some axons in the **olfactory tract** project to the hypothalamus, thalamus, orbitofrontal cortex, and amygdala. The direct projections to the amygdala suggest that smells can have an emotional aspect, since the amygdala is involved in emotional processing. Because the olfactory system has direct input to the limbic system, it is believed that the olfactory system is one of the oldest sensory systems and feeds directly into limbic system responses. Other sensory systems can also have an impact on limbic system function, but these all have indirect inputs by way of thalamic and cortical projections.

Clinical considerations

Bilateral lesions in the **mammillary bodies** can be produced with a vitamin B1 (thiamine) deficiency (**Wernicke-Korsakoff syndrome**) (Jung *et al.*, 2012). These lesions

---

Clinical box 16.3

A specific example that can provide insight into the role of the limbic system on behavior is the case of Charles Whitman. In 1966, Charles Whitman climbed to the top of the University of Texas clock tower and randomly shot 38 individuals, killing 14 people. Prior to his actions, he realized he had a mental disturbance but was unable to find proper treatment. He consulted a psychiatrist and discussed his uncontrollable violent impulses, which included thoughts about randomly shooting people. He was given an appointment for the next week. He attempted to turn himself into the police, but since he had not committed a crime, he was not retained. Interestingly, when reading his journal entries from this time period, it is apparent that he retained his intellect and realized that changes in his behavior had occurred, but he felt powerless to stop acting upon those impulses. During a postmortem autopsy of his brain, a **glioblastoma** was found in the region of the hypothalamus that extended into the temporal lobe, compressing the amygdala. It is hypothesized that this tumor modified his limbic system function and altered his behavior, producing the resulting tragedy.

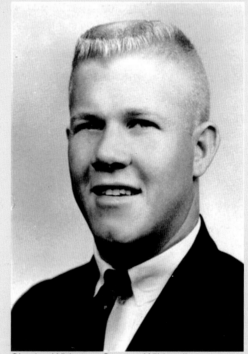

Charles Whitman. Source: Wikipedia

can be found in chronic alcoholics, who develop vitamin deficiencies due to poor dietary habits. These patients generally show apathy, anterograde amnesia, and confabulation (making up a story to fit the circumstances). These patients also have ataxia and can display ophthalmoplegia. While some of the symptoms can be alleviated with the return to proper vitamin B1 levels, others are difficult or impossible to recover.

Interestingly, research has shown that with **prolonged stress**, the amygdala has new neuronal outgrowth, while the hippocampus has neuronal degeneration (Boyle, 2013; Leuner and Shors, 2013). This is believed to produce a heightened response to fear and panic, with a concomitant loss of short-term memory while under prolonged stress. Therefore, stress (e.g., post traumatic stress disorder) and other environmental factors can have pronounced effects on limbic system function.

Case 1

A 38-year-old female accountant, Mrs Audrey Johnson, was involved in an automobile accident where she suffered traumatic brain injury, along with other peripheral injuries. After her other injuries were treated and while she was recovering in the hospital, her husband and family began noticing cognitive changes in Mrs Johnson. She had difficulty finding words, had a programmed speech pattern, and could not recognize some of her family friends when they visited. Her emotional affect became flattened and she did not smile or laugh as she had in the past. She also continuously chewed on toothpicks or other objects and started to behave provocatively with the male health care staff.

Mrs Johnson's husband noted many of these symptoms to the medical staff. Her neurologist, Dr Stephen Curry, suggested that an MRI be obtained to determine if any trauma had occurred. On the MRI, there were indications of diffuse blunt traumatic brain injury, especially in the medial-anterior portion of the temporal lobe (Figure 16.10). Dr Curry hypothesized that Mrs Johnson's amygdalae could have been injured during the car accident, leading to a presentation of **amygdala dysfunction**, Klüver-Bucy syndrome.

After researching the medical literature for descriptions of this rare syndrome (Kusano *et al.*, 2012), Dr Curry discussed his results with Mr and Mrs Johnson. He mentioned that in most instances this type of injury resolves over time. Two months after the accident, Mrs Johnson returned for a follow-up neurological exam. Both she and Dr Curry were pleased to see that the majority of the symptoms associated with Klüver-Bucy syndrome had resolved. Mrs Johnson still had some difficulties with word choice and sentence construction, but overall her recovery from the accident was excellent.

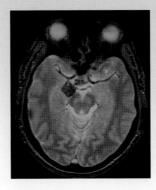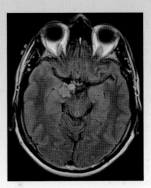

Figure 16.10 Two axial magnetic resonance images of a patient with an amygdala lesion. Note the darker lesion in the right medial temporal region (on the right image) impacting on the amygdala.

Case 2

A 42-year-old single construction worker, Mr James Warren, begins having visual disturbances and problems maintaining his balance. When he falls off a ladder at his job and requires treatment at the emergency room, a third year resident, Dr Mike Vu, collects Mr Warren's history and physical.

When Mr Warren mentions his vision and balance problems, Dr Vu examines him more closely and finds that he has diplopia, occasional nystagmus, and a wide-stanced gait. The resident also notices that Mr Warren provides short answers to his questions and appears apathetic and indifferent to his surroundings. While at first denying any alcohol use, Mr Warren reluctantly admits that he drinks three six-packs of beer per night and is generally not that hungry.

Dr Vu reports to the attending physician and suggests that Mr Warren may have a nutritional disorder: a thiamine (vitamin B1) deficiency due to his excessive alcohol consumption (**Wernicke-Korsakoff syndrome**) (Jung, *et al.*, 2012; Krill and Harper, 2012). The attending physician concurs and suggests that Dr Vu counsel Mr Warren about the disorder.

Dr Vu talks frankly with Mr Warren, describing how low levels of thiamine can cause a disruption in a neural pathway in the brain involving the mammillary bodies. This disruption can produce visual problems, along with balance and walking difficulties. Dr Vu suggests that Mr Warren eats a better diet, that he takes a multivitamin with thiamine, and that he limits his alcohol intake. He also prescribes intramuscular thiamine injections to help restore Mr Warren's thiamine levels.

Mr Warren takes Dr Vu's suggestions seriously and begins to follow his advice. He maintains good nutritional intake and reduces his alcohol intake. Six months later, many of the symptoms have resolved. However, one year later, after a very stressful period in his life, Mr Warren begins drinking again and his proper nutritional intake declines.

Study questions

1. A 58-year-old male patient with a thiamine deficiency who has anterograde amnesia, confabulation, and ataxia could have a lesion in the:
a) amygdala
b) hippocampus
c) mammillary bodies
d) hypothalamus
e) cingulate gyrus

2. A 47-year-old female patient who presents with a loss of fear and an inability to recognize faces could have a lesion in the:
a) amygdala
b) hippocampus
c) mammillary bodies
d) hypothalamus
e) cingulate gyrus

3. A 28-year-old male patient with intractable epilepsy has the medial regions of his temporal lobes removed. After the surgery, he has anterograde amnesia. Which region was damaged by the surgery?
a) amygdala
b) hippocampus
c) mammillary bodies
d) hypothalamus
e) cingulate gyrus

4. The neural region that helps maintain homeostasis is the:
a) amygdala
b) hippocampus
c) mammillary bodies
d) hypothalamus
e) cingulate gyrus

5. The structure anterior to the hippocampus in the temporal lobe is the:
a) amygdala
b) nucleus accumbens
c) fornix
d) hypothalamus
e) cingulate gyrus

 For more self-assessment questions, visit the companion website at
www.wileyessential.com/neuroanatomy

FURTHER READING

For additional information on the limbic system, the following textbooks and review articles may be helpful:

Adolphs R. 2013. The biology of fear. *Curr Biol*, 23(2): R79–R93.

Arias-Carrión O, Caraza-Santiago X, Salgado-Licona S, Salama M, Machado S, Nardi AE, Menéndez-González M, Murillo-Rodríguez E. 2014. Orquestic regulation of neurotransmitters on reward-seeking behavior. *Int Arch Med*, 7: 29–44.

Blumenfeld H. 2002. *Neuroanatomy Through Clinical Cases*. Sinauer Associates, Sunderland, Massachusetts.

Boyle LM. 2013. A neuroplasticity hypothesis of chronic stress in the basolateral amygdala. *Yale J Biol Med*, 86(2): 117–125.

Buijs RM. 2013. The autonomic nervous system: a balancing act. *Handb Clin Neurol*, 117: 1–11.

Buijs RM, Escobar C, Swaab DF. 2013. The circadian system and the balance of the autonomic nervous system. *Handb Clin Neurol*, 117: 173–191.

Felten DL, Shetty A. 2009. *Netter's Atlas of Neuroscience*, 2nd edition. Saunders Elsevier, Philadelphia, Pennsylvania.

Flouris AD. 2011. Functional architecture of behavioural thermoregulation. *Eur J Appl Physiol*, 111(1): 1–8.

Haines DE. 2012. *Neuroanatomy: An Atlas of Structures, Sections and Systems*, 8th edition. Lippincott Williams & Wilkin, Baltimore, Maryland.

Jung YC, Chanraud S, Sullivan EV. 2012. Neuroimaging of Wernicke's encephalopathy and Korsakoff's syndrome. *Neuropsychol Rev*, 22(2): 170–180.

Koelsch S. 2014. Brain correlates of music-evoked emotions. *Nat Rev Neurosci*, 15(3): 170–180.

Kril JJ, Harper CG. 2012. Neuroanatomy and neuropathology associated with Korsakoff's syndrome. *Neuropsychol Rev*, 22(2): 72–80.

Kusano Y, Horiuchi T, Tanaka Y, Tsuji T, Hongo K. 2012. Transient Klüver-Bucy syndrome caused by cerebral edema following aneurysmal subarachnoid hemorrhage. *Clin Neurol Neurosurg*, 114(3): 294–296.

Leuner B, Shors TJ. 2013. Stress, anxiety, and dendritic spines: what are the connections? *Neuroscience*, 251: 108–119.

Moore KL, Dalley AF, Agur AMR. 2014. *Moore Clinically Oriented Anatomy*, 7th edition. Lippincott, Williams & Wilkins, Philadelphia, Pennsylvania.

Patestas MA, Gartner LP. 2006. *A Textbook of Neuroanatomy*. Blackwell Publishing, Malden, Massachusetts.

Schneeberger M, Gomis R, Claret M. 2014. Hypothalamic and brain stem neuronal circuits controlling homeostatic energy balance. *J Endocrinol*, 220(2): T25–T46.

Squire LR. 2009. The legacy of patient H.M. for neuroscience. *Neuron*, 61: 6–9.

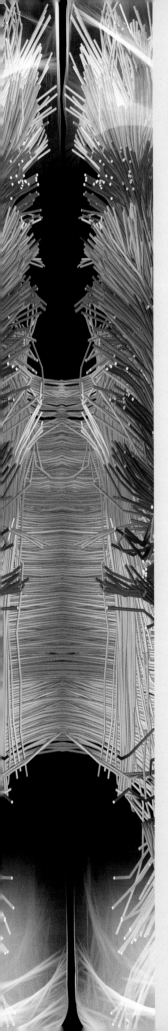

CHAPTER 17
Cortical integration

Learning objectives

1. Describe the functional anatomy of the cerebral cortex.
2. Discuss the interrelationships between the cortical domains.
3. Describe the clinical conditions that affect the cerebral cortex.

Essential Clinical Neuroanatomy, First Edition. Thomas H. Champney.
© 2016 John Wiley & Sons, Ltd. Published 2016 by John Wiley & Sons, Ltd.
Companion website: www.wileyessential.com/neuroanatomy

Introduction

The integration of cortical function occurs when the regions of the cortex communicate with each other. While there is very good evidence that specific cortical functions are localized in specific regions of the cortex, there is also evidence to support a more global or diversified functional component throughout the cortical regions. This can make understanding cortical function more difficult because of the two separate yet interrelated aspects of cortical activity. This chapter will provide a generalized overview of cortical function and some of the deficits that can occur with specific lesions within the cortex.

Anatomical organization of the cortex

Over one hundred years ago, Korbinian Brodmann, a neuroanatomist, carefully examined the regions of the cortex and found specific histological differences in different regions. He numbered each region of cortex that was histologically different and produced a cortical map, with over 50 different regions delineated. This was long before any known functions were attributed to the specific regions and it was only decades later that researchers were able to apply specific functions to these numbered regions (Loukas *et al.*, 2011). **Brodmann's areas**, as they are known today, are used to denote specific areas of cortex that have specific functions (Figure 17.1a and b). For example, the strip of cortex anterior to the central sulcus is referred to as the **precentral gyrus** or Brodmann's area 4 and is functionally attributed to the skeletal motor output of the corticospinal tract. Likewise, the strip of cortex posterior to the central sulcus (referred to as the **postcentral gyrus** or Brodmann's area 3 (along with 1 and 2)) is functionally attributed to the somatosensory input from the thalamus (Figure 17.1c).

When examining the neurohistology of cortical structures, a large variation in the architecture of the cortex can be observed. Some regions of cortex have six well-defined layers of cells and are believed to be the most recent, most sophisticated regions of cortex (neocortex) (Figure 17.2). Other regions have a simpler, three-layered cortex and are believed to be older cortex (archicortex). The majority of the cortex associated with the limbic

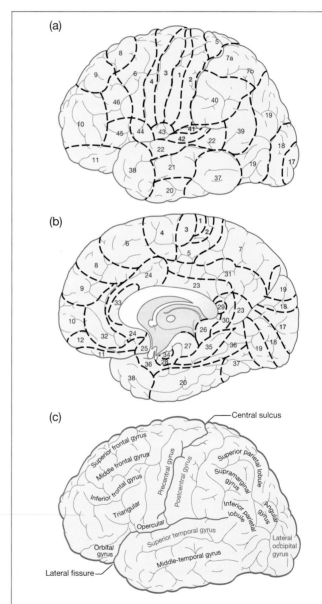

Figure 17.1 A drawing of the lateral (a) and midsagittal (b) surfaces of the brain, with the Brodmann areas denoted. A drawing of the lateral surface of the brain with the specific gyri highlighted (c). Note the precentral gyrus (area 4) has the skeletal motor output, while the postcentral gyrus (area 3) has the somatosensory input.

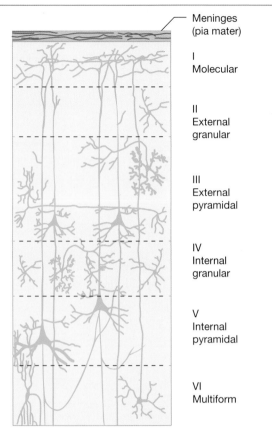

Figure 17.2 A drawing of the six layers of the neocortex. Note the complexity and interactions of the neurons between all six layers.

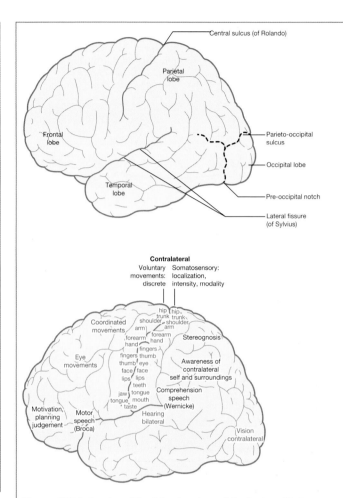

Figure 17.3 A drawing of the lateral surface of the brain, with the lobes of the cortex indicated (a) and the functions attributed to various areas of the cortex (b).

system is archicortex, while the frontal cortex and occipital cortex are neocortex.

Cerebral functional anatomy

The four main areas of cortex have four distinct functional aspects. The **frontal cortex** is responsible for planning motor functions and instigating the primary motor output, along with its prefrontal area which mediates personality and emotional components. The **parietal cortex** is the region for the primary somatosensory (touch, pain, and temperature) input to the cortex and has a major role in integrating and processing all of the sensory inputs. The **temporal cortex** is the primary auditory input/processing region and integrates this sensation with speech and reading functions. The **occipital cortex** is the primary visual input and processing region (Figure 17.3a and b). All of these cortical areas have interactivity both within the same hemisphere and across the cerebral hemispheres. This interactivity has been hypothesized as the means that general **consciousness** is established. Disruption of this interactivity is believed to occur during anesthesia, coma, or other states of unconsciousness.

Cerebral hemisphere localization

Although specific areas of the cortex have specific functional capacities, each of the cerebral hemispheres has its own specific functional attributes. In the **dominant cerebral hemisphere** (usually the left hemisphere in most individuals), language and speech processing takes place, along with analytical reasoning and skilled motor functions. In the **non-dominant cerebral hemisphere**, visual and spatial processing takes place, along with emotional significance and music perception (Figure 17.4). The non-dominant hemisphere also appears to play a role in attention and cognitive awareness.

The functional attributes of these hemispheres have been investigated in patients with hemispheric lesions or with the inability to communicate between hemispheres. Interhemispheric communication occurs primarily through the large **corpus callosum** located superior to the thalamus and deep to the cingulate gyrus. The corpus callosum has thousands of axons that run from one area of the cortex to other areas of the cortex in the opposite hemisphere (Figure 17.5) (Devinsky and Laff, 2003; Gooijers and Swinnen, 2014). Individuals without a corpus callosum have unique clinical symptoms since the hemispheres cannot communicate with each other.

There are also two smaller interhemispheric communication pathways, termed the **anterior** and **posterior commissures**. These are located just anterior and posterior to the corpus callosum and have a small but significant role in cross-hemisphere communication.

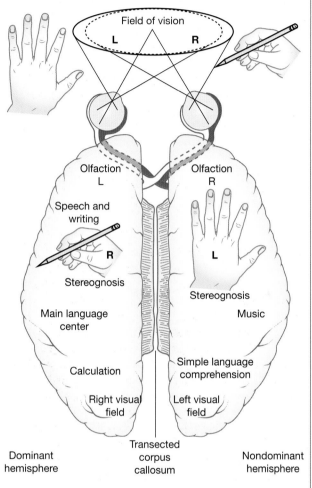

Figure 17.4 A drawing of a superior view of the two hemispheres of the cortex indicating the different functions in each hemisphere. Note the transected corpus callosum that would prevent communication between the hemispheres.

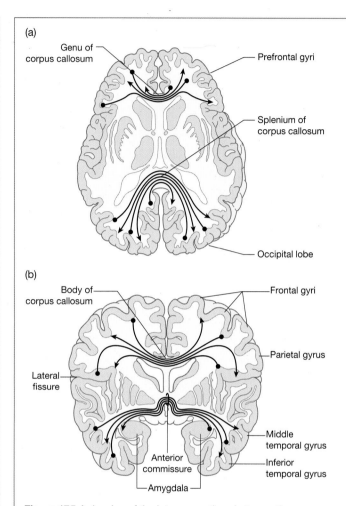

Figure 17.5 A drawing of the interconnections between the hemispheres, with the majority of fibers crossing in the corpus callosum.

Clinical box 17.1

The Neurological Examination and Mental Status Examination

Now that the majority of neuroanatomy has been presented, it is possible to understand how the neurological exam and the mental status exam can be used to test for functional deficits in the nervous system. The neurological exam uses a logical and straightforward approach to testing the different sensory modalities and the motor system. It is used to provide a detailed report on each specific functional component of the nervous system. One comment that should be emphasized is that the neurological exam begins with the first introduction to the patient. The clinician should carefully watch the behavior and mannerisms of the patient, including all motor activities (walking, shaking hands, smiling), as well as cognitive responses to simple questions ("How are you feeling today?").

Another important point to emphasize is that many patients will try to be helpful and do as the clinician suggests, using any "work around" to achieve the task. For example, when asked to follow a finger through space, the patient may move her head instead of her eyes, especially if her eye muscles are weak or dysfunctional. Likewise, if a patient has a dysfunctional trochlear nerve (superior oblique muscle), she may orient her head so that she does not experience diplopia. At the other extreme, if a patient has a memory problem, she may make up answers (**confabulate**) when asked a direct question. For example, when asked why the patient is in the office that day, she may state that she is there to see her brother (an incorrect answer, but she is trying to be helpful, not consciously lying).

Patient history

The exam should begin with the patient's history. A complete history should be obtained, including the chief complaint, its onset, and duration. The handedness of the patient can be relevant since different functions are attributed to different hemispheres of the brain. Family and social history, as well as pharmaceutical, alternative medicinal, and drug history, can be important information to obtain. During the questioning phase of the history, the clinician should listen carefully to the phrasing of the responses. This can provide insight into the hearing and speech capabilities of the patient.

Physical examination

After obtaining the patient's history, a general physical exam should be conducted. The vital signs, cardiovascular status, as well as the eye exam can be especially important. Again, during the physical exam, examination of the fine and gross movements of the patient can provide insight into the motor capabilities of the patient.

Neurological examination

The neurological examination, as part of the physical examination, generally covers six areas: **mental status**, **cranial nerves**, **motor system**, **reflexes**, **cerebellar function**, and **sensation**. Each of these areas is important to asses individually, with a record of competency in each area which can be compared with results from past or future exams.

The **mental status** begins with an assessment of consciousness (the Glasgow Coma Scale can be helpful). Obviously, a comatose patient will have a very different response to many of the tests in the neurological exam. The conscious patient can be tested for his mental status with either the **abbreviated mental test score** or the **mini-mental state examination**. Both of these tests ask the patient to provide specific answers to questions and are graded on a point scale for correct answers. The questions generally ask about time (month, date, and day of the week), about place (specific location, including floor or address), about history (the current president, the date of the World Trade Center attacks), and about the patient (date of birth, number of siblings). The patient is also asked to remember three simple words which are repeated back to the clinician at a later time in the exam. The patient is asked to perform simple calculations (e.g. subtracting seven from one hundred, then seven from the result, then seven from that result) and can also be asked to name specific objects in the room (pen, watch). Clinicians may report a normal patient as "alert and oriented to person, place, and time". When the mental status of the patient is not normal, then more specific results for the tests should be reported (for future comparisons and for other clinicians to be able to interpret the results).

To test the **cranial nerves**, the clinician assesses each of the twelve nerves. Testing olfaction (olfactory (I)) is not commonly performed, although it is known that a change in the sense of smell may be an early indicator of dementia or Parkinsonism. Specific smell tests have been developed for this purpose. Testing vision (optic (II)) is done by an eye exam, along with eye movement tests (oculomotor (III), trochlear (IV), and abducens (VI)). This is also a good opportunity to check pupil dilation and constriction (sympathetic and parasympathetic control) with direct and consensual light responses. Pin prick or feather sensation from the forehead, cheek, and lower jaw test the three divisions of the trigeminal nerve (V), while asking the patient to "bite down strongly", "to squeeze her eyes shut", and "to smile broadly" can test the mastication (trigeminal (V)) and facial muscles (facial (VII)). Taste (facial (VII), glossopharyngeal (IX), and vagus (X)) can be tested by rubbing cotton swabs dabbed in sugar water or lemon juice on the lateral surface of both sides of the tongue. Like olfaction, this test is not commonly performed, but may be valuable in locating specific brain stem lesions or indicating the onset of neurodegenerative diseases. Hearing (vestibulocochlear (VIII)) is tested with auditory stimulation in each ear (snapping fingers, whispered words) and may also be tested with a tuning fork. The vestibular system is not commonly tested at this time, but it can be inferred during coordination and cerebellar tests. If necessary, caloric and nystagmus tests can be performed.

By placing a small cotton swab at the back of the throat, a "gag" reflex can be elicited. This tests the sensory (glossopharyngeal (IX)) and motor (vagus (X)) components of the reflex arc, but can cause discomfort to the patient and may induce vomiting. Asking the patient to say "Ah" and examining the activity of the palate can also test the motor component with less distress. Listening to the patient speak and examining the vocal cords during phonation, can indicate if the vocal muscles (vagus (X)) are functional. Shrugging the shoulders and touching the tip of the jaw to each shoulder tests the spinal accessory nerve (XI). Finally, asking the patient to stick out her tongue and move it from side to side will test the hypoglossal nerve (XII). Recall that the tongue will point towards the side of the lesion, if a weakness exists.

The **motor system** is first tested by observing the patient for any resting motor abnormalities (tremors, fasciculations) and inspecting the muscles for any atrophy or wasting. Muscle tone is tested by passively moving the digits or extremities to determine if any rigidity is present. Cogwheel rigidity can be an indicator of Parkinsonism. Change in muscle tone can also be used to distinguish upper motor lesions from lower motor lesions. Functional testing of muscle groups occurs next. The patient is asked to close her eyes and hold her arms out straight at shoulder height in front of her with her palms up for 30 seconds. Both hands should remain at the same height. This is testing **pronator drift** – the ability to maintain muscle control based on proprioceptive feedback. The patient is also asked to perform repetitive movements, such as touching the tip of each finger to the thumb or foot tapping. This is testing fine motor control. Finally, the strength of individual muscles or muscle groups is tested. This uses a 0–5 scale with "0" being no movement detected, "3" being movement against gravity, but not against resistance, and "5" being normal strength. For example, to test the deltoid muscle, the patient is asked to raise her arm parallel to the floor. If she is able to raise it against gravity, but not against the clinician's mild resistance, then a grade of "3" would be given. Intermediate grades can be given; consistency in grading is an important standard. When multiple muscles or muscle groups are graded, this can lead the clinician to refine the diagnosis to specific myotomes or specific nerves. This requires a detailed knowledge of the nerve roots that supply each muscle or muscle group.

Reflexes are tested in patients by using a reflex hammer to stimulate a tendon and cause an associated muscle contraction. Reflexes are rated on a scale of 0–4+ or 5+. The absence of reflex activity gives a score of "0", while a normal reflex is a "2+". Any reflex above a "3+" is considered an increased deep tendon reflex. Reflexes are normally measured in the jaw (masseter), elbow (biceps brachii and triceps brachii tendons), knee (patellar tendon), ankle (calcaneal tendon), and plantar surface (Babinski). Both sides should be tested to determine that equal reflex activity occurs. Recall that upper motor neuron lesions will result in increased deep tendon reflexes (with a decrease in reflexes acutely after the injury), while lower motor neuron lesions produce a consistent decrease in reflex response.

Cerebellar function is tested in patients by examining their coordination and gait. Recall that the cerebellum, the basal ganglia, the motor cortex, and local spinal cord circuitry are all involved in motor coordination (as are vestibular and visual pathways), so that deficits need to be carefully examined to tease apart which systems are involved. Generally, disorders of coordination and gait are referred to as **ataxia**. These tend to be abnormal involuntary movements that disrupt the normal smooth action observed when a patient performs a simple motor task. If the disorder is limited to the extremities, this is **appendicular ataxia** and suggests that the cerebellar hemispheres are involved, while a disorder of the back, thorax, abdominal, or pelvic muscles is **truncal ataxia** and suggests that midline cerebellar structures are involved.

Patients with cerebellar disorders will often have difficulty with smooth continuous movements and will overshoot or "past point" the intended object. This can be observed by asking a patient to touch the clinician's finger, then touch her own nose, then touch the clinician's finger again (finger-nose-finger test). The intended finger should be placed at the full reach of the patient. The intended finger for the second touch should be moved as she approaches. This can demonstrate overshoot. Any wavering or random motion between the nose and the finger is cause for concern. A similar test can be performed in the lower extremity by asking the supine patient to place the heel of one foot on the opposite knee and then smoothly move the foot down the anterior surface of the leg to the ankle and back to the knee (heel-shin test). Again, observe the motion carefully, looking for any abnormal movements.

Rapid, alternating movements can also be used to test coordination. Ask a patient to use the same hand to touch her index finger to her thumb, then her middle finger to her thumb, then the ring finger to her thumb and then the small finger to her thumb, repeating ther movement as rapidly as possible. Likewise, the patient can sit with her hands on her lap and is asked to flip her hands from prone to supine repeatedly. The inability to perform rapid, alternating movements is **dysdiadochokinesia**.

To test for abnormalities of the trunk muscles, the patient can be asked to walk a few steps, turn around and walk a few steps back. Carefully examine the patient's posture, stability, and stance (foot spacing) prior to walking and then again while she is walking. They should not noticeably change. During walking and turning, examine the smoothness and equality of the gait, how high her feet are raised, and whether there are any abnormal or excessive movements. To further investigate any gait disturbances, the patient can be asked to walk heel to toe in a straight line (tandem gait) or can be asked to walk on her heels or her toes (forced gait). These tests can accentuate any gait disturbances that may be present. Additionally, a patient can be asked to stand upright with her feet close together and then to close her eyes (**Romberg test**). The clinician should be close by and available to catch the patient should she start to fall over. Normally, a patient with intact proprioceptive, vestibular, and cerebellar systems will be able to stand upright with her eyes closed, but if these systems are compromised, then the patient may sway or fall over.

Realize that all of the tests for cerebellar function involve multiple sensory and motor components, so it is necessary to test the other systems separately to indicate that they work appropriately before concluding that a failure of these tests is due solely to cerebellar dysfunction. It is especially important to distinguish between the vestibular, proprioceptive, and cerebellar systems since they have strong interrelated functions.

Testing for general **sensory deficits** involves the use of a pin or feather for pain and light touch, a cool piece of metal (such as the tuning fork) for temperature, the tuning fork for vibratory sense, and a bent paper clip for two-point discrimination. Each of these tests is described in more detail below, but they all rely on the patient giving accurate and appropriate responses. This can be limiting in certain circumstances (e.g. an uncooperative patient, a language or comprehension deficit, or a patient in a coma). Sensory testing should occur with the patient's eyes closed, so that visual information is not used to mask sensory deficits. The testing should be done on both sides of the body, from proximal to distal and should especially concentrate on areas where sensory disturbances are noted. Detailed mapping of sensory losses can indicate if a peripheral nerve or spinal nerve is involved and can indicate the level of a spinal cord lesion based on well-described dermatomal maps (Figure 11.5).

To test for **light touch**, a cotton swab or a feather can be rubbed on the skin to elicit a verbal response from the patient. **Pain** sensation can be determined by having the patient discriminate between the sharp and dull ends of a pin. **Temperature** sensation can be tested by placing the cool metal of the tuning fork on the patient's skin or by using drops of cool and warm water and asking the patient to differentiate between them. **Two-point discrimination** is the ability to determine whether one or two points of a bent paper clip are placed on the skin. It is measured in millimeters between the two points at the limit of the ability to discriminate. The back has a much wider two-point discrimination than the tips of the fingers, based on cutaneous nerve density. Therefore, these tests should be conducted bilaterally, so that differences from one side can be compared to the other side, since regional differences in the skin are normal.

Additional sensory testing includes vibration testing and joint position tests. **Vibration testing** involves the use of a vibrating tuning fork on areas of muscle mass and asking the patient to identify when she feels the vibration stop. **Joint position testing** involves lightly grasping a digit and moving it slightly in one direction, the patient should be able to state in which direction the joint has been moved. This is an especially sensitive sensation, so the joint does not need to be moved a large distance for a normal patient to be able to indicate a change.

Recall that testing for **special sensory deficits** occurred during the cranial nerve tests (specifically cranial nerves I (smell), II (vision), VIII (hearing and balance), and VII/IX/X (taste)). To test for **cortical sensory losses**, it must first be established that the peripheral sensory systems are functioning normally. With normal peripheral senses intact, the patient is asked to close her eyes and identify a letter or number that is drawn on the palm of each hand (graphesthesia). The patient can also be asked to close her eyes and identify a common object (such as a key or a bottle cap) when it is placed in each hand (**stereognosis**). Inability to identify the written letter or the object (even though the patient can "feel" both of them) usually indicates a lesion in the contralateral sensory cortex. Finally, with the patient's eyes closed, the patient can be asked to identify where she is being touched – either singly or simultaneously (tactile extinction). The hand can be touched singly or both hands touched simultaneously. A normal patient should be able to state that one hand or both hands are being touched. A patient with a cortical lesion (producing hemineglect) will not recognize the simultaneous touch on the contralateral side.

While the previous description of the neurological exam may appear quite long and highly detailed, experienced clinicians conduct a few of the tests indicated and then, if areas of concern are noted, can probe in those specific areas with more detailed tests. It is recommended that when learning the neurological exam it be practiced often on normal colleagues, so that the novice can form a baseline for normal responses to many of the tests. This will allow a better interpretation of an abnormal response when examining a patient. An excellent and detailed description of the neurologic exam is provided in Blumenfeld (2002) (neuroexam.com).

Prior to the advent of computed tomography and magnetic resonance imaging (Chapter 18), the neurological examination was the most important diagnostic tool for determining the site of lesions. Now it is used as an adjunct with imaging modalities to determine the extent and debilitation of a neurologic deficit. It is also valuable to trace the time course of a diagnosis; do the results from the exam get better or worse over time? This can indicate that other areas of the central nervous system have adapted and taken on functional roles that were lost due to the lesion. This is one of the most remarkable aspects of the nervous system – the ability to regain neural function by reorganization of specific brain regions (**neuroplasticity**) (Galarza et al., 2014).

Clinical considerations

Deficits in specific regions of the cortex can produce unique clinical presentations. For example, a lesion in Brodmann's areas 44 and 45 (**Broca's area**) leads to a pronunciation aphasia referred to as **Broca's aphasia**. Likewise, a lesion in Brodmann's area 22 (**Wernicke's area**) leads to a comprehension aphasia referred to as **Wernicke's aphasia** (Figure 17.6). A patient with Broca's aphasia has little or no comprehension problems, but has difficulty speaking and can be very frustrated with the inability to find and form coherent sentences. The patient with Wernicke's aphasia, on the other hand, has little difficulty in producing words and sentences, but speaks incoherently or in gibberish because of the comprehension difficulties. Both of these patients have aphasias (speech difficulties), but their clinical presentation is quite different (Ziegler *et al.*, 2012).

Note that there is an important white matter tract in the cortex that connects Wernicke's area with Broca's area: the **arcuate fasciculus** (Figure 17.6). This tract is important in coordinating fluent speech and when lesioned can produce aphasia. It is also important to preserve Broca's and Wernicke's areas during brain surgery, so that the patient does not have these aphasias induced surgically. Prior to surgery, a patient will have a functional magnetic resonance test (Figure 17.7) to delineate the actual distribution of these areas which can then be avoided during surgery.

Cerebral cortex lesions due to tumors or stroke can impact on the ability to perform a motor function in response to a verbal direction (**apraxia**). When asking a patient to perform a specific motor task ("brush your hair" or "salute the flag"), the patient has difficulty performing the requested action. Apraxia can occur with a variety of cortical lesions and can be seen in patients with aphasias. Cortical lesions can also produce other specific cognitive deficits, including the inability to read (**alexia**) or the inability to write (**agraphia**). These losses can occur singly in patients or in conjunction with aphasias or apraxias (Basso *et al.*, 2011).

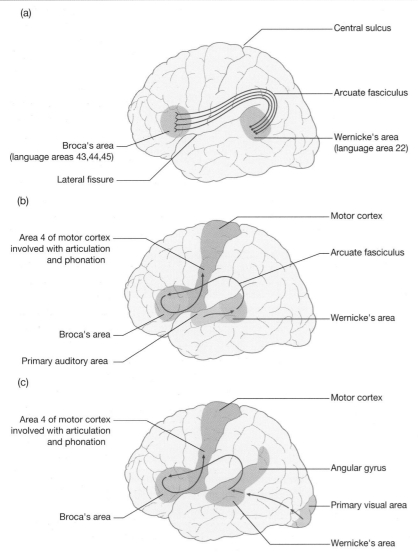

(a)

Central sulcus

Arcuate fasciculus

Wernicke's area (language area 22)

Broca's area (language areas 43,44,45)

Lateral fissure

(b)

Area 4 of motor cortex involved with articulation and phonation

Broca's area

Primary auditory area

Motor cortex

Arcuate fasciculus

Wernicke's area

(c)

Area 4 of motor cortex involved with articulation and phonation

Broca's area

Motor cortex

Angular gyrus

Primary visual area

Wernicke's area

Figure 17.6 A drawing of the interconnections between Wernicke's and Broca's language areas on the dominant hemisphere (arcuate fasciculus) (a). Note that when an individual is asked to repeat a word that is heard (b) or say a word that is read (c) the information passes from the primary sensory cortex to Wernicke's area then to Broca's area prior to the motor cortex.

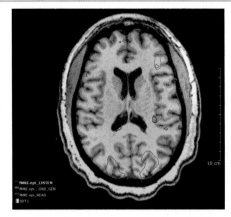

Figure 17.7 Functional magnetic resonance imaging of a patient with epilepsy to determine the localization of Broca's and Wernicke's areas. The red areas were activated when the patient was asked to read a passage, while the blue areas were activated when the patient was asked to listen to a spoken passage.

Patients with a large lesion in the right parietal cortex can exhibit a lack of recognition for the left side of their body (**hemi-neglect syndrome**) (Jacobs *et al.*, 2012; Vuilleumier, 2013). They do not recognize the left side of their body and they may neglect visual and other sensory information from the left side of their awareness (**sensory neglect**). They can also have a **motor neglect** in which they will not use the muscles on the affected side (even though they may have sensation from the affected side). There can be a **combined neglect** (both a sensory and motor neglect). Perhaps the most interesting is a **conceptual neglect** in which the individual does not recognize the affected side of the body as their own and states that no problem exists (anosognosia). These individuals may see their arm on the affected side and declare that it is someone else's arm. Hemi-neglect is found predominantly on the left side of the body, because, for unknown reasons, there are more redundant neural connections from the right parietal cortex to the left parietal cortex, so that lesions on the left side of the cortex are less likely to produce neglect. The opposite interaction is not as strong, so that right parietal cortex lesions are more likely to result in neglect. Testing patients for hemi-neglect can be complex and requires careful examination to determine if the patient has a sensory or motor deficit prior to testing for neglect.

While the deficits described above generally produce effects on one side of the body (or have localized lesions to a particular area of the brain), there are also global neural deficits that occur, such as hallucinations, epilepsy, delirium, and dementia. **Hallucinations**, both auditory and visual, can occur when the specific sensory region of the cortex has altered neural activity that creates the perception of a sound or vision that does not exist. In some patients with general brain psychosis, auditory hallucinations can occur due to activation of a wide range of brain regions. When hallucinations are localized to a specific brain region, then surgical treatments may be available. However, without a specific locale for the hallucinations, many patients are prescribed drugs that have a general depressant effect on the nervous system in the hopes of reducing the hallucinations.

Epilepsy, like hallucinations, can have a similar global occurrence. It can occur after trauma to the brain, after drug use, or without any known causative event. It usually originates in one region of the brain as a spike in neural activity which can then radiate throughout the entire brain. This increased neural activity may produce an "aura" of sensory perception (smell, sound, or vision) which can rapidly progress to seizures (a short period of increased global cortical activity). In some cases, this increased activity leads to convulsions (involuntary, uncoordinated muscle activity). These are generalized tonic-clonic seizures or grand mal seizures. Interestingly, some epilepsy patients have increased brain activity that produces a loss of awareness with no motor activity and a blank, vacant stare. These are absence or petit mal seizures. In both instances, there is increased brain activity (which can be measured by an electroencephalogram (EEG)), but which produces opposite behavioral responses. Most patients receive pharmacologic treatment to lessen the chance for seizures to occur – usually GABAergic drugs or general depressants – but these can have notable side effects. When the onset of the epileptic activity can be localized to a specific brain region, surgical treatments may be available (Galarza *et al.*, 2014).

When patients become confused, agitated, and hallucinate, they can be classified as having **delirium**. Usually, this is a rapid, acute response to a biochemical alteration in brain function produced by an exogenous compound (toxin, drug, or unique foodstuff). This can be treated by clearing the blood of the causative agent. Delirium can also occur with a major infection or with head trauma. Treating the causative factor can usually reduce or eliminate the resulting delirium.

Patients can present with a loss of memory or other cortical functions that become worse over time. These are referred to as **dementia**, which can be subdivided into numerous subtypes based on the cause, the time frame, or the location of the disturbance. Treatments can vary, depending on the type of dementia, with some causes having little or no treatment. **Alzheimer's disease** is a well-known degenerative type of dementia that can be very debilitating.

Alzheimer's disease is classified as a senile dementia that is observed in older individuals. There is a form that occurs before the age of 60 (early onset Alzheimer's disease) that can have a genetic basis, but the more common form occurs in individuals over 60 years old (late onset Alzheimer's disease). It is characterized by memory disturbances, a decrease in cognitive skills, as well as emotional and personality changes (De-Paula *et al.*, 2012). These changes occur gradually over time and usually begin with typical forgetfulness, continue as mild cognitive impairment, and then progress to symptoms which interfere with daily activities. This is a chronic progressive disorder that eventually removes an individual's independence and personality.

The cause of Alzheimer's disease is not known, although in some cases there is a genetic component. For example, individuals with Down's syndrome (who have three copies of chromosome 21) develop early onset Alzheimer's disease (at around 40 years of age). The brains of patients with advanced Alzheimer's disease are decreased in size with a specific loss of gray matter in the cortex and hippocampus. They have increased space in the sulci of the cortex and increased size of the ventricles. They also have unique histopathological structures (senile plaques and neurofibrillary tangles). **Senile plaques** are made of amyloid proteins (beta amyloid) and apolipoprotein E. The beta amyloid is a breakdown product of amyloid precursor protein, a transmembrane protein. The role of specific genes and enzymes in the over production (or reduced clearance) of the components of senile plaques has been described, although a complete understanding of their formation is not known. **Neurofibrillary tangles** are composed of tau proteins, an accumulation of microtubule associated proteins that are hyperphosphorylated. While these structures are found in post-mortem brain samples from patients with Alzheimer's disease, the exact role they play in initiating or propagating the disease is still not known.

There are no cures for Alzheimer's disease and the treatments available attempt to limit the progression of the disease. There are medications that alter cholinergic function which can have an effect on disease progression, but there are no well-established, robust treatments or preventative mechanisms. This is an area of extensive research. The prognosis for a patient with Alzheimer's disease is poor, with an average of seven years from diagnosis until death.

Summary

While the gross neuroanatomy of the human brain has been well described, the location of cell bodies and white matter tracts are well established, and the basic sensory and motor functions are well understood, many of the higher levels of neural function (e.g. consciousness, decision making, and expression of personality) are still not well

---

Clinical box 17.2

Schizophrenia and autism, in contrast to other neurologic conditions, are not as well understood. They can both be described by specific behaviors and by psychiatric diagnostic criteria, but the underlying cellular deficits are not known. Both of these disorders are believed to have complex genetic components and to occur throughout the brain with no specifically targeted neuroanatomical component.

Schizophrenia is a cognitive disassociation between what is "real" and not "real" that involves disrupted thought processes and emotional disturbances. Individuals with schizophrenia can have difficulty thinking clearly and acting normally. They may experience hallucinations, delusions, and attention deficits. The cause and cellular mechanisms of schizophrenia are unknown, but it appears to involve disruptions in many genes and neurotransmitters (Dauvermann *et al.*, 2014). Generally, symptoms first appear as a teenager and increase over time. The only treatments available, at present, are antipsychotic medications that modify central dopamine or serotonin receptor activation and produce side effects, such as sleepiness, slowed thought processes, and weight gain. Long-term use of antipsychotics may produce tardive dyskinesia – an involuntary motor disorder. The prognosis for schizophrenia can be poor, with an increase in other clinical problems (depression), decreased life span, and increased suicide rates.

Autism is a neurologic developmental disorder whose cause is poorly understood. It produces characteristic behavioral responses in young children. Children with autism tend to have difficulty with language and with interactions with others. There can be a wide diversity of symptoms, ranging from low-functioning to high-functioning individuals. There appears to be a genetic component, although other causes are also considered (Anagnostou and Taylor, 2011). At one time, it was thought that vaccinations could cause autism. This has been strongly refuted and one of the proponents for this cause was shown to have committed fraud and research misconduct (Holton *et al.*, 2012). There are no specific treatments for the underlying cause of autism, but therapy and behavioral programs can help autistic children develop to their fullest potential, while providing families with guidance. Medications may be used to help modify excessive behaviors. The prognosis for a child with autism is highly dependent on the level of functioning that the child can achieve.

characterized. This will require detailed research in the future, with the use of increasingly refined imaging techniques, such as functional magnetic resonance imaging. These techniques will allow investigators to determine the areas of the brain that are involved in these higher cognitive functions, although it will also be necessary to have a more detailed understanding of cellular and axonal interactions in these areas.

Case 1

A 62-year-old chiropractor, Dr Robert Branson, was on vacation with his wife in Puerto Vallarta, Mexico, when, after dinner, he experienced a sharp headache and collapsed. He was rushed to the local emergency room where he regained consciousness a few hours later. He was confused and disoriented, with speech difficulties. During his physical examination, it was found that Dr Branson was unable to move his left lower extremity and had a sensory loss below the waist on the left side.

The emergency room physicians, believing that a **stroke** had occurred (Table 17.1), gave Dr Branson aspirin to help prevent further blood clots and kept him quiet with his head lower than his body to encourage reperfusion of the damaged tissue. Within the next 48 hours, Dr Branson was medically transported to a stroke unit in his hometown of St Louis, Missouri.

In the stroke unit, Dr Branson had an MRI (with MRI angiography), which indicated that an occlusion had occurred in his right **anterior cerebral artery** (Figure 17.8). Since the stroke blocked the majority of circulation in his right anterior cerebral artery, he lost blood supply to his right interhemispheric cortical surfaces, resulting in sensory and motor deficits (Toyoda, 2012). The loss of blood supply also affected the personality centers of the frontal cortex, along with the orbitofrontal cortex. This resulted in a diminished, muted personality and a loss of flavor sensation. Dr Branson found that food had specific "tastes" (sweet, sour, savory) but he could not identify the food he ate by taste alone.

With time and rehabilitation, Dr Branson regained much of his sensory loss below the waist and his flavor appreciation returned. His personality and speech deficits improved, but, sadly, he was only able to regain approximately 30% of his motor control. He continues his physical therapy with the hope of regaining more motor function.

Table 17.1 Key principles for assessing the clinical effects of cerebral stroke

1. Three main arteries supply the cortex (Figure 2.8):
   a) The anterior cerebral artery supplies the anterior/medial surface of the frontal cortex.
   b) The middle cerebral artery supplies the lateral (temporal/parietal) surface of the cortex.
   c) The posterior cerebral artery supplies the posterior (occipital) surface of the cortex.
2. The cerebral hemisphere controls the opposite (contralateral) side of the body.
3. The motor and sensory homunculi (Figures 11.8 and 11.13) have similar distributions on the precentral and postcentral gyri, respectively. Losses on the lateral aspects of these gyri affect the face and upper limb, while losses on the medial aspect (interhemispheric surface) of these gyri affect the lower limb.
4. Fine motor control or fine sensory discrimination (e.g. in the hands) has a greater cortical surface area than regions with less control or discrimination (e.g. the back).
5. Left hemisphere strokes are more likely to produce language deficits, while right hemisphere strokes are more likely to produce visuospatial deficits (neglect).

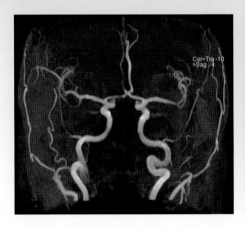
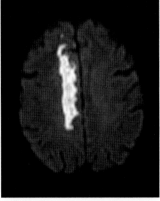

Figure 17.8 Magnetic resonance imaging of a patient with a right anterior cerebral artery stroke (infarct). Note that the right anterior cerebral artery is much smaller than the left in the magnetic resonance angiogram. The hyperintense area in the image on the right is the region of cortical loss produced by the infarct.

Case 2

A 45-year-old computer technician, Mr Allen Dean, is an avid rock climber. During one climb, he lost control, fell twenty feet and hit the right side of his head on a rock outcropping. His friends responded quickly, stopped the bleeding, and carried him to their car for transport to a local hospital. In the hospital, he was monitored closely and had a CT of his head.

The CT scan indicated that Mr Dean had a small fracture in the right temporal bone of the skull with damage to the overlying skin and subcutaneous tissue. The physician in charge of the emergency room, Dr Varsha Burke, examined the CT carefully and discussed the findings with Mr Dean, who had regained consciousness a few hours earlier.

One day later, Mr Dean was still disoriented and he had difficulty speaking. His sentences were short and he had difficulty finding words. When a neurologist,

Dr Caroline Govea, examined Mr Dean, she surmised that he had a pronunciation aphasia, **Broca's aphasia**. She suggested that Mr Dean have an MRI to determine if his brain had suffered a contusion in the accident. When examining the MRI carefully, Dr Govea saw an injury to the lateral part of the left temporal lobe – the opposite side from the injury. She concluded that Mr Dean had a **contrecoup injury**: an injury on the opposite side of the initial impact (the **coup**), possibly due to the brain impacting the skull during the trauma (Figure 17.9) (Asha'Ari *et al.*, 2011).

Dr Govea suggested that over time the injury could heal and that Mr Dean's aphasia could be resolved. A few weeks after the accident, Mr Dean's speech was notably improved. He would occasionally experience headaches and periods of disorientation, but these also began to recede.

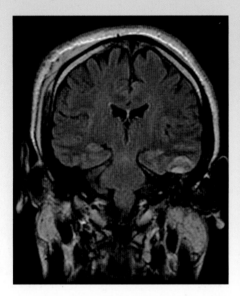 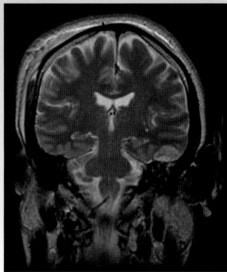

Figure 17.9 Frontal magnetic resonance images of a patient with a coup-contrecoup injury. Note the wound with subcutaneous swelling in the upper right portion of the skull (coup) and the damage to the lower left temporal lobe (contrecoup).

Case 3

Although not a typical case study, the following description of an actual event can be a valuable learning tool. United States Congress member, Gabrielle Giffords, was shot in the head at point blank range in 2011. The bullet passed through her skull and brain on the left side producing numerous neurological deficits. She made a remarkable recovery and her ability to regain function is a testament to her hard

work, her excellent care, and the ability of her brain to reroute and rewire (Figure 17.10).

With neuroanatomical knowledge from this text, consider Mrs Gifford's injury and the neurological losses that would be associated with damage to the left side of her brain. Would motor and sensory deficits be found on her right or left side? What visual deficits might she possess? Could she have speech difficulties and, if so, how would they present?

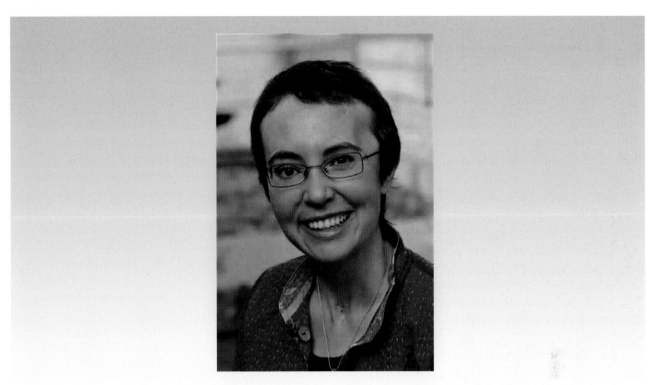

Figure 17.10 Former congressional member, Gabrielle Giffords, who was shot through the left side of her head and has made a remarkable recovery. Source: P.K. Weiss/Released by United States Congress.

Study questions

1. A 42-year-old female patient with fluent speech that is nonsensical could have a lesion in the:
a) frontal cortex (Broca's area – area 44/45)
b) temporal cortex (Wernicke's area – area 22)
c) parietal cortex (area 4)
d) occipital cortex (area 17)
e) parietal cortex (area 1)

2. If a 65-year-old male begins to add more salt and pepper to his food and displays short, small lapses in his memory, a physician should consider the onset of:
a) Broca's aphasia
b) Wernicke's aphasia
c) Alzheimer's disease
d) Huntington's chorea
e) Parkinson's disease

3. Which of the following pairings is incorrect?
a) occipital cortex – vision
b) temporal cortex – hearing
c) precentral gyrus – skeletal muscle motor control
d) postcentral gyrus – general sensation
e) cingulate gyrus – intelligence

4. A 27-year-old female patient presents to the emergency room in an agitated state believing that bats are flying into her hair. A friend of the patient states that she recently tried some wild mushrooms. The patient is experiencing:
a) dementia
b) delirium
c) apraxia
d) agnosia
e) aphasia

5. After a stroke, a 58-year-old male patient presents with an inability to recognize anything in his left field of vision or on the left side of his body. He states that he feels "perfectly fine" and that nothing is wrong. The patient may have had a stroke in the:
a) right cortex, producing hemi-neglect
b) left cortex, producing hemi-neglect
c) right cortex, producing dementia and delirium
d) left cortex, producing dementia and delirium
e) left cerebellum, producing dysdiodochokinesia

For more self-assessment questions, visit the companion website at
www.wileyessential.com/neuroanatomy

FURTHER READING

For additional information on cortical integration, the following textbooks and review articles may be helpful:

Anagnostou E, Taylor MJ. 2011. Review of neuroimaging in autism spectrum disorders: what have we learned and where we go from here. *Mol Autism*, 2(1): 4(1–9).

Asha'Ari ZA, Ahmad R, Rahman J, Kamarudin N, Ishlah LW. 2011. Contrecoup injury in patients with traumatic temporal bone fracture. *J Laryngol Otol*, 125(8): 781–785.

Basso A, Cattaneo S, Girelli L, Luzzatti C, Miozzo A, Modena L, *et al.*, 2011. Treatment efficacy of language and calculation disorders and speech apraxia: a review of the literature. *Eur J Phys Rehabil Med*, 47(1): 101–121.

Blumenfeld H. 2002. *Neuroanatomy Through Clinical Cases*. Sinauer Associates, Sunderland, Massachusetts.

Dauvermann MR, Whalley HC, Schmidt A, Lee GL, Romaniuk L, Roberts N, *et al.*, 2014. Computational neuropsychiatry – schizophrenia as a cognitive brain network disorder. *Front Psychiatry*, 5: 30(1–19).

De-Paula VJ, Radanovic M, Diniz BS, Forlenza OV. 2012. Alzheimer's disease. *Subcell Biochem*, 65: 329–352.

Devinsky O, Laff R. 2003. Callosal lesions and behavior: history and modern concepts. *Epilepsy Behav*, 4(6): 607–617.

Felten DL, Shetty A. 2009. *Netter's Atlas of Neuroscience*, 2nd edition. Saunders Elsevier, Philadelphia, Pennsylvania.

Galarza M, Isaac C, Pellicer O, Mayes A, Broks P, Montaldi D, *et al.*, 2014. Jazz, guitar, and neurosurgery: the Pat Martino case report. *World Neurosurg*, 81(3–4): 651. e1–7.

Gooijers J, Swinnen SP. 2014. Interactions between brain structure and behavior: the corpus callosum and bimanual coordination. *Neurosci Biobehav Rev*, 43C: 1–19.

Haines, DE. 2011. *Lippincott's Illustrated Q&A Review of Neuroscience*. Lippincott, Williams and Wilkins, Baltimore, Maryland.

Haines DE. 2012. *Neuroanatomy: An Atlas of Structures, Sections and Systems*, 8th edition. Lippincott Williams & Wilkin, Baltimore, Maryland.

Holton A, Weberling B, Clarke CE, Smith MJ. 2012. The blame frame: media attribution of culpability about the MMR-autism vaccination scare. *Health Communication*, 27(7): 690–701.

Jacobs S, Brozzoli C, Farnè A. 2012. Neglect: a multisensory deficit? *Neuropsychologia*, 50(6): 1029–1044.

Loukas M, Pennell C, Groat C, Tubbs RS, Cohen-Gadol AA . 2011. Korbinian Brodmann (1868–1918) and his contributions to mapping the cerebral cortex. *Neurosurgery*, 68(1): 6–11.

Moore KL, Dalley AF, Agur AMR. 2014. *Moore Clinically Oriented Anatomy*, 7th edition. Lippincott, Williams & Wilkins, Philadelphia, Pennsylvania.

Patestas MA, Gartner LP. 2006. *A Textbook of Neuroanatomy*. Blackwell Publishing, Malden, Massachusetts.

Toyoda K. 2012. Anterior cerebral artery and Heubner's artery territory infarction. *Front Neurol Neurosci*, 30: 120–122.

Vuilleumier P. 2013. Mapping the functional neuroanatomy of spatial neglect and human parietal lobe functions: progress and challenges. *Ann NY Acad Sci*, 1296: 50–74.

Ziegler W, Aichert I, Staiger A. 2012. Apraxia of speech: concepts and controversies. *J Speech Lang Hear Res*, 55(5): S1485–1501.

CHAPTER 18
Imaging essentials

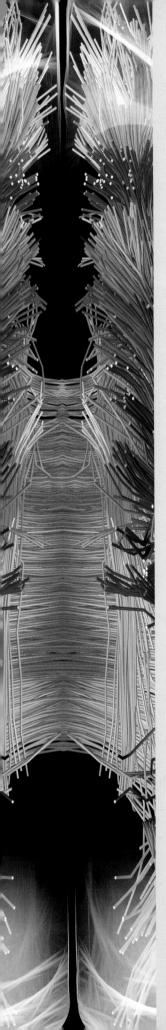

Learning objectives

1. Describe the types of imaging used in neuroanatomy.
2. Describe the clinical conditions that can be observed with neuroimaging.

Essential Clinical Neuroanatomy, First Edition. Thomas H. Champney.
© 2016 John Wiley & Sons, Ltd. Published 2016 by John Wiley & Sons, Ltd.
Companion website: www.wileyessential.com/neuroanatomy

Introduction

Determining structural and functional abnormalities in the brain has advanced tremendously over the past 30 years. In the past, the brain was a "black box" in the skull with the only means for examination being a view into the interior of the eye.

Radiography of the skull and brain was an advancement that provided some indication of tumor location or other abnormalities, but was a crude measure. In order to improve plain film radiographic imaging, physicians would inject air into the ventricles or would inject contrast-enhancing dyes into the bloodstream (both of which increased the contrast between the soft tissue of the brain and the fluid in the vessels). These techniques presented hazards to the patients and only provided slightly improved resolution.

With the development of **computerized tomography (CT)**, **magnetic resonance imaging (MRI)**, and their enhancements, clinicians today can see details of neuroanatomy unheard of twenty years ago. Likewise, with further refinement, these technologies allow detailed, fine resolution of neural structures.

Neuroanatomical imaging

Radiography

The first means of imaging the brain was the use of plain film radiography. This technique utilizes an X-ray beam that passes through the tissue of interest and impacts on photographic film or on a specialized electronic detector. The denser the tissue, the fewer X-rays pass through and the "whiter" the tissue appears on the film or detector. Therefore, metal or bone will appear "white" on a radiograph (**radiodense**), while air will appear "black" (**radiolucent**). Intermediate density tissues (blood, muscle, brain) will appear as various shades of gray.

The soft tissue of the brain has similar density with the blood vessels, ventricles, and cerebrospinal fluid. In addition, the brain is encased in a hard, bony skull. Both of these facts make it quite difficult to image neuropathologies with plain film radiography (Figure 18.1). Interestingly, physicians would use the location of the **pineal gland** as a radiological marker, since it calcifies with age (making it radiodense) and is normally located in the midline. Any deviation of the pineal in a plain film radiograph would suggest that a tumor or other space filling structure had rearranged the normal neural architecture. Plain film radiography is rarely used in neuroimaging today, since it has been supplanted by techniques that produce higher quality images with better tissue resolution.

Utilizing the same physical properties of plain film radiology, while incorporating computerized processing of multiple images, the development of **computerized tomography (CT)** allows for better imaging of the brain. This technology revolutionized radiology and was especially beneficial to neuroimaging, since the interior of the brain could be seen in much finer detail. The basic description of CT is the rapid acquisition of many radiographic images from numerous viewing angles (360 degrees), compiled by a computer to construct a two-dimensional image of a section of the body. This image has the same "look and feel" of a normal radiograph, with bone being radiodense and air being radiolucent. Since this image is computer generated, it can be modified to highlight specific radiodensities (windows). Bone densities ("bone windows") (Figure 18.2a) can be used to highlight fractures, while soft tissue densities

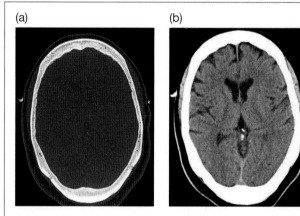

Figure 18.2 (a) A computerized tomography (CT) view of the skull utilizing the "bone window." Notice the fine detail of the bones of the skull, but the poor resolution of the brain (although a faint shadow of the ventricles and the location of the pineal gland can be observed). This view is especially beneficial in determining skull fractures. (b) The same computerized tomography (CT) view of the skull as Figure 18.2a utilizing the "brain window." Notice the poor detail of the bones of the skull, but the much better resolution of the brain, including the ventricles, sulci, gyri, and the location of the pineal gland. This view is especially beneficial in determining vascular deficits and tumors.

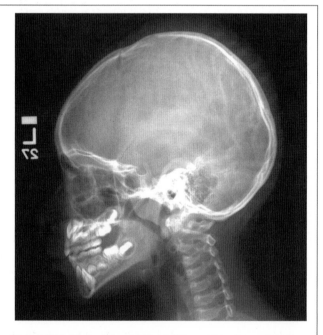

Figure 18.1 A lateral view of the skull in a child using a plain film radiograph. Notice the lack of fine tissue resolution of the brain.

(a)

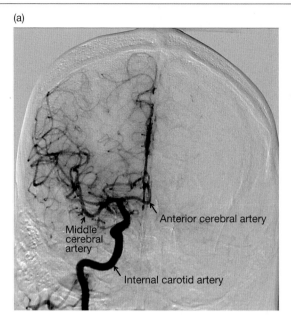

(b)

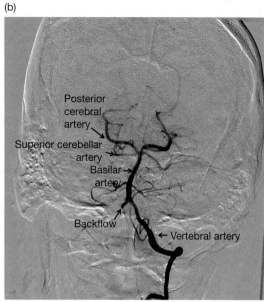

Figure 18.3 (a) A normal angiogram of the internal carotid artery. Note the tortuous nature of the internal carotid artery, along with its two major branches, the middle cerebral artery and the anterior cerebral artery. (b) A normal angiogram of the vertebral artery. Note the formation of the basilar artery from the vertebral arteries (there is backflow of contrast material into the opposite vertebral artery). The terminal branches of the basilar artery can also be observed: the superior cerebellar artery and the posterior cerebral artery. Recall that the oculomotor nerve (III) passes between the superior cerebellar and posterior cerebral arteries.

("brain windows") (Figure 18.2b) can be used to highlight differences in brain tissue (e.g. normal versus tumor). This increases the diagnostic potential of CT over normal radiography. The prevalence of CT scanners is so widespread that virtually all patients with a suspected head injury receive a CT during their emergency room visit.

Recall that the standard orientation utilized by clinicians for axial (horizontal) imaging is that posterior is at the bottom of the field, with anterior at the top of the field, and the patient's right side on the left aspect of the field. This is usually described as the clinician standing at the foot of the bed looking at the patient on his back. In addition, the standard orientation for frontal (coronal) imaging is that the patient would be looking at the clinician (with the patient's right side on the left aspect of the field).

In order to examine details of the cerebral blood vessels, specific contrast dyes can be injected into the vessel to increase its radiodensity (**angiography**). The flow of the contrast agent can be followed through the arterial system into the capillary beds and then into the venous system by obtaining a series of timed radiographic images (using normal radiography, fluoroscopy, or a CT scanner) (Figure 18.3a and b). The capillary perfusion in the brain is difficult to follow, since the blood-brain barrier excludes the contrast dye. These images can, however, be quite useful in determining if a stroke has occurred and the extent of damage (the areas of ischemia, the point of blockage). In addition, the size and extent of aneurysms can be visualized, along with other vascular defects or anomalies (Figure 18.4).

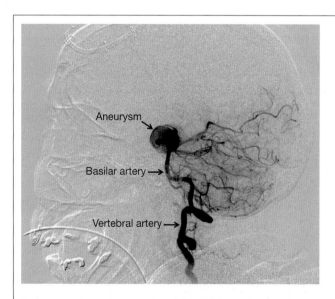

Figure 18.4 An angiogram of the vertebral artery, with an aneurysm at the termination of the basilar artery. Note the basilar artery and the vertebral artery from the lateral oblique view. Consider how this aneurysm could impact on the extraocular muscles of this patient due to compression of the adjacent oculomotor nerve (III).

This technique can be quite beneficial for determining cerebrovascular problems, but it does involve the intravenous administration of a foreign substance (which can be toxic to the kidneys).

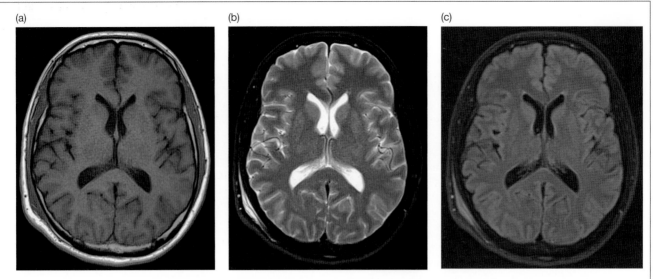

Figure 18.5 (a) A normal magnetic resonance image (MRI) of the brain in the T1 format. Note the "bright" skin and bone marrow and the "dark" bones of the skull. Also, note that the blood and cerebrospinal fluid are hypointense, while the soft tissue of the brain is hyperintense. (b) A normal magnetic resonance image (MRI) of the same section of brain in the T2 format. Note that the blood and cerebrospinal fluid are hyperintense, while the soft tissue of the brain is relatively hypointense. The hyperintense area in the lower left region of the field is due to recent bleeding from an injury. (c) A normal magnetic resonance image (MRI) of the same section of brain in the FLAIR (fluid attenuated inversion recovery) format. Note that the blood and cerebrospinal fluid are now hypointense.

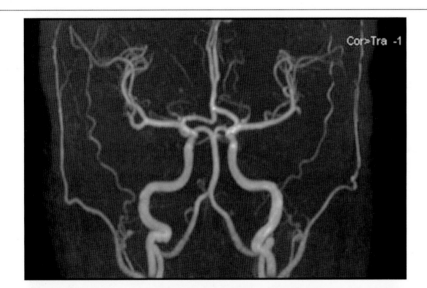

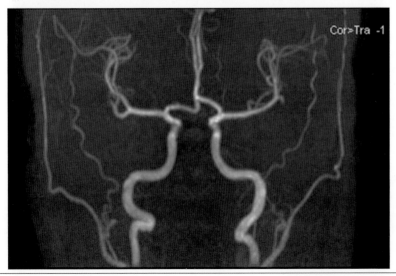

Figure 18.6 A normal magnetic resonance image (MRI) of the brain using the angiography format (MRA). In the upper panel, note the complete view of the cerebral blood supply, while in the lower panel the posterior (vertebral) circulation has been subtracted.

Magnetic resonance imaging

Within a few years of the development of CT, another imaging technique was developed that was able to visualize the brain without the use of ionizing radiation. This technique, **magnetic resonance imaging (MRI)**, uses very powerful magnets to align the hydrogen atoms in molecules. When the atoms are held in alignment by the magnets, they are then pulsed with electromagnetic radio waves. This causes a change in their orientation and they give off a small pulse of radio frequency energy. This pulse of radio energy is measured and used to construct images of the tissue. This is a very simplified explanation of a highly complex procedure that requires many magnets, numerous radio frequency pulses, highly sensitive detection devices, and computers to both run and process the results.

In a simple sense, the activity of the hydrogen atoms present in various tissues is different, producing a typical MRI that will have "dark" bone and air (low hydrogen activity) and "bright" soft tissue (high hydrogen activity). These are usually referred to as **hypointense** and **hyperintense**, respectively. Since the image is computer generated, there are a number of ways to modify or enhance the view of the tissue. By using a different combination of measurement factors, the same view of the tissue can be observed in different formats. For example, in a **T1 MRI** format, fluid (blood, cerebrospinal fluid) is hypointense, while soft tissue (brain) is comparatively hyperintense (Figure 18.5a). In the same section of the brain, but presented in the **T2 MRI** format, the fluids are hyperintense while the soft tissue is comparatively hypointense (Figure 18.5b). The **FLAIR** (fluid attenuated inversion recovery) MRI format represses the fluid signal (fluid is hypointense), but provides good imaging of soft tissues (Figure 18.5c). Comparing these three images side by side can provide clinicians with the ability to diagnose masses in the brain (solid tumors versus ischemic tissue versus fluid-filled cysts). An additional MRI technique, which requires different scanning parameters, can generate images that display blood vessels (**MR angiography**) (Figure 18.6). These are comparable with normal angiograms, but are non-invasive (no use of contrast agents). Finally, contrast agents can be used in MRI in a similar manner as found in conventional radiology. These agents are not radiodense, but are proton dense and when injected will produce hyperintensity in the vessels or tissues (Figure 18.7). The most common MRI contrast agent is **gadolinium**, which is highly toxic, so it is bound to a carrier compound, preventing its ability to cross the blood-brain barrier. If, during a gadolinium-enhanced MRI, the agent is seen in brain tissue this can be an indication that the blood-brain barrier is disrupted.

Refinements of MRI technology have yielded high resolution scans of the body with specifically notable improvements in neuroimaging. The resolution of the images is superior to CT and the ability to "fine tune" them gives the technique a much broader range of use. The use of MRI in neuroimaging allows visualization of the interior of the skull in remarkable detail, providing a virtual "window into the brain".

Functional imaging

As the preceding tools (CT and MRI) were developed to provide static images of neuroanatomical structures, it was realized that these tools could also be used to examine the functional aspects of tissues. For example, by using MRI to measure blood flow or oxygenation to specific regions of the brain, the functional activation of those regions can be determined. This is referred to as **functional MRI** (fMRI) (Figure 18.8). By asking a patient to perform a specific function at multiple intervals while undergoing an MRI scan, a clinician can see which portion of the cortex is activated when performing the function. This can be valuable prior to brain surgery to localize specific regions that should be avoided or spared during the surgery (Pittau, *et al.*, 2014). It can also be used as a research tool to understand functional dynamics in the cerebral cortex.

Two additional functional imaging techniques are available and they both require the use of fast decaying radioisotopes. The first technique is **positron emission tomography** (PET), which detects the localization of a radiolabeled substance that is administered to a patient (Morbelli and Nobilli, 2014;

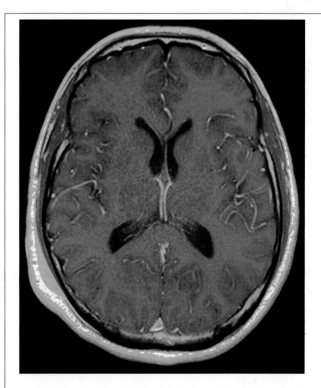

Figure 18.7 A normal magnetic resonance image (MRI) of the same brain as Figure 18.5 in the T1 format with gadolinium contrast agent. Note the "bright" skin and bone marrow and the "dark" bones of the skull. Also, note that the blood vessels are now hyperintense due to the presence of the contrast agent.

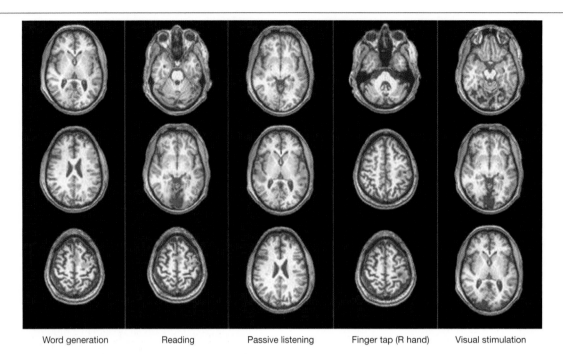

Word generation   Reading   Passive listening   Finger tap (R hand)   Visual stimulation

Figure 18.8 A normal functional magnetic resonance image (fMRI) of the brain from a patient undergoing pre-surgical assessment for task-specific functions. Note the various areas of the brain that are active during specific tasks. This allows surgeons to avoid these areas during surgical removal of tumors or epileptic tissue.

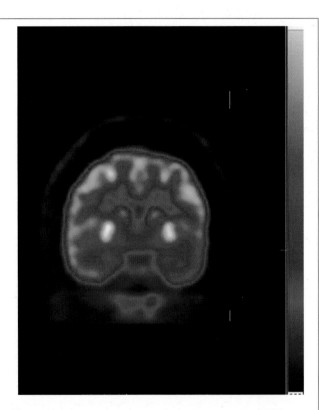

Figure 18.9 A normal positron emission spectroscopy (PET) image of the brain. Note the relatively poor resolution of this technique which localizes glucose utilization in the brain with radioactively labeled glucose molecules.

Torigian, *et al.*, 2013). For example, a radiolabeled precursor for dopamine can be given to a patient and then the radioactivity of specific brain regions that synthesize dopamine can be observed. More common metabolic compounds, like radiolabeled glucose, can also be used to localize functional brain activity (Figure 18.9). Because these radiolabeled compounds have short half-lives, they are usually made in close proximity to the detector and this requires dedicated, expensive machinery. This places a large limitation on the number and distribution of PET scanners. The second technique is **single photon emission computed tomography** (SPECT), which detects gamma rays emitted by a radioactive substance injected into a patient. In typical brain imaging, a radioactive technetium or iodine coupled with a compound of interest is injected into a patient. The gamma radiation from the radioactive compound is detected and processed to produce a computer generated image (Figure 18.10). This technique can be used, like PET, to localize functional activity in the brain. SPECT is primarily used for the determination of dementia, for traumatic brain injury, and for the localization of seizures. It can also be used to localize dopamine activity in the brains of Parkinson's patients (Figure 18.10). SPECT is used more widely than PET because the radioisotopes are more easily generated and have a longer half-life. The machinery necessary to detect and produce the images is also more readily available, since it can be used with other nuclear medicine procedures. Both of these functional imaging techniques require the administration of radioactive materials to patients, which can produce detrimental side effects.

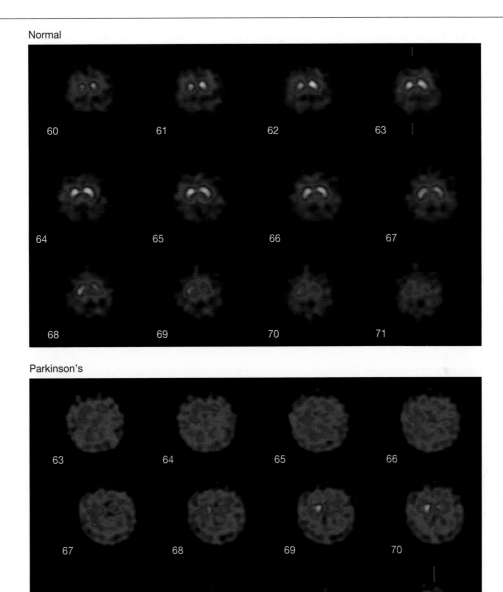

Normal

60   61   62   63

64   65   66   67

68   69   70   71

Parkinson's

63   64   65   66

67   68   69   70

71   72   73   74

Figure 18.10 A series of single photon emission computed tomography (SPECT) images of the dopamine transporter (DaT) in the brain. Note the use of this technique to localize dopamine utilization in the brain of both a normal patient and a patient with Parkinson's disease.

Ultrasound

The use of **ultrasound** is primarily used in a pregnant woman to examine the development of her child. It also has multiple uses in cardiology. Ultrasound has the advantage of being non-invasive, without the use of radioisotopes, as well as being portable and inexpensive to operate. Its use in neuroimaging is generally limited to measurement of cerebral artery blood flow (transcranial Doppler or carotid ultrasonography). This can be helpful when a rapid assessment of neurovascular problems, such as strokes or aneurysms, is required and access to a CT or MRI is unavailable. Ultrasound can also be used in babies prior to the closure of their fontanels, since these openings provide an acoustic window into the brain. Once the fontanels close, however, the bones of the skull block the use of ultrasound. The detail and resolution of ultrasound images is of much lower quality than those seen with CT or MRI (Blondiaux and Garel, 2013).

Clinical considerations

Since plain films are rarely used in neuroimaging today, clinicians generally choose between CT or MRI when determining the type of imaging to suggest for use in their patients. Overall, MRI provides superior tissue resolution and has the increased ability to distinguish clinical entities (tumors, cysts, vascular damage). However, MRI scanners are not as readily available as CT scanners, take longer to operate, can be problematic in patients with pacemakers or other internal metallic components, can be claustrophobic, and are more expensive. CT scanners are used in emergency situations for rapid examination of the brain when delays in treatment can produce serious complications (such as after an acute stroke). CT can also detect skull fractures and acute bleeding more easily.

One of the major advances with the use of computerized imaging (both in CT and MRI) is the ability to scan through a series of cross sections, coronal sections, or even oblique sections that allow a three-dimensional view of the brain. This computerized three-dimensional construct can then be rotated and viewed from multiple angles, providing clinicians with an excellent view of the region of interest.

This is an exciting time to learn neuroanatomy, with the current state of neuroimaging allowing more detailed location of clinical deficits (aneurysms, tumors, infarcts). A clinician can use the results of the neurological exam to predict a preliminary diagnosis and then neuroimaging can substantiate this diagnosis. Neuroimaging also allows surgeons the ability to remove damaged tissue, while reducing the impact on adjacent normal tissue.

Case 1

A 68-year-old mechanical engineer, Tim Masters, begins experiencing seizures after an automobile accident. He meets with a neurologist, Dr Sydney Charif, who recommends an MRI to evaluate his brain structure. Mr Masters undergoes an MRI and Dr Charif discusses the results with him. Dr Charif does not see any noticeable changes or differences in Mr Master's MR images. He then suggests that another MRI study be performed in which the activity of the neurons can be determined. He suggests a functional MRI (fMRI) that measures the amount of oxygen utilization by the regions of the brain as a surrogate for neural activity (Pittau, et al., 2014).

The results of the fMRI suggest that the medial aspects of the temporal lobe of the brain have altered oxygen utilization which may make them more sensitive to seizure initiation. All of this information is discussed with Mr Masters and it is determined that he will try to control the seizures with anti-epileptic medications before he considers surgery. The medications do help to control the seizures, but they come with side effects. Mr Masters feels depressed and lethargic when on the medications.

Case 2

A 35-year-homemaker, Mrs Beverly Willis, is six months pregnant and begins experiencing repeated, painful headaches. Her personal physician suggests she have an MRI to help rule out some causes of her headaches. Her physician believes this is a much safer way to examine her brain without the use of radiation, which could be harmful to her child.

When discussing the results of her MRI with her physician, Mrs Willis is informed that there are no noticeable changes in her brain and that the neuroanatomy appears normal. Her physician suggests that Mrs Willis makes sure she does not become dehydrated, her blood pressure is monitored to prevent any increases and, if she experiences any more headaches, to lie down in a darkened room and use deep breathing relaxation methods.

Study questions

1. Which of the following is a non-radiographic, non-invasive means of imaging the brain?
a) plain film radiography
b) angiography
c) computed tomography (CT)
d) magnetic resonance imaging (MRI)
e) positron emission tomography (PET)

2. A physician suspects an elderly patient at a nursing home has had a small stroke. He is unable to transport her to a local hospital, but would like to quickly determine if her carotid blood flow is impaired. He can use _____ to obtain a basic view of her carotid arteries.
a) positron emission tomography
b) ultrasound
c) plain film radiography
d) magnetic resonance imaging
e) computed tomography

3. When a patient has functional magnetic resonance neuroimaging performed, the scan is depicting the:
a) specific neurotransmitter activity in the region of interest
b) actual firing of specific classes of neurons in the region of interest

c) blood flow or oxygenation to the region of interest
d) quantity of neurotransmitter in neurons in the region of interest
e) direct glucose metabolism of neurons and glia in the region of interest

4. When a physician in a major metropolitan hospital needs a scan of a patient's brain for a diagnosis of the presence of a slow growing tumor, the best choice would be:
a) plain film radiography
b) single photon emission computed tomography
c) positron emission tomography
d) computed tomography
e) magnetic resonance imaging

5. Which of the following is NOT a consideration when comparing the use of computed tomography with magnetic resonance imaging in a patient with unresolved headaches?
a) the patient has a 20-year-old pacemaker implanted in his chest.
b) the patient is claustrophobic and unable to remain immobile for more than a few minutes
c) the patient may be in the acute phase of a stroke
d) the patient's insurance will cover CT imaging, but not MRI imaging
e) the patient is pregnant and should avoid ionizing radiation

For more self-assessment questions, visit the companion website at
www.wileyessential.com/neuroanatomy

FURTHER READING

For additional information on neuroimaging, the following textbooks and review articles may be helpful:

Blondiaux E, Garel C. 2013. Fetal cerebral imaging – ultrasound vs. MRI: an update. *Acta Radio,* 54(9): 1046–1054.

Blumenfeld H. 2002. *Neuroanatomy Through Clinical Cases.* Sinauer Associates, Sunderland, Massachusetts.

Felten DL, Shetty A. 2009. *Netter's Atlas of Neuroscience,* 2nd edition. Saunders Elsevier, Philadelphia, Pennsylvania.

Haines DE. 2012. *Neuroanatomy: An Atlas of Structures, Sections and Systems,* 8th edition. Lippincott Williams & Wilkin, Baltimore, Maryland.

Moore KL, Dalley AF, Agur AMR. 2014. *Moore Clinically Oriented Anatomy,* 7th edition. Lippincott, Williams & Wilkins, Philadelphia, Pennsylvania.

Morbelli S, Nobili F. 2014. Cognitive reserve and clinical expression of Alzheimer's disease: evidence and implications for brain PET imaging. *Am J Nucl Med Mol Imaging,* 4(3): 239–247.

Pittau F, Grouiller F, Spinelli L, Seeck M, Michel CM, Vulliemoz S. 2014. The role of functional neuroimaging in pre-surgical epilepsy evaluation. *Front Neurol,* 5(31): 1–16.

Torigian DA, Zaidi H, Kwee TC, Saboury B, Udupa JK, Cho ZH, *et al.* 2013. PET/MR imaging: technical aspects and potential clinical applications. *Radiology,* 267(1): 26–44.

Answers to study questions

Chapter 1

1. c) A CT has the standard arrangement that you are standing at the end of a patient's bed looking up at the patient who is lying on his back. Therefore, you would be looking at an inferior view with posterior (dorsal) at the bottom of the field and anterior (ventral) at the top of the field. When the symptoms are on the same side as the lesion this is an ipsilateral effect.

2. a) The precentral gyrus is the region where motor output leaves the cortex to descend to the brain stem. The postcentral gyrus is the location of somatosensory input to the cortex. The cingulate gyrus is involved in the limbic system. The superior temporal gyrus is the location of auditory input to the cortex. The calcarine gyrus is the site of visual input to the cortex.

3. e) Oligodendrocytes are responsible for myelination of axons in the central nervous system, while Schwann cells are responsible for myelination of the peripheral axons. Astrocytes provide nutrition and support to the neurons, as well as establishing the blood-brain barrier. Ependymal cells line the ventricular system and microglia act as resident phagocytes in the central nervous system.

4. e) The pineal gland is part of the epithalamus, the third component to the diencephalon. The cingulate gyrus is part of the telencephalon. The midbrain is derived from the mesencephalon and is part of the brain stem. The pituitary gland is not considered part of the central nervous system even though axons from the hypothalamus project into the posterior pituitary. The cerebellum is a separate part of the brain that is derived from the metencephalon, along with the pontine portion of the brain stem.

5. See the following table.

Name	Function	Exit skull	Lesion effects
Olfactory (I)	Sensory	Cribriform plate	Loss of smell
Optic (II)	Sensory	Optic foramen	Loss of vision
Oculomotor (III)	Motor	Superior orbital fissure	Loss of motor control to five muscles of the orbit and parasympathetic innervation to the iris (sphincter pupillae muscle)
Trochlear (IV)	Motor	Superior orbital fissure	Loss of superior oblique muscle
Trigeminal (V)	Both	Superior orbital fissure, foramen rotundum, foramen ovale	Loss of sensation from the face, nasal cavity, and oral cavity; loss of muscles of mastication (plus four other muscles)
Abducens (VI)	Motor	Superior orbital fissure	Loss of lateral rectus muscle
Facial (VII)	Both	Internal acoustic meatus	Loss of facial musculature; salivary secretion from the submandibular and sublingual glands; loss of lacrimal secretion; loss of taste from the anterior ⅔ of the tongue
Vestibulocochlear (VIII)	Sensory	Internal acoustic meatus	Loss of hearing; loss of balance, equilibrium
Glossopharyngeal (IX)	Both	Jugular foramen	Loss of sensation from the pharynx; loss of taste from the posterior ⅓ of tongue; loss of stylopharyngeus muscle
Vagus (X)	Both	Jugular foramen	Loss of parasympathetic control to the heart, lungs, and digestive tract (to left colic flexure); loss of motor control to the larynx; loss of sensation from the larynx
Spinal accessory (XI)	Motor	Jugular foramen	Loss of ipsilateral trapezius and sternocleidomastoid muscles
Hypoglossal (XII)	Motor	Hypoglossal canal	Loss of ipsilateral tongue musculature

Essential Clinical Neuroanatomy, First Edition. Thomas H. Champney.
© 2016 John Wiley & Sons, Ltd. Published 2016 by John Wiley & Sons, Ltd.
Companion website: www.wileyessential.com/neuroanatomy

Chapter 2

1. b) Hydrocephalus is due to an increase in pressure in the ventricular system created by too much cerebrospinal fluid. This could be due to a blockade in the system at some point, to overproduction at the choroid plexus, or to inadequate drainage from the arachnoid granulations.

2. f) A spinal tap collects cerebrospinal fluid from the subarachnoid space. The needle should be inserted below the third lumbar vertebra in order to avoid damaging the spinal cord (which usually ends by the second lumbar vertebra).

3. a) The anterior communicating artery is a single, unpaired artery that connects the right and left anterior cerebral arteries. The paired posterior communicating arteries connect the posterior cerebral arteries with the internal carotid arteries on each side. The lateral communicating artery does not exist.

4. d) The oculomotor (III), trochlear (IV), and abducens (VI) nerves all pass through the cavernous sinus, which when compromised would impact on the movement of the ocular muscles. Paralysis of the facial muscles and tinnitus are generally associated with facial nerve (VII) disturbances, but the facial nerve does not pass through the cavernous sinus. Likewise, lesion of the optic nerve (II) would lead to loss of vision, but the optic nerve does not pass through the cavernous sinus. The third portion of the trigeminal nerve (V) (mandibular division) innervates the muscles of mastication, but it also does not pass through the cavernous sinus even though the other two divisions of the trigeminal nerve do pass through the sinus.

5. e) In an epidural hematoma, a vessel ruptures that is external to the dura mater. The only vessel in the choices provided that is external to the dura is the middle meningeal artery. All of the other vessels are either integral to the dura (inferior sagittal sinus) or are internal to the dura (great cerebral vein, posterior cerebral artery and the anterior communicating artery).

6. From Figure 2.8, the cross hatched area is the region that would be lost with a stroke in the left anterior cerebral artery. If the stroke occurred prior to the cerebral arterial circle, then collateral blood supply from other arterial branches may be able to compensate for the blocked blood vessel and the cortical losses could be minimized. A stroke that occurs after the cerebral arterial circle, where there are limited anastomotic connections, would produce much greater functional losses.

Chapter 3

1. c) The nervous system develops from the ectoderm as a layer of expanded cell division above the notochord.

2. a) The spinal cord has an alar plate which will develop into the posterior (dorsal) horn with somatosensory functions. The

(a)

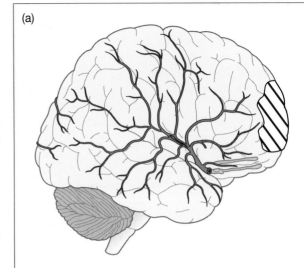

(b)

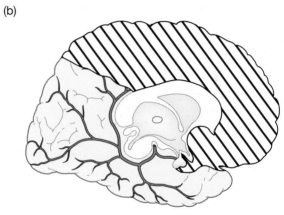

Figure 2.8. Lateral (a) and sagittal (b) views of the brain with its associated blood supply. Notice the distribution of the three cerebral arteries (anterior, middle, and posterior) and the regions of the brain where the vessels meet ("watershed" areas).

spinal cord's basal plate develops into the anterior (ventral) horn with voluntary motor functions.

3. e) Ependymal cells develop from neuroepithelial cells and do not develop from neural crest cells. They do not, therefore, go through an epithelial to mesenchymal transition.

4. b) Folic acid is required for proper development of the neural tube. Children born to mothers with low folic acid levels can develop spina bifida and meningoceles.

5. a) Neural development occurs throughout a women's pregnancy, so at no time during the pregnancy should she consume alcohol. Alcohol consumption during pregnancy can lead to fetal alcohol syndrome.

Chapter 4

1. c) There are eight cervical nerves and only seven cervical vertebrae. The first cervical nerve exits above the first cervical vertebra (between the occiput of the skull and the atlas (first cervical vertebra). This order continues until the eighth cervical nerve, which exits between the seventh cervical vertebra and the first thoracic vertebra. From this point inferiorly, each spinal nerve exits below its associated vertebra.

2. a) The posterior (dorsal) columns carry first order sensory axons from the periphery to second order sensory cell bodies located in nuclei in the caudal medulla oblongata. Their cell bodies are located in the posterior (dorsal) root ganglia of the spinal nerves. The axons stay on the same side of the body where they originated (ipsilateral).

3. b) The posterior (dorsal) columns contain only ascending tracts, while the anterior (ventral) columns contain only descending tracts. The lateral columns contain two ascending tracts and two descending tracts. There are no central or rostral columns.

4. b) The anterior (ventral) horns of gray matter contain the lower motor neuronal cell bodies that control voluntary skeletal muscle. Since the majority of skeletal muscle is in the upper and lower extremities, the anterior horns in the cervical and lumbar regions are enlarged to contain the extra neuronal cell bodies necessary to innervate this increased amount of skeletal muscle.

5. c) The preganglionic sympathetic cell bodies are located in the lateral column of the spinal cord in the thoracic and upper lumbar regions (T1–L2/3). There are also preganglionic parasympathetic cell bodies located in the lateral column of the sacral region (S2–S4). There are no autonomic cell bodies in the cervical or the coccygeal regions of the spinal cord.

Chapter 5

1. c) The nucleus gracilis contains the second order sensory cell bodies for fine touch and proprioception from the lower extremity on the same side of the body (ipsilateral). The axons from the nucleus gracilis will decussate in the caudal medulla oblongata and form the medial lemniscus.

2. b) The spinothalamic tract arises in the spinal cord from the second order sensory axons for pain and temperature that have decussated across the spinal cord soon after they synapsed in the posterior (dorsal) horn. Therefore, a lesion of the spinothalamic tract in the spinal cord or the brain stem produces contralateral deficits.

3. c) The hypoglossal nerve (XII) controls the tongue musculature on the same side of the body (ipsilateral). If the nerve is lesioned, the patient is unable to protrude the tongue on that side of the body and, therefore, the tongue points to the side of the lesion. The hypoglossal nerve (XII) is the only cranial nerve to leave the brain stem from the preolivary sulcus.

4. b) The corticospinal tract as it travels through the medulla oblongata produces a ridge on the ventral surface named the pyramid. The pyramid ends as the corticospinal tract decussates and enters the lateral column of the spinal cord. Therefore, a lesion of the pyramid in the medulla oblongata would produce a contralateral loss of voluntary motor control.

5. f) The nucleus ambiguous contains the lower motor neuronal cell bodies that control the voluntary motor control for the muscles of the pharynx and larynx. The axons from these cell bodies travel ipsilaterally through the glossopharyngeal (IX) and vagus (X) nerves.

Chapter 6

1. c) The trigeminal nerve (V) carries the general sensation, pain, and temperature axons from the face to the brain stem. The first order cell bodies are located in the trigeminal ganglion (similar to the posterior (dorsal) root ganglion). The trigeminal nerve (V) has three branches: the ophthalmic division covers the skin of the forehead, the upper and lateral eye, the maxillary division covers the skin of the lower eye, the upper lip, and the cheek, the mandibular division covers the lower lip, chin, lateral cheek/jaw, and the skin anterior to the ear. The mandibular division also supplies the motor control to the muscles of mastication (along with four other smaller muscles).

2. d) The abducens nerve (VI) supplies the lateral rectus muscle, which moves the eye laterally. The trigeminal nerve (V) carries all of the sensory innervation from the face along with the motor supply to the muscles of mastication. The facial nerve (VII) supplies the muscles of facial expression, but does not supply any of the extraocular muscles. The oculomotor nerve (III) supplies the majority of the extraocular muscles, while the trochlear nerve (IV) supplies one extraocular muscle, the superior oblique muscle.

3. c) A lesion in the pons in the vicinity of the abducens nucleus could also damage the facial nerve (VII) axons as they arch around the nucleus to exit from the lateral pontomedullary junction. This would produce a loss of motor control to the ipsilateral muscles of facial expression.

4. b) The trigeminal nerve (V) carries the general sensation, pain, and temperature axons from the face to the brain stem. The first order cell bodies are located in the trigeminal ganglion (similar to the posterior (dorsal) root ganglion). The trigeminal nerve (V) has three branches: the ophthalmic division covers the skin of the forehead, the upper and lateral eye; the maxillary division covers the skin of the lower eye, the upper lip, and the cheek; the mandibular division covers the lower lip, chin, lateral cheek/jaw, and the skin anterior to the ear. The mandibular division also supplies the motor control to the muscles of mastication (along with four other smaller muscles).

5. b) The medial lemniscus carries the second order sensory fibers from the contralateral side of the body below the neck. The cell bodies for these fibers originate in the nucleus gracilis or cuneatus in the caudal medulla. The fibers decussate in the medulla and ascend up the brain stem to eventually reach the thalamus. Therefore, a lesion in the medial lemniscus in the brain stem will produce a loss of general sensation (although not pain and temperature) from the contralateral side of the body.

Chapter 7

1. b) The oculomotor nerve (III) controls four extraocular muscles (superior rectus, medial rectus, inferior rectus, and inferior oblique), along with the levator palpebrae superioris muscle. In addition, it carries the preganglionic parasympathetic innervation to the ciliary ganglion, which will eventually control the constrictor pupillae muscle of the iris. Therefore, a patient with a lesion of the oculomotor nerve (III) will present with a drooping eyelid, the eye deviated laterally (due to unopposed action from the lateral rectus muscle) and slightly inferiorly (unopposed action of the superior oblique muscle). In addition, the pupil will be dilated because of unopposed sympathetic innervation (impaired parasympathetic innervation).

2. d) The trochlear nerve (IV) controls one extraocular muscle, the ipsilateral superior oblique muscle. It arises posteriorly from the midbrain, courses anteriorly around the midbrain to enter the cavernous sinus. It passes through the sinus to enter the orbit through the superior orbital fissure.

3. e) The tectum of the midbrain contains the periaqueductal gray along with the corpora quadrigemina (the superior and inferior colliculi). The superior and inferior colliculi are relay nuclei for visual and auditory pathways, respectively.

4. e) The cerebral peduncles in the midbrain contain the corticospinal, corticobulbar, and corticopontine axons. These are upper motor neurons that supply, respectively, the skeletal muscles of the trunk and extremities, the skeletal muscles of the face and head, and the cortical axons to the pons, which will then project to the cerebellum.

5. d) The lateral lemniscus contains auditory sensory fibers from the cochlear nuclei that ascend through the lateral brain stem to synapse in the inferior colliculus. A lesion of the lateral lemniscus would have an effect on hearing, but this would not be located to only one side, since many of the auditory projections from the cochlear nuclei are bilateral.

Chapter 8

1. c) The thalamus is the main collection of relay nuclei bringing information to the cortex. Virtually all sensory information and motor control information synapses in the thalamus and is then forwarded to the cortex. The general sensory information from the surface of the body decussates prior to entering the thalamus, so a thalamic lesion produces deficits on the contralateral side of the body.

2. e) The thalamus has numerous component parts that have specific inputs. Two of the best known are the medial geniculate and lateral geniculate that are thalamic relay nuclei for hearing and vision, respectively.

3. c) The hypothalamus is a collection of nuclei that control water intake, food intake, body temperature, and many other homeostatic mechanisms, including basal metabolic rate.

4. a) The ophthalmic artery arises from the internal carotid artery and enters the orbit through the optic canal with the optic nerve (II). Therefore, if the artery increases in size it can place pressure on the optic nerve (II) in the canal leading to visual deficits. In addition, the ophthalmic artery gives off the central retinal artery that enters the optic nerve to supply the retina. If this artery is damaged, blindness can occur.

5. e) The sensation of smell is one of the few neural inputs that can reach the cortex directly without utilizing thalamic relay nuclei. This may be one reason why smells can be so evocative and emotion-laden.

Chapter 9

1. a) The final cortical output for motor signals occurs in Broadman's area 4 of the cortex at the posterior end of the frontal cortex, just anterior to the central sulcus (the precentral gyrus). The frontal cortex just anterior to the precentral gyrus (area 6) is also involved in skeletal muscle motor control.

2. a) The interventricular foramina drain each of the lateral ventricles into the third ventricle. If one of the foramen was closed, then the cerebrospinal fluid produced in the lateral ventricle by the choroid plexus would have nowhere to drain and pressure could increase in the ventricle.

3. d) The hippocampus is one component of the limbic system and is involved in new memory consolidation. The caudate nucleus, putamen, globus pallidus, and subthalamic nuclei are all part of the basal ganglia.

4. c) The corpus callosum is a very large commissure, with thousands of axons interconnecting one hemisphere of the brain with the other. Loss of the corpus callosum by trauma or by surgery can produce a split brain patient.

5. c) The temporal cortex is responsible for primary auditory input and processing these auditory signals into recognizable sounds and words. Lesions in parts of the temporal cortex can produce difficulties with comprehension.

Chapter 10

1. c) Climbing fibers are specialized fibers that arise from the inferior olive in the medulla oblongata and enter the cerebellum to synapse at the deep cerebellar nuclei (with excitatory stimulation) as well as wrapping around the Purkinje cell dendrites in the cerebellar cortex (with excitatory input).

2. e) The output from the cerebellar cortex that projects to the deep cerebellar nuclei is from inhibitory Purkinje cell axons. These inhibitory axons interact with the excitatory stimulation from the climbing and mossy fibers to balance the final cerebellar output from the deep cerebellar nuclei.

3. a) The cerebellum controls motor output on the same side of the body (ipsilateral effects). This is due to having direct ipsilateral inputs or having double decussated inputs. Likewise, the output from the cerebellum decussates as it projects to the thalamus/cortex, modifying firing in the contralateral cortex. The firing in the contralateral cortex will decussate as it descends to the body, leading to effects occurring on the opposite side of the body as the cortex, but the same side of the body as the cerebellum.

4. b) The cortex provides input to the cerebellum by way of the corticopontine fibers that synapse in the pons of the brain stem. The neurons in the pontine nuclei then decussate and enter the cerebellum through the middle cerebellar peduncle as mossy fibers. The cerebellar output to the cortex leaves the deep cerebellar nuclei and exits through the superior cerebellar peduncle, where it decussates before synapsing in the red nucleus or travelling through the midbrain to the thalamus.

5. c) The lateral cerebellar cortex is involved in motor planning activity, while the intermediate cerebellar cortex helps to control distal extremity motor activity. The midline (vermis) of the cerebellar cortex controls trunk and proximal extremity motor activity. Each of these cortical areas project to specific deep cerebellar nuclei: the lateral cerebellar cortex to the dentate nuclei, the intermediate cerebellar cortex to the emboliform and globose (interposed) nuclei, and the midline (vermis) to the fastigial nuclei.

Chapter 11

1. e) The fasciculus gracilis carries the fine touch and proprioceptive sensory information from below the waist to the brain stem. These are ipsilateral, first order sensory axons with their cell bodies in the posterior (dorsal) root ganglion.

2. a) The spinothalamic tract carries the second order pain and temperature sensory fibers from the posterior (dorsal) horn of the spinal cord to the thalamus. The first order fibers enter the posterior (dorsal) horn of the spinal cord on the same (ipsilateral) side and then synapse. The second order fibers decussate across the spinal cord through the anterior white commissure and ascend in the opposite (contralateral) spinothalamic tract.

3. a) The lateral corticospinal tract descends in the spinal cord containing upper motor neurons. These neurons will innervate lower motor neurons in the anterior (ventral) horn that drive skeletal muscles on the same (ipsilateral) side of the body. Since the lesion occurs in upper motor neurons, the patient will present with a Babinski sign and increased deep tendon reflexes.

4. c) The cerebral peduncle contains upper motor, corticospinal fibers that are descending from the cortex to the spinal cord. These fibers cross over (decussate) in the medulla oblongata, so that fibers in the right cerebral peduncle will eventually synapse in the left anterior (ventral) horn of the spinal cord. Therefore, lesions of the cerebral peduncles will cause skeletal motor losses on the opposite (contralateral) side from the lesion.

5. a) The medial lemniscus contains second order, fine touch sensory fibers that have their cell bodies in the nucleus cuneatus or nucleus gracilis of the medulla oblongata. The fibers decussate after leaving the nucleus, so that the fine touch sensations from the left side of the body ascend in the right (contralateral) medial lemniscus.

Chapter 12

1. b) The optic nerves carry vision from each eye, which partially crosses over in the optic chiasm, so that each optic tract contains the visual information from the opposite visual field. This means that the nasal portion of one visual field and the temporal portion of the opposite visual field are carried in the same optic tract. A lesion in the optic tract results in loss of vision from the opposite (contralateral) visual field, producing homonymous hemianopsia.

2. a) In order for the pupil to respond to light, both the optic nerve (II) (bringing in the light information) and the oculomotor nerve (III) (sending out the motor signal) must be intact. The light information is sent bilaterally to both nuclei of Edinger-Westphal, so that normally both eyes respond to light shone in only one eye. A direct effect on pupil size indicates that both the optic nerve (II) and the oculomotor nerve (III) on that side are intact. A consensual effect on pupil size indicates that the optic nerve (II) from the side that was exposed to the light is intact and that the oculomotor nerve (III) on the opposite side driving pupillary constriction is also intact.

3. c) The left occipital cortex is responsible for vision from the right visual field. The axons controlling pupillary light reflexes synapse in the tectum of the midbrain and are not altered by a lesion in the cortex.

4. c) The ciliary body is the site of aqueous humor production, which then circulates through the posterior chamber, the pupil, and the anterior chamber to drain in the canal of Schlemm at the corneo-scleral junction.

5. d) The direct connection between the retinal photoreceptors and the ganglion cells is the bipolar cell. The amacrine cells and horizontal cells can modify the signal transduction from the photoreceptors through the bipolar cells to the ganglion cells. This indicates that modification of the visual signal is already occurring in the layers of the retina.

Chapter 13

1. b) The internal acoustic meatus is the foramen in the temporal bone where the facial nerve (VII) and the vestibulocochlear nerve (VIII) enter the skull after leaving the brain stem. Any mass in that area, such as an acoustic neuroma, can produce compression deficits in these nerves.

2. c) The superior temporal gyrus in the temporal lobe is the primary cortical area for auditory projections from the medial geniculate.

3. e) The lateral lemniscus carries auditory information from the cochlear nuclei to the inferior colliculus and the medial geniculate. The lateral lemniscus carries bilateral auditory information from both sets of cochlear nuclei, so lesions do not produce ipsilateral or contralateral deficits.

4. d) The otoliths are small stone-like structures that rest on the top of hair cells in the utricle/saccule portion of the vestibular system. As linear acceleration begins, the otoliths are resistant to motion and the hair cells bend as the "body" moves away from the otoliths. Once a top speed is achieved and acceleration ceases, the otoliths and the body are at the same speed and the hair cells are in a neutral position again. During deceleration, the otoliths continue forward, bending the hair cells in the opposite direction.

5. e) The medial longitudinal fasciculus is responsible for integrating the three motor nuclei responsible for eye motion (oculomotor (III), trochlear (IV), and abducens (VI)). In addition, the fasciculus integrates vestibular information and the control of neck musculature to integrate eye motion with the body's position in space and with head and neck position. The production of nystagmus by the eye muscles can be a direct influence of the vestibular system's input.

Chapter 14

1. a) The olfactory nerves (I) pass through the cribriform plate of the ethmoid bone when transiting from the nasal epithelium in the superior aspect of the nasal cavity to the olfactory bulb.

2. e) The lingual branch of the mandibular division of the trigeminal nerve (V3) brings general sensation and taste sensation from the anterior two-thirds of the tongue into the trigeminal nerve (V) and the facial nerve (VII) respectively.

3. d) Taste fibers can be carried by the facial nerve (VII), the glossopharyngeal nerve (IX), and the vagus nerve (X), with

their first order sensory cell bodies located in sensory ganglia associated with each nerve. All of these fibers enter the brain stem and converge on the rostral solitary nucleus (gustatory nucleus) where they synapse on second order sensory cell bodies. The second order sensory fibers for taste ascend through the brain stem to synapse in the thalamus.

4. f) Taste and smell sensory information converge in the orbitofrontal cortex to provide a mechanism to appreciate flavors processed by both sensations. This interaction can be used to determine if the flavor is pleasurable or distasteful and whether this food product was encountered in the past.

5. d) The medial olfactory tract provides smell information to the opposite (contralateral) olfactory bulb, so that both olfactory bulbs are in possession of the same smell sensations. This creates a bilateral projection of smell to both sides of the brain.

Chapter 15

1. c) The subthalamic nucleus is part of the inhibitory feedback loop in the indirect pathway and is not part of the direct pathway. There are direct inputs to the internal globus pallidus from the putamen and caudate (striatum) and there are indirect inputs from these same structures through the external globus pallidus and the subthalamic nucleus. The balance of firing through these two pathways impacts on the tonic inhibitory output of the internal globus pallidus to the thalamus.

2. a) A decrease in the tonic inhibitory output from the internal globus pallidus to the thalamus produces an increase in neural excitation from the thalamus to the cortex. This can lead to an increase in motor activity (a hyperkinetic disorder).

3. e) If muscle atrophy occurs due to denervation of the skeletal muscles, this means that the lower motor neurons (those actually innervating the muscle) are involved. The cell bodies for these neurons are found in the anterior (ventral) horn of the spinal cord. The axons exit the spinal cord via the anterior (ventral) roots to enter the spinal nerves and distribute to the peripheral muscles.

4. d) The facial nerve (VII) innervates the muscles of facial expression on the same (ipsilateral) side of the face. If all of the muscles on one side of the face are affected, then the lesion has occurred peripherally in the facial nerve (VII) on that side. If the muscles of the forehead are spared from the lesion, then the lesion has occurred centrally and is from the opposite side (contralateral) of the muscle loss.

5. a) The caudate nucleus and the putamen, when combined together, can be referred to as the striatum. The putamen and the globus pallidus, when combined together, can be referred to as the lenticular nuclei.

Chapter 16

1. c) Lesions in the mammillary bodies can produce anterograde amnesia, confabulation, and ataxia, called Wernicke-Korsakoff syndrome. These lesions can be found in alcoholics or other individuals that do not have adequate nutrition, especially those with decreased thiamine (vitamin B1).

2. a) The amygdala is found in the anterior portion of the temporal lobe (anterior to the hippocampus). It is involved in facial recognition, as well as attaching emotions (such as fear) to objects. Patients with amygdala lesions (Klüver-Bucy syndrome) display flattened emotions, lack of fear, hyperorality, and hypersexuality.

3. b) The hippocampus is found in the medial and central regions of the temporal lobe and is connected to other portions of the limbic system by way of the fornix and the parahippocampal gyrus. The hippocampus is responsible for consolidating new declarative memories, so that a lesion of the hippocampus prevents the acquisition of new memories (anterograde amnesia) without altering the recall or storage of old memories.

4. d) The hypothalamus is a collection of many small nuclei that measure and maintain set points for numerous physiologic processes, including body temperature, basal metabolic rate, food intake, water balance, blood sugar levels, and hormone balance. These processes help to maintain physiological homeostasis.

5. a) The amygdala is situated anterior to the hippocampus in the temporal lobe.

Chapter 17

1. b) Wernicke's aphasia is a comprehension aphasia in which patients can speak fluently and with relative ease, but the content of their speech is disordered or nonsensical. This can occur due to lesions in the temporal cortex, especially those near Brodmann's area 22.

2. c) One of the first noticeable losses in patients with Alzheimer's disease is a decline in their sense of smell. Food begins to taste bland and the patients add more seasoning. As the disease progresses, short lapses in memory can occur, followed by longer and more pronounced memory loss.

3. e) Intelligence is not found in any one portion of the cerebral cortex. It is believed to be a distributed neural function throughout the cortex. The cingulate gyrus is a part of the limbic system and has an integrated connection with the hippocampus and the thalamus.

4. b) Delirium is an agitated state in patients who may experience hallucinations. This can occur due to biochemical modifications in brain neurochemistry.

5. a) A patient with hemi-neglect generally has a loss of recognition on the side opposite from the lesion (contralateral). A right cortical lesion can produce a hemi-neglect on the left side of the body. Hemi-neglect is seen predominantly on the left side of the body.

Chapter 18

1. d) Magnetic resonance imaging (MRI) utilizes powerful magnets to align the hydrogen atoms in water molecules. Once aligned, these atoms can be deflected by a pulse of radiofrequency energy which causes a small change in energy output when the atoms reset. This energy change can be detected and imaged. This procedure is non-invasive and does not use ionizing radiation.

2. b) Ultrasound is an inexpensive, portable means for assessing carotid artery structure and blood flow. It is non-invasive and does not require the patient to be transported to a hospital or medical center.

3. c) Functional MRI measures the blood flow or oxygenation to the brain and this can be used as a correlate for the functional activity of that region in the brain. It does not allow the direct determination of neuronal firing, neurotransmitter activity, or glucose metabolism in the brain.

4. e) The imaging technique that provides the best tissue resolution for tumor determination is magnetic resonance imaging. It is less invasive, without the use of radioisotopes or radiation. While computed tomography may provide an indication of a tumor's presence, magnetic resonance imaging in T1, T2, and FLAIR formats can provide much more detailed information on the tumor's location and structure, although with a greater cost.

5. d) Although the cost of MRI may be higher than the cost of CT, this should not be a limiting factor when diagnosing brain disorders. Pacemakers and other metallic implants may be problematic with the magnets necessary for MRI scanning. To obtain an MRI, a patient generally has to remain quiet in an enclosed tube for many minutes, so claustrophobic or fidgety patients could be problematic. In acute cerebrovascular incidents, the use of CT over MRI may be warranted since it can provide valuable information more quickly.

Answers to figures

Answer to Figure 4.8

Green lesion: loss of ipsilateal fine touch from the lower extremity due to lesion of the first order sensory axons in the fasciculus gracilis.

Blue lesion: loss of ipsilateral skeletal motor activity below this spinal level due to lesion of the upper motor axons in the lateral corticospinal tract.

Red lesion: loss of contralateral pain and temperature below this spinal level due to lesion of the second order sensory axons in the spinothlamic tract. There may also be vestibulospinal tract and reticulospinal tract deficits, but these can be difficult to quantify due to the nature of the loss and the redundancy of the signal distribution. Note that the lower motor axons for that spinal segment are also passing through the site of the lesion to enter the anterior roots; therefore, there could be a segmental loss of voluntary motor supply to that specific myotome.

Yellow lesion: loss of anterior descending columns (vestibulospinal, reticulospinal, tectospinal, and anterior corticospinal). This may produce poor spinal cord coordination of movement and regulation of trunk musculature with difficulty identifying ipsipateral or contralateral effects.

Answer to Figure 5.17

Yellow lesion: loss of contralateral skeletal motor control due to loss of the pyramid (corticospinal tract).

Purple lesion: loss of ipsilateral skeletal motor control for muscles innervated by the glossopharyngeal (IX) and vagus (X) nerves due to lesion of the nucleus ambiguous. Cardiac muscle innervation may also be affected, as well as preganglionic parasympathetic fibers of passage for the vagus (X) nerve.

Blue lesion: loss of ipsilateral skeletal muscle control to the tongue (hypoglossal nucleus) as well as the ipsilateral preganglionic parasympathetic contribution of the vagus (X) nerve due to loss of the dorsal motor nucleus of the vagus.

Gray lesion: loss of ipsilateral taste sensation due to lesion of the tract and solitary nucleus.

Answer to Figure 6.19

Yellow lesion: loss of ipsilateral facial muscles due to a loss of the facial nerve (VII) (may also have the loss of lacrimal, submandibular, and sublingual gland function, and taste from anterior ⅔ of tongue). There could also be some loss of pontocerebellar fibers to the middle cerebellar peduncle (although difficult to notice clinically).

Green lesion: loss of pain, temperature, and general sensation from the contralateral face and body due to a lesion of the spinothalamic tract, trigeminothalamic tract, and medial lemniscus. Also, ipsilateral loss of lateral rectus muscle due to loss of abducens (VI) axons passing through the region.

Blue lesion: loss of ipsilateral facial muscles due to loss of the facial nerve (VII) as it passes around the abducens nucleus (which would also produce the ipsilateral loss of the lateral rectus muscle).

Red lesion: loss of contralateral motor control to the skeletal muscles of the body due to lesion of the corticospinal tract. There may also be loss of skeletal motor control to cranial nerves inferior to the lesion (due to loss of corticobulbar axons) as well as some loss to the cerebellum (due to loss of corticopontine and pontocerebellar axons).

Black lesion: loss of output from cerebellum to the red nucleus, thalamus, and cortex (due to a lesion of the superior cerebellar peduncle). This could produce deficits in learned motor activities and motor error correction.

Answer to Figure 7.9

Blue lesion: loss of cerebral peduncle produces contralateral loss of skeletal motor activity in the head and body due to loss of corticospinal, corticobulbar, and corticopontine axons.

Yellow lesion: loss of unilateral substantia nigra produces signs of Parkinsonism. More details are available in Chapter 15.

Green lesion: loss of superior colliculus produces defects in the pupillary light reflex and may impact on eye coordination with head and neck movements. More details are available in Chapter 12.

Red lesion: loss of medial lemniscus, trigeminothalamic tract, and spinothalamic tract produces contralateral loss of general sensation (touch, pain, and temperature) from the face, head, and body due to loss of second order somatosensory axons.

Answer to Figure 11.21

Blue: lateral corticospinal tract; loss of skeletal motor function (upper motor neurons) ipsilateral below this level.

Essential Clinical Neuroanatomy, First Edition. Thomas H. Champney.
© 2016 John Wiley & Sons, Ltd. Published 2016 by John Wiley & Sons, Ltd.
Companion website: www.wileyessential.com/neuroanatomy

Black: fasciculus gracilis; loss of fine touch, vibration from ipsilateral lower extremity (first order sensory neurons).

Green: anterior commissure; loss of pain and temperature bilaterally at this level (second order sensory neurons).

Yellow: anterior columns; contralateral loss of descending visual, balance, and autonomic input below this level.

Red: spinothalamic tract (perhaps spinocerebellar tract); loss of pain and temperature from contralateral side below this level (second order sensory neurons) (perhaps some proprioceptive loss).

Answer to Figure 11.22

Blue: pyramid in medulla; loss of upper motor neurons produces contralateral skeletal muscle loss below the neck.

Green: nucleus gracilis; loss of fine touch, vibration from ipsilateral lower extremity (second order sensory cell bodies).

Black: medial lemniscus; loss of fine touch, vibration from contralateral side of body (second order sensory axons). Also, loss of corticospinal fibers decussating across medulla to lateral corticospinal tract producing ipsilateral motor loss. Perhaps loss of the trigeminothalamic tract just lateral to lesion; loss of pain and temperature from the contralateral face (second order sensory axons).

Yellow: spinal nucleus (and tract) of trigeminal; loss of pain and temperature from ipsilateral face (first order sensory neurons).

Red: spinothalamic tract; loss of pain and temperature from contralateral side of body (second order sensory axons).

Answer to Figure 11.23

Blue: pyramid in medulla; loss of upper motor neurons produces contralateral muscle loss below the neck.

Green: hypoglossal nucleus; loss of motor control to ipsilateral tongue (lower motor neuron cell bodies).

Black: medial lemniscus; loss of fine touch, vibration from contralateral side of body (second order sensory axons). Also, perhaps the trigeminothalamic tract just lateral to lesion; loss of pain and temperature from contralateral face (second order sensory axons).

Yellow: medial longitudinal fasciculus; altered eye muscle/neck muscle coordination.

Red: spinothalamic tract; loss of pain and temperature from contralateral side of body (second order sensory axons).

Answer to Figure 11.24

Blue: corticospinal fibers in pons; loss of upper motor neurons produces contralateral muscle loss below the neck. Also, some loss of corticobulbar fibers to cranial nerves perhaps leading to

pharynx, larynx, and tongue muscle deficits. Perhaps loss of ipsilateral abducens nerve (VI) due to fibers of passage (lower motor axons).

Green: abducens nucleus; loss of motor control to lateral rectus muscle of eye (diplopia) (lower motor neuron cell bodies). Perhaps loss of ipsilateral face nerve (VII) due to fibers of passage (lower motor axons).

Black: medial lemniscus; loss of fine touch, vibration from contralateral side of body (second order sensory axons). Also, perhaps the trigeminothalamic tract just lateral to lesion; loss of pain and temperature from contralateral face (second order sensory axons). Perhaps loss of ipsilateral abducens nerve (VI) due to fibers of passage.

Yellow: medial longitudinal fasciculus; altered eye muscle/neck muscle coordination. Perhaps loss of ipsilateral face nerve (VII) due to fibers of passage (lower motor axons).

Red: spinothalamic tract; loss of pain and temperature from contralateral side of body (second order sensory axons).

Answer to Figure 11.25

Blue: corticospinal fibers in pons; loss of upper motor neurons produces contralateral muscle loss below the neck. Also, some loss of corticobulbar fibers to cranial nerves perhaps leading to pharynx, larynx, and tongue muscle deficits, as well as loss of decussating pontocerebellar fibers.

Green: superior cerebellar peduncle; loss of primary cerebellar output (as well as some spinocerebellar input) leading to motor coordination difficulties. Perhaps also balance/vertigo difficulties (Chapter 10).

Black: medial lemniscus; loss of fine touch, vibration from contralateral side of body (second order sensory axons). Also, perhaps the trigeminothalamic tract just posterior to lesion; loss of touch, pain, and temperature from contralateral face (second order sensory axons).

Yellow: medial longitudinal fasciculus; altered eye muscle/neck muscle coordination.

Red: spinothalamic tract; loss of pain and temperature from contralateral side of body (second order sensory axons).

Answer to Figure 11.26

Blue: corticospinal fibers in cerebral peduncle (midbrain); loss of upper motor neurons produces contralateral muscle loss below the neck. Also, loss of corticobulbar fibers to cranial nerves (V, VII, IX, X, and XII) leading to jaw, face, pharynx, larynx, and tongue muscle deficits, as well as loss of corticopontine fibers (to cerebellum).

Green: inferior colliculus; central hearing deficits (Chapter 13).

Black: medial lemniscus; loss of fine touch, vibration from contralateral side of body (second order sensory axons). Also, perhaps the trigeminothalamic tract just posterior to lesion; loss of touch, pain, and temperature from contralateral face (second order sensory axons).

Yellow: trochlear nucleus; contralateral loss of superior oblique muscle in eye (diplopia) (lower motor neuron cell bodies).

Red: spinothalamic tract; loss of pain, and temperature from contralateral side of body (second order sensory axons).

Answer to Figure 11.27

Blue: corticospinal fibers in cerebral peduncle (midbrain); loss of upper motor neurons produces contralateral muscle loss below the neck. Also, loss of corticobulbar fibers to cranial nerves (V, VII, IX, X, and XII) leading to jaw, face, pharynx, larynx, and tongue muscle deficits, as well as loss of corticopontine fibers (to cerebellum).

Green: red nucleus; cerebellar deficits, perhaps contralateral motor coordination difficulties (Chapter 10).

Yellow: substantia nigra; loss of motor coordination (Parkinsonism) (Chapter 15).

Answer to Figure 11.28

Blue: internal capsule; loss of upper motor neurons produces contralateral muscle loss below the neck. Also, loss of corticobulbar fibers to cranial nerves (V, VII, IX, X, and XII) leading to jaw, face, pharynx, larynx, and tongue muscle deficits, as well as loss of corticopontine fibers. Also loss of third order sensory neurons from thalamus to cortex producing contralateral sensory loss.

Green: hippocampus; limbic system loss (primarily memory consolidation) (Chapter 16).

Black: thalamus; loss of sensory input (touch, pain, and temperature) from contralateral head, face, and body as well as loss of cerebellar, limbic, and hypothalamic input.

Yellow: cortical gray matter; loss of all sensation from specifc area of the face (homunculus).

Red: cortical gray matter; loss of all sensation from specifc area of the upper extremity (homunculus).

Answer to Figure 11.29

Blue: posterior limb of internal capsule; loss of upper motor neurons produces contralateral muscle loss to head, face, and body. Also loss of third order sensory neurons from thalamus to cortex producing contralateral sensory loss.

Green: basal ganglia; central motor control loss (motor coordination difficulties) (Chapter 15).

Black: thalamus; loss of sensory input (touch, pain, and temperature) from contralateral head, face, and body, as well as loss of cerebellar, limbic, and hypothalamic input.

Yellow: cortical gray matter; loss of vision from contralateral visual field (Chapter 12).

Red: pineal gland; loss of melatonin secretion (Chapter 8).

Answer to Figure 15.10

Blue = putamen, yellow = caudate nucleus, red = globus pallidus, green = subthalamic nucleus.

Glossary

Abducens nerve (VI) The sixth cranial nerve arises from a nucleus in the pons, exits inferiorly and medially at the pontomedullary junction, passes into the cavernous sinus and enters the orbit through the superior orbital fissure. It innervates one ocular muscle, the lateral rectus.

Abducens nucleus The lower motor neuronal cell bodies for the sixth cranial nerve found in the posterior aspect of the caudal pons. It innervates one ocular muscle, the lateral rectus.

Acoustic neuroma A glioblastoma (tumor) found in the internal acoustic meatus that can impact on the function of the facial nerve (VII) and vestibulocochlear nerve (VIII).

Afferent Axons that project into the nervous system, bringing sensory information from the periphery.

Alar plate The region of the mantle layer in the developing spinal cord that is nearest the roof plate and will develop into the sensory, posterior (dorsal) horn of the spinal cord.

Alcoholic cerebellar degeneration A decline in cerebellar function due to excessive, long-term alcohol intake.

Allodynia The sensation of painful responses from non-painful stimuli.

Alzheimer's disease An age-associated, neurodegenerative disease characterized by a loss of memory and cognitive deficits (dementia). It is associated with the histological development of neurofibrillary tangles and amyloid senile plaques.

Ampulla A dilated region at the end of each semicircular canal in the inner ear that contains neuroepithelial receptor cells in a gelatinous structure. During acceleration, the fluid in the canal bends the stereocilia of the receptor cells.

Amygdala A collection of nuclei at the anterior end of the hippocampus in the medial temporal lobe that are involved in the limbic system, emotions, and the recognition of fear.

Amyotrophic lateral sclerosis (Lou Gehrig's disease) A degenerating motor disease that affects both upper motor and lower motor neurons.

Anatomic view The inferior view of a horizontal section of the brain or spinal cord, with the anterior (ventral) side down and the posterior (dorsal) side up. This is the historical view that has been used for decades by neuroanatomists.

Anencephaly A defect in the development of the anterior neural tube, leading to little or no telencephalon formation.

Angiography The use of specific contrast dyes that are injected into blood vessels and then radiographic images are obtained detailing the course and distribution of the vessel.

Annulus fibrosus The outer fibrous ring of the intervertebral disc.

Anosmia The loss of smell, usually due to damage of the olfactory neurons, olfactory bulbs, or olfactory tract.

Anterior cerebral artery A terminal branch of the internal carotid artery that arches over the corpus callosum supplying the medial surface of the cortex in the anterior region of the interhemispheric fissure.

Anterior columns Descending tracts in the anterior spinal cord (anterior corticospinal, reticulospinal, vestibulospinal, and tectospinal).

Anterior commissure A small white matter tract for communication between the cortical hemispheres, located antero-inferior to the corpus callosum.

Anterior communicating artery A short anastomotic artery between the right and left anterior cerebral arteries.

Anterior corticospinal tract The descending motor tract in the anterior spinal cord that carries upper motor axons from the cortex to the anterior horn of the spinal cord to control skeletal musculature of the trunk.

Essential Clinical Neuroanatomy, First Edition. Thomas H. Champney.
© 2016 John Wiley & Sons, Ltd. Published 2016 by John Wiley & Sons, Ltd.
Companion website: www.wileyessential.com/neuroanatomy

Anterior (ventral) horn The portion of the gray matter in the spinal cord that contains the large alpha motor neurons, controlling skeletal muscles and the associated motor interneurons.

Anterior inferior cerebellar artery A branch from the basilar artery that supplies the lower portion of the cerebellum.

Anterior olfactory nucleus A collection of sensory nerve cell bodies located in the olfactory tract whose axons project into the contralateral olfactory bulb.

Anterior (ventral) root(lets) The extension of the motor axons from the neural cell bodies in the anterior horn out of the anterior surface of the spinal cord that course laterally to join with the posterior root(lets) to form the spinal nerve.

Anterior (ventral) spinocerebellar tract A double decussating, ipsilateral tract carrying unconscious proprioception that ascends up the lateral spinal cord to enter the cerebellum thorough the superior cerebellar peduncle as mossy fibers.

Anterior white commissure A small central region in the spinal cord adjacent to the central canal in which the second order pain and temperature axons decussate to the contralateral side to form the spinothalamic tract.

Anterograde amnesia The inability to form new, declarative memories. It is associated with the loss of the hippocampus.

Antidiuretic hormone A neuroendocrine hormone released from the posterior pituitary that mediates water balance by acting at the collecting ducts of the kidney.

Aphasia The inability or difficulty in comprehending and/or producing speech.

Apraxia The inability or difficulty in performing a motor function when given a verbal command.

Aqueous humor The fluid that circulates from the posterior chamber of the eye, through the pupil to the anterior chamber of the eye. It is produced by the ciliary body and drains into the canal of Schlemm.

Arachnoid granulations Tufts of arachnoid mater that project into the dural venous sinuses for drainage of the cerebrospinal fluid.

Arachnoid mater A thin, spider web-like connective tissue between the dura mater and the pia mater that creates a space for cerebrospinal fluid to flow.

Arcuate fasciculus A white matter tract that connects Wernicke's and Broca's areas, integrating the production of coordinated and fluent speech.

Area postrema A collection of cell bodies adjacent to the dorsal motor nucleus of the vagus in the medulla oblongata that is outside of the blood-brain barrier. It is also referred to as the emetic center.

Ascending tract A collection of axons found in the peripheral white matter of the spinal cord that travel through the spinal cord to reach the brain stem, cerebellum, or brain.

Astrocyte The glial cell in the central nervous system that provides nutritional and metabolic support for the neurons. It also participates in the blood-brain barrier.

Ataxia Uncoordinated movement or unsteady gait that can be associated with cerebellar disorders.

Athetosis Slow, writhing motions seen in some disorders of the basal ganglia. This can be a common finding in individuals with cerebral palsy.

Auditory tube The connection between the middle ear cavity and the upper pharynx that allows for equalization of air pressure in the middle ear.

Autism A neurologic developmental disorder that produces characteristic behavioral responses usually related to language and social interactions.

Autonomic nervous system The portion of the nervous system that controls involuntary, unconscious actions utilizing smooth or cardiac muscle. It modifies cardiac, respiratory, digestive, and reproductive function.

Axon The projection of the neuron that carries information from the cell body to its target.

Axon hillock The pale staining region of the neuronal cell body at the beginning of the axon. This region does not absorb typical stains due to the increased presence of microtubules.

Axoplasmic transport The flow of compounds, proteins, and organelles through the length of the axon. Anterograde flow is from the cell body to the axon terminal, while retrograde flow is from the terminal to the cell body.

Babinski sign
A marker of upper motor neuron damage that involves the flaring of the toes after running an object along the sole of the foot. In normal individuals, the toes will curl under with this stimulus.

Ballismus
Violent, flailing and flinging motions of the extremities seen in disorders of the basal ganglia. This can be seen in patients with excessive chorea.

Basal ganglia
The brain nuclei located lateral to the internal capsule and thalamus, which help initiate and control motor activity. They are composed of the striatum (caudate nucleus and putamen) as well as the globus pallidus.

Basal plate
The region of the mantle layer in the developing spinal cord that is nearest the floor plate and will develop into the motor, anterior (ventral) horn of the spinal cord.

Basilar artery
Formed by the fusion of the vertebral arteries, ascends up the anterior surface of the brain stem to terminate as the posterior cerebral arteries.

Basilar membrane
The thick cellular structure that separates the scala media and the scala tympani in the cochlea. It contains the neuroepithelial receptor cells that are deflected against the tectorial membrane during sound reception.

Basket cells
Interneurons in the molecular layer of the cerebellum.

Berry (saccular) aneurysm
A globe or sphere-like expansion of a cerebral arterial vessel that can place pressure on adjacent structures or rupture unexpectedly.

Bipolar neurons
These are neurons with a single dendrite and a single axon. They are found in the olfactory mucosa, inner ear, and the retina.

Bitemporal (heteronymous) hemianopsia
A lesion in the optic chiasm that produces a loss of vision in both of the temporal (lateral) portions of the visual fields.

Blood-brain barrier
A thick protective layer on the blood vessels in the central nervous system that limits the transfer of large proteins and cells. It is composed of type 1 capillary endothelial cells, along with the foot processes of astrocytes.

Brain stem
The superior (rostral) extension of the spinal cord, containing nuclei of cranial nerves, nuclei for basic neural functions, and white matter tracts. It is subdivided into the medulla oblongata, the pons, and the midbrain.

Broca's area
A region of the inferior lateral portion of the left frontal lobe (Brodmann's areas 44 and 45) that is associated with producing speech (pronunciation aphasia – Broca's aphasia).

Brodmann's areas
A cortical map of histologically different regions of the brain that have unique functional roles.

Brown-Séquard syndrome
A hemisection of the spinal cord in which touch, proprioception, and skeletal motor function are lost ipsilaterally from the site of the lesion inferiorly, while pain and temperature sensations are lost contralaterally.

Caloric test
A vestibular system test in which a patient has warm or cold water placed in the external auditory meatus. During the test, the patient's eyes are examined for nystagmus. In a normal individual, cold water will produce nystagmus in the opposite direction from the irrigated ear, while warm water will produce nystagmus in the same direction as the irrigated ear.

Canal of Schlemm
A drainage point for aqueous humor along the corneo-scleral junction of the eye.

Cataract
The increased opacity of the lens of the eye that usually occurs with age, producing a decrease in vision and visual acuity.

Cauda equina
The collection of descending spinal nerve rootlets inside a dura mater enclosure (lumbar cistern) in the lower lumbar region of the vertebral column.

Caudate
A portion of the striatum that begins at the anterior end of the putamen, arches superiorly, posteriorly, and laterally to end in the temporal lobe. It is part of the basal ganglia which controls motor activity.

Cavernous sinus
A dural venous sinus formed at the lateral side of the sella turcica (pituitary) in the middle cranial fossa, draining the ophthalmic vein anteriorly and the superior and inferior petrosal sinuses posteriorly. The internal carotid artery and the oculomotor nerve (III), trochlear nerve (IV), abducens nerve (VI), and two divisions of the trigeminal nerve (V) pass through the sinus.

Cephalic flexure
A bend in the developing midbrain (mesencephalon) that will persist into adulthood as the midbrain flexion.

Central canal
The cerebrospinal fluid-filled tube in the center of the spinal cord lined by ependymal cells.

Central nervous system
The portion of the nervous system that is inside of the vertebral column and skull. This includes the brain and spinal cord, with a dura mater covering, and contains both groups of neuronal cell bodies, along with axonal tracts.

Central tegmental tract
An ascending tract in the brain stem of second order sensory axons from the gustatory portion of the solitary nucleus to the thalamus. It is located anterior and lateral to the cerebral aqueduct and fourth ventricle.

Central sulcus
A laterally-oriented groove in the cortex that separates the frontal and parietal regions of the cortex.

Cerebellum
The brain region, with unique foliated morphology, located superior and posterior to the brain stem and inferior to the occipital cortex. It is involved in balance, coordination, motor skills, and motor planning.

Cerebral aqueduct (of Sylvius)
The cerebrospinal fluid-filled tube that runs through the midbrain connecting the third ventricle and the fourth ventricle and is lined by ependymal cells.

Cerebral arterial circle (of Willis)
An anastomosis of arteries around the inferior surface of the diencephalon that connects the vertebral-basilar system with the internal carotid arteries from both sides.

Cerebral cortex
The superficial surface of the telencephalon that contains gray matter hills (gyri) and valleys (sulci).

Cerebral palsy
A developmental disorder of the motor control regions of the brain, leading to large, permanent, non-progressive motor symptoms.

Cerebral peduncles
The large white matter tracts on the anterior surface of the midbrain that contain the descending corticospinal, corticopontine, and corticobulbar tracts.

Cerebrocerebellum
The region of the cerebellum that receives input from the cerebral cortex, notably the lateral portion of the cerebellum.

Cerebrospinal fluid
A plasma-like fluid that circulates throughout the central nervous system allowing the brain to "float" in a protective fluid. It is produced in the choroid plexus in the ventricles of the brain, circulates around the brain and spinal cord and is drained through arachnoid granulations into dural venous sinuses.

Cervical flexure
A bend in the developing hindbrain (rhombencephalon).

Cervical nerves
The eight spinal nerves which exit between the occiput of the skull and the seventh cervical vertebra.

Chiari malformation
A disorder in which the lower portion of the cerebellum (tonsil) extends into the foramen magnum, placing pressure on the adjacent medulla oblongata/spinal cord and restricting cerebrospinal fluid flow.

Chorea
Dance-like, involuntary motions of the body that are usually produced by basal ganglia or extrapyramidal disorders.

Choroid
The layer of the eye next to the retina that contains large quantities of melanin for excess light absorption, as well as numerous blood vessels for nutritional supply to the retina.

Choroid plexus
A collection of ependymal cells in the cranial ventricles that produce cerebrospinal fluid.

Ciliary body
The circular structure in the anterior portion of the eye, lateral to the iris and the lens that contains the ciliary muscle, the suspensory ligaments (zonule fibers) of the lens, and the cells that produce aqueous humor.

Ciliary muscle
Circular smooth muscle in the ciliary body that surrounds the lens and when contracted allows the lens to naturally round up. When relaxed, the muscle creates tension in the suspensory ligaments of the lens which flatten the lens.

Ciliary ganglion
The postganglionic parasympathetic cell bodies for innervation of the sphincter pupillae and ciliary muscles in the eye. It is found on the lateral side of the optic nerve in the orbit and receives its preganglionic parasympathetic innervation from the oculomotor nerve (III).

Cingulate gyrus
The ridge of cortical tissue just superior to the corpus callosum. It is part of the limbic system.

Circumventricular organ
Neural tissue close to the ventricles that does not have the usual blood-brain barrier protection.

Climbing fibers
Axons from the inferior olivary nuclei in the medulla oblongata that enter the cerebellum and project to both the deep cerebellar nuclei and to the dendrites of the Purkinje cells.

Clinical view
The inferior view of a horizontal section of the brain or spinal cord with the posterior side down and the anterior side up. This is the standard view that is used for all neurological imaging.

Cochlea The spiral-shaped acoustic sensory structure located in the temporal bone.

Cochlear nuclei Two nuclei (anterior and posterior) in the lateral aspect on each side of the caudal pons and rostral medulla oblongata that receive ipsilateral, first order, auditory axons from the spiral ganglia in the cochlea. The axons from these nuclei project bilaterally to the superior olive and the inferior colliculus by way of the lateral lemniscus.

Combined neglect The inability to recognize or react to sensory information, as well as the inability to use skeletal muscles from one side or one region of the body. This is a combined sensory and motor neglect.

Computed tomography (CT) The use of multiple radiologic images to construct a computer generated, two-dimensional image of the body.

Conceptual neglect The conscious inability to recognize one side or one region of the body.

Confabulate Providing incorrect or wrong answers to direct questions in order to be helpful, not consciously lying.

Confluence of the sinuses A joining of the superior sagittal and straight dural venous sinuses that drains into the transverse sinuses at the point where the falx cerebri meets the tentorium cerebelli.

Consensual pupillary light reflex The ability of the pupil of the eye to contract when light is shone into the opposite (contralateral) eye.

Contralateral Occurring on the opposite side of the body.

Contrecoup injury Damage to the brain on the opposite side of a force-induced injury. This occurs when the brain rebounds to the opposite wall within the skull after a forceful impact to the head.

Conus medullaris The narrowing of the distal end of the spinal cord.

Cornea The avascular, transparent, curved structure on the anterior surface of the eye that refracts the light that enters the eye.

Corpora quadrigemina The four hills on the posterior surface of the midbrain composed of the superior and inferior colliculi.

Corpus callosum A large myelinated tract of axons that connect the two hemispheres of the brain. It extends from the anterior commissure to the posterior commissure just superior to the thalamus.

Corticobulbar tract A descending motor tract that carries upper motor axons from the cortex to the motor nuclei associated with cranial nerves in the brain stem.

Corticopontine tract A descending motor tract that carries upper motor axons from the cortex to the pontine nuclei. Axons from the pontine nuclei project to the contralateral cerebellar hemisphere.

Corticospinal tract A descending motor tract in the brain stem that carries upper motor axons from the cortex to the anterior horn of the spinal cord.

Coup injury Damage to the brain at the site of a force-induced injury.

Cranial nerves Twelve nerves associated with the brain or brain stem identified by roman numerals (I–XII).

Cribriform plate The superior portion of the ethmoid bone that has numerous small openings through which the olfactory nerves pass.

Dandy-Walker syndrome A congenital cerebellar disorder with an associated increase in the size of the fourth ventricle. Motor dysfunction, as well as symptoms of hydrocephalus, are common.

Decussation The crossing over of axons from one side of the spinal cord or brain stem to the opposite side.

Deep cerebellar nuclei The set of nuclei that are the final output pathway from the cerebellum, composed of the dentate, interposed, and fastigial nuclei.

Delirium A short-term, confused, disoriented, or agitated state of consciousness usually produced by an exogenous compound altering neural biochemistry.

Dementia A long-term abnormal decline in cognitive function usually associated with memory loss, problem solving, and language ability (a neurocognitive disorder).

Dendrite The projections of the neuron that bring information into the cell body.

Dentate gyrus A subdivision of the hippocampus that receives the majority of cortical input to the hippocampus. It is composed of cortex (archicortex) that only has three cellular layers.

Dentate nuclei The lateral deep cerebellar nuclei associated with the lateral portion of the cerebellum involved in motor planning.

Dermatome map A diagram of a human with the sensory distribution of the spinal nerves indicated for referencing the spinal level of a lesion of the spinal cord.

Descending tract A collection of axons in the peripheral white matter of the spinal cord that travel from the brain stem, cerebellum, or cortex into the spinal cord.

Diabetes insipidus A loss of the posterior pituitary neurons that produce antidiuretic hormone, leading to polydipsia and polyuria.

Diencephalon The portion of the central nervous system between the midbrain of the brain stem and the telencephalon (cortical structures). It is composed of the hypothalamus, thalamus, and epithalamus (pineal and habenula).

Dilator pupillae muscle Radiating bands of longitudinal smooth muscle in the iris which, when sympathetically contracted, increase the size of the pupil allowing more light to enter the eye.

Direct pathway A neural circuit in the basal ganglia that is excitatory to the motor cortex and involves the striatum and globus pallidus.

Direct pupillary light reflex The ability of the pupil of the eye to contract when light is shone into that eye.

Dominant cerebral hemisphere The side of the brain (usually the left side) that is involved in language and speech processing, analytical reasoning, and skilled motor functions.

Dorsal motor nucleus of the vagus (X) The preganglionic parasympathetic cell bodies for the vagus nerve (X) located just lateral to the hypoglossal nucleus in the medulla oblongata.

Dura mater A thick, protective connective tissue layer loosely covering the brain and spinal cord.

Dural venous sinus A venous structure formed by folds of dura mater surrounding the brain. These bring venous blood from the brain to the jugular foramen where the internal jugular vein begins.

Dysdiadochokinesia The inability of a patient to perform a rapidly alternating motion, such as flipping the hands rapidly from prone to supine. This can be associated with cerebellar disorders.

Efferent Axons that project out of the nervous system, bringing motor information to the periphery.

Emboliform nuclei A subset of nuclei in the interposed nuclei of the cerebellum.

Endolymph The specialized fluid found inside the membranous labyrinth in the inner ear of the temporal bone.

Ependymal cells The columnar epithelial cells lining the ventricles and central canal in the brain and spinal cord. In specialized areas, they are congregated as choroid plexus and produce cerebrospinal fluid.

Epidural hematoma A blood clot produced by a break in a meningeal artery (usually the middle meningeal artery) that depresses the dura mater against the brain, producing a smooth-sided, egg-shaped structure.

Epidural space A fat and vein filled space just superficial to the dura mater in the vertebral column. This is a potential space in the cranium where the dura mater is normally adherent to the bone.

Epilepsy A spontaneous increase in neuronal firing over a region of the brain that can produce a range of symptoms from loss of awareness to convulsions, depending on the extent and severity of the firing.

Epithalamus The supero-posterior portion of the diencephalon that contains the habenula, posterior commissure, and the pineal gland.

External capsule A white matter tract in the cerebral hemisphere that is lateral to the basal ganglia, which allows for interaction among the different areas of cortex in each hemisphere.

Facial nerve (VII) The seventh cranial nerve arises from nuclei in the pons, has axons which arch superiorly around the abducens nucleus before exiting laterally from the pontomedullary junction. It then enters the internal acoustic meatus, passes multidirectionally through the temporal bone giving off branches, before exiting out of the stylomastoid foramen to supply the facial muscles. It innervates the facial muscles, as well as supplying parasympathetic innervation to the lacrimal gland, submandibular, and sublingual glands. It also carries taste fibers from the anterior two-thirds of the tongue.

Facial nucleus — The lower motor neuronal cell bodies for the seventh cranial nerve found in the central portion of the caudal pons. Its axons arch superiorly around the abducens nucleus before exiting laterally from the pontomedullary junction to eventually innervate the facial muscles.

Falx cerebri — A layer of dura mater that is found between the cerebral hemispheres. It contains the inferior and superior sagittal dural venous sinuses.

Fasciculations — A random, coarse set of muscle contractions that can occur after lower motor neuron lesions.

Fasciculus cuneatus — Laterally placed, ascending axons in the posterior columns of the spinal cord that carry first order fine touch and proprioceptive sensory information from the upper extremity.

Fasciculus gracilis — Medially placed, ascending axons in the posterior columns of the spinal cord that carry first order fine touch and proprioceptive sensory information from the lower extremity.

Fastigial nuclei — The medial set of deep cerebellar nuclei associated with the vermis and flocculonodular lobe.

Fetal alcohol syndrome — A developmental disorder due to alcohol consumption by the mother during pregnancy resulting in characteristic facial dysmorphology and decreased intellectual development.

Fibrous tunic — The protective outer layer of the eye composed of the sclera and the cornea.

First order neurons — The sensory neurons that bring a specific sensation from the periphery to the central nervous system. Their peripheral processes begin at a receptor and their central processes synapse at second order neurons. They are typically pseudounipolar or bipolar neurons.

Flocculonodular lobe — A small lobe of the cerebellum that runs across its inferior surface. It regulates balance and vestibular ocular reflexes.

Floor plate — The area of the developing neural tube that is closest to the notochord and furthest from the ectoderm surface.

Folia — The narrow, tightly folded outer gray matter in the cerebellum.

Foramen magnum — The large opening in the base of the skull that allows passage of the spinal cord/medulla oblongata and the vertebral arteries into the cranial cavity.

Forebrain — The anterior of the three brain vesicles of the neural tube that will subsequently develop into the telencephalon (cerebral cortex/limbic system/basal ganglia) and the diencephalon (hypothalamus/thalamus/epithalamus). It can also be referred to as the prosencephalon.

Fornix — An arching white matter tract of the diencephalon that connects the hippocampus with the mammillary bodies.

Fourth ventricle — The diamond-shaped, cerebrospinal, fluid-filled space posterior to the pons and medulla, and anterior to the cerebellum.

Fovea centralis — The central portion of the macula lutea of the retina that is very thin and contains an increased concentration of cone cells for the highest visual acuity.

Frontal cortex — The portion of the brain that is anterior to the central sulcus and behind the forehead. It has roles in personality and motor planning.

Frontal plane — A section of the brain from superior to inferior and perpendicular to the floor as if the patient "walked into a door". This is also called a coronal section.

Functional magnetic resonance imaging (fMRI) — The use of a magnetic resonance imager to determine the functional aspects of specific areas of the brain, due to metabolic changes in those regions during activation.

Ganglion — A group of neuronal cell bodies found in the peripheral nervous system.

Ganglion cells — Specific neuronal cells of the outer retina whose axons project into the brain by way of the optic nerves and optic tracts.

Geniculate ganglion — A collection of first order pseudounipolar sensory cell bodies for taste sensation from the anterior two-thirds of the tongue associated with the facial nerve (VII). A small general sensory component from the external ear may also be involved.

Glaucoma — Increased intraocular pressure in the anterior chamber of the eye, usually due to increased production or decreased drainage of aqueous humor.

Glia The cells that provide nutrition, protection, and structural support to the neurons. These include the astrocytes, oligodendrocytes, the microglia, and the Schwann cells.

Glioblastoma A tumor of glia cells that can expand and place pressure on adjacent neural structures, altering their function.

Globose nuclei A subset of nuclei in the interposed nuclei of the cerebellum.

Globus pallidus A portion of the basal ganglia that controls motor activity. It can be divided into an internal and external segment, both of which are lateral to the internal capsule and the thalamus.

Glossopharyngeal nerve (IX) The ninth cranial nerve arises from receptors in the pharynx, auditory tube, and middle ear. These axons enter the skull through the jugular foramen and enter the medulla oblongata in the postolivary sulcus to synapse at specific nuclei. It carries general sensation from the pharynx, auditory tube, and middle ear, as well as taste sensation from the posterior one-third of the tongue. It also innervates one pharyngeal muscle; the stylopharyngeus.

Golgi cells Interneurons in the granule cell layer of the cerebellum.

Granule cells Interneurons in the granule cell layer of the cerebellum.

Granule cell layer The innermost, deep gray matter layer of the cerebellar cortex that contains Purkinje cell axons, granule cells, and other interneurons.

Gray matter The portion of the central nervous system that contains neuronal cell bodies, dendrites, and axons.

Gyrus A ridge or raised portion in the cerebral cortex enabling a larger surface area of gray matter.

Habenula A portion of the epithalamus in the diencephalon that is involved in negative reward, limbic system function.

Hallucinations The perception of sensory input (usually sounds or visions) that does not actually exist.

Helicotrema The distal-most point in the spiral turns of the cochlea where the scala vestibuli joins the scala tympani.

Hemiballismus Violent flailing and flinging motions of the extremities on one side of the body. This can be seen in patients with lesions of the contralateral subthalamic nucleus.

Hemi-neglect syndrome The inability to recognize or use one entire side of the body.

Hindbrain The posterior of the three brain vesicles of the neural tube that will develop into the metencephalon (pons/cerebellum) and the myelencephalon (medulla oblongata). It can also be referred to as the rhombencephalon.

Hippocampus A specialized collection of neurons in the medial aspect of the temporal lobe that has a unique convoluted appearance. It is part of the limbic system and is involved in new declarative memory consolidation.

Homeostasis The control of normal physiologic function (body temperature, water balance, food intake, metabolism) across a changing environment.

Homonymous hemianopsia A lesion in the optic tract that produces a loss of vision in the temporal (lateral) portion of one visual field and the nasal (medial) portion of the other visual field. The lesion would be on the side of the nasal field loss.

Homunculus The specific anatomical (somatotopic) distribution of function over a region in the brain that can be described as a small human displayed over that region.

Horizontal plane A cross section of the brain or spinal cord in the anterior to posterior direction and parallel to the floor in the upright or anatomical position. It is also called a transverse or cross-sectional plane.

Huntington's disease (chorea) An autosomal dominant, hyperkinetic disease in which patients produce random, spontaneous motions. This is due to an imbalance in basal ganglia function produced by neurodegeneration of the striatum.

Hydrocephalus An increase in the size of the cerebral ventricles due to increased production (or decreased drainage) of cerebrospinal fluid.

Hyperkinetic disorder Spontaneous, involuntary motor movements commonly due to basal ganglia dysfunction. Huntington's disease and choreas are types of hyperkinetic disorders.

Hyperreflexia An increase in the deep tendon reflexes of muscles. This condition can be associated with upper motor neuron lesions.

Hypertonia An increase in muscle tone that can be associated with upper motor neuron lesions.

Hypoglossal canal An opening in the antero-lateral aspect of the occipital bone just superior to the foramen magnum allowing the passage of the hypoglossal nerve (XII).

Hypoglossal nerve (XII) The twelfth cranial nerve arises from the hypoglossal nucleus in the medulla oblongata, exits from the preolivary sulcus and leaves the skull through the hypoglossal canal to innervate the muscles of the tongue.

Hypoglossal nucleus The lower motor cell bodies for the hypoglossal nerve (XII) located in the postero-medial aspect of the medulla oblongata.

Hypokinetic disorder Difficulty initiating or controlling voluntary motor movements commonly due to basal ganglia dysfunction. Parkinson's disease is one type of hypokinetic disorder.

Hyporeflexia A decrease in the deep tendon reflexes of muscles. This condition can be associated with a lower motor neuron lesion.

Hypothalamus A bilateral collection of nuclei inferior to the thalamus in the diencephalon on either side of the midline third ventricle. It is responsible for homeostasis, including hormone secretion, water and food intake, body temperature, and autonomic regulation.

Hypotonia A widespread decrease in muscle tone that can be associated with cerebellar disorders or lower motor neuron lesions.

Incus The second middle ear ossicle that mechanically transduces sound from the malleus (first ear ossicle) to the stapes (third ear ossicle).

Indirect pathway A neural circuit in the basal ganglia that is inhibitory to the motor cortex and involves the striatum, globus pallidus, and the subthalamic nuclei.

Inferior cerebellar peduncle A large white matter tract connecting the medulla oblongata and the cerebellum, composed primarily of afferent fibers bringing information into the cerebellum from the vestibular nuclei, spinal cord, and brain stem.

Inferior colliculus A collection of cell bodies in the posterior midbrain (tectum) that act as a relay nucleus for hearing.

Inferior olives Bilateral bulges on the anterior surface of the medulla oblongata just lateral to the pyramids. These are relay nuclei providing climbing fiber cerebellar input.

Inferior petrosal sinus A dural venous sinus draining from the cavernous sinus to the jugular foramen along the lateral border of the clivus.

Inferior sagittal sinus A dural venous sinus formed at the inferior border of the falx cerebri that drains into the straight sinus.

Inferior salivatory nucleus Preganglionic parasympathetic cell bodies in the pontomedullary region that provide axons to the ipsilateral otic ganglion, mediating salivary secretion from the parotid gland.

Infundibulum The neural tract that connects the hypothalamus to the posterior pituitary along with hypothalamo-hypophyseal blood vessels. It is also called the pituitary stalk.

Inner nuclear layer The nerve cell layer of the retina between the inner plexiform layer and the outer plexiform layer. It contains bipolar, amacrine, and horizontal cell bodies.

Inner plexiform layer The nerve fiber layer of the retina between the ganglion cell layer and the inner nuclear layer. It contains neural processes from bipolar cells in the inner nuclear layer.

Insular cortex A portion of cortex deep to the lateral fissure involved in a number of integrated association functions, including an area for taste and smell sensations that identify and catalog complex flavors.

Integrative Axons that project within the nervous system providing communication between different parts of the nervous system. These are sometimes called relay or association fibers.

Intercavernous sinus A dural venous sinus that connects the right and left cavernous sinuses.

Interhemispheric fissure The deep valley that runs midsagittally between the two halves of the brain.

Intermediate portion of the cerebellum The region of the cerebellum between the vermis and the lateral portion that is responsible for motor control of the distal extremities.

Internal acoustic meatus The foramen in the posterior cranial fossa in which the facial nerve (VII) enters the temporal bone and the vestibulocochlear nerve (VIII) exits the temporal bone.

Internal capsule A large white matter tract in the center of each cerebral hemisphere that carries afferent axons from the thalamus to the cortex, as well as efferent motor axons from the cortex to the brain stem and spinal cord.

Internal carotid artery A branch of the common carotid artery that enters the skull through the carotid canal, passes through the cavernous sinus, gives off the ophthalmic artery, before terminating as the middle cerebral and anterior cerebral arteries.

Internal jugular vein Begins at the jugular foramen with drainage from the sigmoid sinus and the inferior petrosal sinus. It runs through the neck, with the common carotid artery and the vagus nerve (X) to terminate in the brachiocephalic vein.

Interneurons The neural cells that act as relays between sensory and motor neurons for reflex activation and for integration of complex functions.

Interposed nuclei Deep cerebellar nuclei located between the dentate and fastigial nuclei which contain the emboliform and globose nuclei.

Interventricular foramen (of Monro) The opening that connects each lateral ventricle with the third ventricle.

Intervertebral discs The connective tissue shock absorber found between the bodies of two vertebrae.

Intervertebral foramen A small opening formed by two vertebrae through which the spinal nerve exits the spinal (vertebral) canal.

Involuntary motor Efferent motor axons that project to smooth or cardiac muscle for unconscious (autonomic) control of activity.

Ipsilateral Occurring on the same side of the body.

Iris The colored circular structure in the eye that extends from the antero-lateral border to a small circular opening, the pupil. The iris limits the amount of light that can enter the eye by increasing or decreasing the size of the pupil.

Jugular foramen An opening in the inferior aspect of the posterior cranial fossa of the skull that transmits the glossopharyngeal nerve (IX), the vagus nerve (X), and the spinal accessory nerve (XI), along with the origin of the internal jugular vein.

Klüver-Bucy syndrome A rare disorder that includes bilateral loss of the amygdala in the anterior temporal lobes, leading to a flattened emotional affect, hyperorality, and a loss of recognition of objects, especially those associated with fear.

Lateral columns Ascending sensory (spinocerebellar and spinothalamic) and descending motor (lateral corticospinal and rubrospinal) tracts in the lateral spinal cord.

Lateral corticospinal tract The descending motor tract in the spinal cord that carries upper motor axons from the contralateral cortex to the anterior horn of the spinal cord.

Lateral fissure A deep groove on the lateral surface of the brain that runs from anterior to posterior. It separates the temporal lobe from the parietal and frontal lobes of the cortex. It is also called the Sylvian fissure.

Lateral foramen (of Luschka) An opening at the lateral extent of the fourth ventricle that allows cerebrospinal fluid to leave the ventricular system to circulate in the subarachnoid space.

Lateral geniculate A specific relay nucleus of the posterior thalamus that is associated with vision, whose axons project to the primary visual cortex in the occipital lobe.

Lateral horn The portion of the gray matter in the spinal cord that contains the preganglionic autonomic cell bodies that control involuntary motor activity.

Lateral lemniscus A collection of sensory fibers associated with hearing that have their cell bodies in the cochlear nuclei, ascend through the brain stem to synapse in the inferior colliculus.

Lateral portion of the cerebellum The lateral region of the cerebellum that is responsible for motor planning.

Lateral ventricle The cerebrospinal fluid-filled space that extends beneath each hemisphere of the cortex. It has anterior, posterior, and inferior horns that extend under the frontal, occipital, and temporal lobes, respectively.

Lemniscus A generic term for a collection of second order sensory axons.

Lens The transparent oval-shaped structure deep to the pupil of the eye that modifies the refraction of incoming light depending on its thickness. The thickness of the lens is altered by the surrounding ciliary muscle.

Lenticular nuclei
The combined nuclei of the putamen and globus pallidus that appear as a set of three oval-shaped "lenses" on coronal section.

Lenticulostriate arteries
A series of small branches of the middle cerebral artery that supply the basal ganglia and the internal capsule.

Limbic system
A collection of brain nuclei and tracts associated with the diencephalon and deep portions of the telencephalon. It is involved in memory consolidation, emotions, autonomic regulation, reward, and homeostasis.

Lipofuscin
A collection of cellular waste found in cell bodies of long-lived cells, such as neurons.

Locus coeruleus
A collection of noradrenergic cell bodies found in the postero-medial pons that distribute their axons throughout the brain stem and cortex.

Long term potentiation
The ability of specific neurons, notably in the hippocampus, to retain their firing pattern for extended periods of time.

Lower motor neurons
The cell bodies and axons that ipsilaterally innervate specific skeletal muscles. Typically, the cell bodies are found in the anterior horn of the spinal cord with axons that project through anterior roots and spinal nerves to reach their specific muscles.

Lumbar cistern
The large, cerebrospinal fluid-filled dural sac at the distal end of the spinal cord that contains the cauda equina of spinal nerve rootlets. A lumbar puncture draws cerebrospinal fluid from this cistern.

Lumbar nerves
The five spinal nerves which exit below the first through the fifth lumbar vertebra.

Lumbar puncture
A procedure in which a needle is inserted into the lumbar cistern to sample cerebrospinal fluid. It is also known as a spinal tap.

Macula
A structure in the utricle or saccule of the inner ear that contains neuroepithelial receptor cells in a gelatinous structure, with otoliths embedded in the outer surface. During acceleration, the fluid in the utricle or saccule moves the gelatinous structure, bending the stereocilia of the receptor cells.

Macula lutea
The region of the retina that is thinner and contains an increased concentration of cone cells for greater visual acuity. In the center of the macula lutea is the fovea centralis.

Magnetic resonance imaging (MRi)
The use of powerful magnets and radio waves to modify the state of hydrogen atoms, producing a computer-generated, highly detailed internal image of the body.

Main sensory nucleus of trigeminal (V)
The second order sensory cell bodies for fine touch from the face, found in the central portion of the rostral pons. It sends its second order axons across to the contralateral side to ascend in the trigeminothalamic tract.

Malleus
The first middle ear ossicle that mechanically transduces sound from the tympanic membrane to the incus. The tensor tympani muscle can reduce the vibrations induced at the malleus.

Mammillary bodies
Two round projections that extend from the inferior surface of the diencephalon just posterior to the infundibulum. They are part of the limbic system interconnections between the hippocampus and the thalamus. A nutritional deficiency in Vitamin B1 can alter their function (Wernicke-Korsakoff).

Mammillothalamic tract
A white matter axonal tract connecting the mammillary bodies and the anterior thalamus that is part of the Papez circuit in the limbic system.

Mandibular division of the trigeminal nerve (V₃)
The third branch of the trigeminal nerve that carries first order sensory axons from the skin of the jaw and chin, lower teeth, tongue and oral cavity to the main sensory nucleus of the trigeminal and the spinal nucleus of the trigeminal. This nerve also carries the lower motor axons from the motor nucleus of the trigeminal to the four muscles of mastication and four additional muscles.

Mantle layer
The layer of cells in the developing spinal cord that is closest to the neural tube and will develop into gray matter.

Marginal layer
The layer of cells in the developing spinal cord that is farthest from the neural tube and will develop into white matter.

Massa intermedia
A small bridge of neural tissue that connects the thalamus across the midline third ventricle.

Maxillary division of the trigeminal nerve (V$_2$)
The second branch of the trigeminal nerve that carries first order sensory axons from the skin of the cheek, upper teeth, lateral surface of the nose, and lower nasal cavity to the main sensory nucleus of the trigeminal and the spinal nucleus of the trigeminal.

Mechanical hearing defects
A loss of hearing due to damage in the outer ear or middle ear that prevents the conduction of sound from the air through the tympanic membrane and the middle ear ossicles.

Medial forebrain bundle
A collection of ascending and descending axons that connect anterior brain regions with the brain stem. This pathway mediates the pleasure/reward system by connecting the ventral tegmental area with the nucleus accumbens.

Medial geniculate
A specific relay nucleus of the posterior thalamus that is associated with hearing that projects to the primary auditory cortex in the temporal lobe.

Medial lemniscus
Second order sensory axons for fine touch sensation and conscious proprioception that ascend contralaterally through the brain stem to synapse in the thalamus.

Medial longitudinal fasciculus
A medially placed relay tract in the brain stem that bilaterally coordinates the three motor nuclei that control the muscles of each eye, as well as the vestibular system and the upper neck musculature.

Medulla oblongata
The inferior (caudal) end of the brain stem with the prominent pyramids. It is associated with cranial nerves IX (glossopharyngeal), X (vagus), XI (spinal accessory), and XII (hypoglossal).

Melatonin
A small neuroendocrine hormone derived from serotonin and produced by the pineal gland that influences circadian rhythms and sleep.

Membranous labyrinth
The sac-like structure found inside the osseous labyrinth of the temporal bone that contributes to the cochlea and the vestibular apparatus.

Ménière's disease
A disease of the inner ear in which overproduction of endolymphatic fluid leads to disturbances in balance and hearing.

Meninges
Three protective connective tissue layers that surround the brain and spinal cord: the dura mater, arachnoid mater, and the pia mater.

Meningocele
A variant of spina bifida, with a cyst-like protrusion of meninges extending posteriorly.

Meningomyelocele
A more severe form of spina bifida in which a portion of the spinal cord extends into the meningocele.

Mental status
The level of cognitive awareness and function usually assessed with a test that determines if the patient is alert and oriented to person, place, and time.

Mesencephalic nucleus of trigeminal (V)
The first order pseudounipolar cell bodies for proprioception from the muscles of mastication found in the central portion of the midbrain. It provides central projections to the motor nucleus of the trigeminal (V) for reflex action.

Mesencephalon
A portion of the developing brain stem that will become the midbrain.

Metencephalon
A portion of the developing brain stem that will become the pons and cerebellum.

Microcephaly
A defect in the development of the anterior neural tube leading to reduced telencephalon formation and a smaller than normal brain.

Midbrain
The superior (rostral) end of the brain stem with the prominent cerebral peduncles. It is associated with cranial nerves III (oculomotor) and IV (trochlear). It is also the middle of the three embryologic brain vesicles of the neural tube that develops from the mesencephalon.

Midbrain flexure
The anteriorly-directed, ninety degree bend in the brain stem at the midbrain which positions anteriorly placed structures inferiorly and posteriorly placed structures superiorly.

Middle cerebellar peduncle
A large white matter tract connecting the pons and the cerebellum, composed primarily of pontocerebellar fibers whose cell bodies are in the contralateral pons and whose axons enter the cerebellum as mossy fibers.

Middle cerebral artery
A terminal branch of the internal carotid artery that courses laterally into the lateral fissure to supply portions of the parietal, temporal, and frontal cortices.

Middle meningeal artery
A branch of the maxillary artery that enters the skull through the foramen spinosum to supply the dura mater covering the temporal and parietal lobes of the cortex.

Microglia
A glial cell in the central nervous system that is phagocytic, providing immunologic protection.

Molecular layer
The outermost, superficial gray matter layer of the cerebellar cortex that contains Purkinje cell dendrites, parallel fibers, and interneurons.

Mossy fibers
The majority of the axons that enter the cerebellum and project to the deep cerebellar nuclei, the granule cells, and the Golgi cells.

Motor cortex
The region of the posterior frontal cortex (precentral gyrus and premotor area) that contains the neuronal cell bodies of the upper motor neurons. These neurons send axons to interneurons and lower motor neurons in the brain stem and spinal cord.

Motor neglect
The inability to consciously recognize and use the muscles from one side or one region of the body.

Motor nucleus of trigeminal (V)
The lower motor neuronal cell bodies for the fifth cranial nerve that are found in the central portion of the middle pons. It innervates the four muscles of mastication (temporalis, masseter, medial and lateral pterygoids), along with four other muscles (anterior belly of digastric, mylohyoid, tensor tympani, and tensor veli palatini).

Multipolar neuron
This is the typical large neuron with many dendrites and a single long axon found throughout the nervous system.

Myelencephalon
A portion of the developing brain stem that will become the medulla oblongata.

Myelinated axon
A neuronal projection with a multi-wrapped myelin coat produced by the cell membrane of the glial support cell. This produces faster and more consistent signal transmission.

Nervus intermedius
The portion of the facial nerve (VII) that carries the preganglionic parasympathetic and sensory components that is separate from the motor components.

Neural crest cells
Primitive neural plate cells that leave the posterior surface of the neural plate and migrate throughout the developing embryo.

Neural hearing defects
A loss of hearing due to damage in the inner ear, brain stem, or cortex. This could include damage to the neuroepithelial receptor cells, the spiral ganglion, the cochlear nucleus, the inferior colliculus, the medial geniculate, or the primary auditory cortex.

Neural plate
The fast growing ectodermal cells above the notochord that will develop into the neural tube.

Neural tube
The folded neural plate cells that produce a tube of ectodermally-derived cells above the notochord which will develop into the brain and spinal cord.

Neural tunic
The innermost layer of the eye that contains the retina.

Neuroepithelial (hair) cells
Sensory receptor cells with sterocilia that bend with fluid motion and are used to detect sound in the cochlea, as well as acceleration and gravity in the vestibular apparatus.

Neurofibrillary tangles
Complexes of hyperphosphorylated tau proteins and microtubule associated proteins found in the brains of patients with Alzheimer's disease.

Neuron
The main cellular component of the nervous system. It consists of a cell body (soma), cellular projections that bring information to the cell body (dendrites), and a cellular projection that sends information out of the cell body (axon).

Neuroplasticity
The ability of patients to regain neural functions after substantial loss, due to a rewiring or rerouting of functions in the central nervous system. This can also occur during neurodevelopment and may occur normally throughout life.

Nissl substance (bodies)
The collection of polyribosomes and rough endoplasmic reticulum in the neuronal cell body that stains darkly with typical histological preparations.

Node of Ranvier
The gap along an axon between the myelin coats of two glial cells. This allows the neural signal to jump from node to node by saltatory conduction.

Non-dominant cerebral hemisphere
The side of the brain (usually the right side) that is involved in visual and spatial processing, emotional context, and music perception.

Notochord
The endodermally-derived cells that are found in the midline of the embryo and will develop into the vertebral column.

Nucleus A group of neuronal cell bodies found in the central nervous system.

Nucleus ambiguous Lower motor neuronal cell bodies in the central portion of the medulla oblongata that send their axons to skeletal muscles in the palate, pharynx, and larynx associated with the glossopharyngeal (IX) and vagus (X) nerves.

Nucleus cuneatus Second order sensory cell bodies in the postero-lateral aspect of the medulla oblongata that synapse with first order axons, carrying fine touch and conscious proprioception from the upper extremity. The axons from this nucleus ascend through the brain stem in the contralateral medial lemniscus to synapse in the thalamus.

Nucleus gracilis Second order sensory cell bodies in the postero-medial aspect of the medulla oblongata that synapse with first order axons, carrying fine touch and conscious proprioception from the lower extremity. The axons from this nucleus ascend through the brain stem in the contralateral medial lemniscus to synapse in the thalamus.

Nucleus of Edinger-Westphal Preganglionic parasympathetic cell bodies associated with the oculomotor nerve (III), responsible for pupil constriction and accommodation that are located adjacent to the oculomotor nucleus in the rostral midbrain.

Nucleus pulposus The inner gelatinous portion of the intervertebral disc.

Nucleus solitarius (solitary nucleus) Second order sensory cell bodies in the central portion of the caudal pons and rostral medulla oblongata that synapse with first order axons carrying taste from the tongue, visceral sensory input, as well as chemoreceptive input from the cardiovascular system (carotid body and carotid sinus). Some axons from this nucleus ascend through the brain stem in the central tegmental tract to synapse in the thalamus.

Nystagmus An oscillating eye motion in which the eyes move rapidly in one direction and then return more slowly in the opposite direction.

Occipital cortex The portion of the brain that is posterior to the parietal cortex and superior to the cerebellum. It is involved in visual processing.

Oculomotor nerve (III) The third cranial nerve arises from nuclei in the midbrain, exits inferiorly and medially between the cerebral peduncles, passes between the posterior cerebral and superior cerebellar arteries, through the cavernous sinus and the superior orbital fissure to gain access to the orbit. It innervates five ocular muscles and carries preganglionic, parasympathetic axons to constrict the pupil and ciliary muscle.

Oculomotor nucleus The motor cell bodies for the third cranial nerve that are found adjacent to the medial longitudinal fasciculus and the periaqueductal gray in the rostral midbrain.

Olfactory bulbs Second order sensory cell bodies for smell, located on the basal surface of the brain anteriorly. They are found adjacent to the crista galli and cribriform plates of the ethmoid bone.

Olfactory nerve (I) The first cranial nerve arises in the nasal mucosa and extends through the cribriform plate into the olfactory bulb. It is purely sensory for smell.

Olfactory tracts The second order axons from the olfactory bulbs that project to the contralateral olfactory bulb as well as to the primary olfactory cortex.

Oligodendrocyte The glial cell in the central nervous system that produces the myelin coat for the axons.

Ophthalmic artery A branch of the internal carotid artery that provides the central retinal artery as well as the contents of the orbit.

Ophthalmic division of the trigeminal nerve (V_1) The first branch of the trigeminal nerve that carries first order sensory axons from the forehead, eyelids, orbit, ridge of the nose, and upper nasal cavity to the main sensory nucleus of the trigeminal and the spinal nucleus of the trigeminal.

Ophthalmic vein The venous drainage of the orbit that can drain posteriorly to the cavernous sinus or anteriorly through the facial vein.

Optic canal The opening in the sphenoid bone that connects the orbit with the cranial cavity. It carries the optic nerve (II) and the ophthalmic artery.

Optic chiasm The crossing over point of the two optic nerves (II) in which the nasal visual field axons cross to the contralateral optic tract, while the temporal visual field axons remain in the ipsilateral optic tract.

Optic disc   The region of the retina in which the ganglion cell axons leave to form the optic nerve, while the central retinal artery enters the eye to supply the retina. This is the "blind spot" of the retina.

Optic nerve (II)   The second cranial nerve that runs from the back of the globe of the eye to the optic chiasm. It carries visual sensation from each eye.

Optic nerve fiber layer   The outermost layer of the retina that contains the axons from the ganglion cells which project into the optic nerve (II), through the optic chiasm and into the optic tract.

Optic radiations   The axonal projections from the lateral geniculate nucleus that project to the occipital cortex.

Optic tract   The axons from ganglion cells in both eyes carrying the contralateral visual field that project from the optic chiasm to the lateral geniculate.

Optic vesicles   Developmental outgrowths of the diencephalon that will become the eyes.

Orbitofrontal cortex   A region of the frontal cortex just superior to the orbit that acts as an integrated association area for emotion and reward in conscious decision making. It has also been implicated in the pleasantness of taste and flavor.

Osseous labyrinth   The hollow space inside the temporal bone that houses the cochlea and the vestibular apparatus.

Otic placodes   The ectodermal developmental structures that become the cochlea and vestibular apparatus.

Otoliths   Crystalline structures embedded in the surface of the gelatinous portion of the macula in the utricle and saccule of the inner ear.

Outer plexiform layer   The nerve fiber layer of the retina between the inner nuclear layer and the photoreceptor cell layer. It contains neural processes from bipolar cells in the inner nuclear layer.

Oval window   A membrane-lined opening in the temporal bone that communicates between the middle ear and the inner ear. The footplate of the stapes fills this space and sound vibrations in the stapes cause the footplate to transfer these vibrations to the fluid-filled inner ear.

Oxytocin   A neuroendocrine hormone released from the posterior pituitary that mediates parturition and lactation in females, as well as social trust/bonding.

Papez circuit   A historical looped circuit in the limbic system connecting the hippocampus, fornix, mammillary bodies, thalamus, and cingulate gyrus.

Parahippocampal gyrus   The cortical region surrounding the hippocampus in the temporal lobe. It is the posterior continuation of the cingulate gyrus.

Parallel fibers   Processes from the granule cells in the cerebellum that run perpendicular to the Purkinje cell dendrites in the molecular layer of the cerebellar cortex.

Parasympathetic nervous system   The subdivision of the autonomic nervous system that responds during feeding and sleeping (rest and digest). It depresses heart rate and respiration while increasing digestive function.

Parasthesia   An altered response of the somatosensory system, including tingling or burning sensations.

Parietal cortex   The portion of the brain that is posterior to the central sulcus and anterior to the occipital cortex. It is found on the lateral side of the head above the ears. It contains the postcentral gyrus and has roles in sensory processing.

Parkinson's disease   A neurodegenerative, hypokinetic motor disease of basal ganglia dysfunction that is produced by decreased dopamine levels in the substantia nigra.

Periaqueductal gray   A distributed collection of cell bodies that surrounds the cerebral aqueduct in the midbrain.

Perilymph   A plasma-like fluid that fills the space between the membranous labyrinth and the osseous labyrinth in the inner ear of the temporal bone.

Peripheral nervous system   The portion of the nervous system that is outside of the vertebral column and skull. It includes the cranial and spinal nerves with afferent and efferent axons from the skin and muscles, the sensory ganglia associated with the cranial and spinal nerves, the sympathetic chain, along with the postganglionic cell bodies and axons of the autonomic nervous system, as well as the peripheral sensory receptors.

Photoreceptor cell layer
The nerve cell layer of the retina between the outer plexiform layer and the pigment epithelium. It contains the cell bodies of the photoreceptive cells along with the photoreceptive elements (the rods and cones).

Pia mater
A thin connective tissue layer firmly adherent to the brain and spinal cord.

Pigment epithelium
The innermost layer of the retina that contains cells that support and nourish the photoreceptive elements (the rods and cones), as well as absorb stray light.

Pineal gland
A small pine-coned shaped gland projecting posteriorly from the superior diencephalon. It secretes melatonin in response to the light-dark cycle.

Pituitary adenoma
A tumor in the pituitary gland that can produce endocrine dysfunction along with visual disturbances due to pressure from the tumor on the optic nerve (II), optic chiasm, or oculomotor nerve (III).

Pituitary gland
A small gland located inferior to the hypothalamus in the sella turcica, with an endocrine portion (anterior pituitary) and a neural portion (posterior pituitary). It secretes many regulatory hormones.

Poliomyelitis
A virus induced (poliovirus) lower motor neuron disease leading to muscle wasting and atrophy.

Pons
The large middle portion of the brain stem with the prominent middle cerebellar peduncles. It is associated with cranial nerves V (trigeminal), VI (abducens), VII (facial), and VIII (vestibulocochlear).

Pontocerebellar tract
Axons from the pontine nuclei that decussate across the pons to enter the contralateral middle cerebellar peduncle and ascend into the cerebellum as mossy fibers.

Pontomedullary junction
The border between the pons and the medulla oblongata of the brain stem.

Positional test
A vestibular system test in which a patient sits up with her eyes open and is then rapidly moved backwards into a lying down position with her head rotated 90 degrees. The patient's eyes are examined for nystagmus and the test may be repeated a few times to determine if habituation occurs.

Positron emission tomography (PET)
A radiological imaging technique that involves the specific anatomical localization of a radiolabeled compound that was administered to the patient.

Postcentral gyrus
A laterally-oriented ridge of cortical tissue on the posterior side of the central sulcus. It contains the cortical neurons that receive specific regional distribution of somatosensation from the body (sensory homunculus).

Posterior cerebral artery
The terminal branch from the basilar artery that supplies the occipital lobe of the cortex.

Posterior (dorsal) columns
Ascending sensory tracts in the posterior spinal cord that carry ipsilateral fine touch and proprioceptive axons to the thalamus.

Posterior commissure
A small white matter tract for communication between the cortical hemispheres located postero-inferior to the corpus callosum.

Posterior communicating artery
A short anastomotic artery between the middle cerebral artery and the posterior cerebral artery.

Posterior (dorsal) horn
The portion of the gray matter in the spinal cord that contains some second order sensory cell bodies and associated sensory interneurons.

Posterior inferior cerebellar artery
A branch from the vertebral artery that supplies the lower portion of the cerebellum.

Posterior (dorsal) root(lets)
The central projection of sensory axons from the pseudounipolar cell bodies in the posterior (dorsal) root ganglion into the posterior surface of the spinal cord to enter the posterior (dorsal) horn.

Posterior (dorsal) root ganglia
The location of the pseudounipolar cell bodies of the first order sensory neurons that bring peripheral sensory information into the central nervous system.

Posterior (dorsal) spinocerebellar tract
An ipsilateral tract carrying unconscious proprioception that ascends up the lateral spinal cord to enter the cerebellum through the inferior cerebellar peduncle as mossy fibers.

Postolivary sulcus
The lateral groove between the inferior olive and the body of the medulla oblongata. The glossopharyngeal nerve (IX) and vagus nerve (X) travel through this sulcus.

Post-polio syndrome
A decline in skeletal muscle function with increasing age, due to a polio-induced loss of healthy lower motor neurons years before.

Precentral gyrus
A laterally-oriented ridge of cortical tissue on the anterior side of the central sulcus. It contains the upper motor neurons for regionally specific, skeletal muscle activity (motor homunculus).

Preganglionic parasympathetic
The nerve cell bodies found in the lateral horn of the spinal cord (S2–S4) or the brain stem. The spinal cord neurons send their axons along the ventral root to join the spinal nerve and eventually synapse at postganglionic parasympathetic cell bodies. The brain stem neurons send their axons on cranial nerves to eventually synapse at ganglia containing postganglionic parasympathetic cell bodies.

Preganglionic sympathetic
The nerve cell bodies found in the lateral horn of the spinal cord (T1–L2) that send their axons along the ventral root to join the spinal nerve and eventually synapse at ganglia containing postganglionic sympathetic cell bodies.

Preolivary sulcus
The medial groove between the pyramid and the inferior olive on the anterior surface of the medulla oblongata. The hypoglossal nerve (XII) travels through this sulcus.

Primary auditory cortex
The region of the temporal lobe of the cortex that receives direct sound information from the medial geniculate. It is found in Brodmann's areas 41 and 42.

Primary olfactory cortex
The piriform and periamygdaloid cortex that receives direct smell information from the olfactory bulbs.

Primary visual cortex
The region of the occipital lobe of the cortex that receives direct visual information from the lateral geniculate. It is found in Brodmann's area 17.

Pronator drift
The ability to maintain proper muscle control with only proprioceptive feedback. This is tested by asking the patient to close her eyes, raise her arms to shoulder height, and keep them straight in front of her body for 30 seconds.

Pseudounipolar neuron
This is a sensory neuron that has a peripheral process and a central process. The cell bodies are found in peripheral ganglia, such as the posterior (dorsal) root ganglia.

Pterygopalatine ganglion
The postganglionic parasympathetic cell bodies for innervation of the lacrimal gland and the glands of the nasal cavity. It is found in the pterygopalatine fossa and receives its preganglionic parasympathetic innervation from the facial nerve (VII).

Purkinje cells
Large multipolar neurons that provide the final, inhibitory output from the cerebellar cortex to the deep cerebellar nuclei.

Purkinje cell layer
The middle gray matter layer of the cerebellar cortex that contains the large Purkinje cell soma.

Putamen
A portion of the striatum found lateral to the internal capsule and thalamus as well as medial to the insular cortex. It is part of the basal ganglia which controls motor activity.

Pyramids
Two parallel ridges on the anterior surface of the medulla oblongata that contain the corticospinal tracts.

Quadrantanopia
A lesion in a part of the optic radiations that produces a loss of vision in one quarter of both visual fields. A left superior quadrantanopia is due to a lesion in the contralateral (right) inferior optic radiations.

Rachischisis
A severe form of spina bifida in which the neural tube does not close and dysfunctional neural tissue is found in place of skin over the vertebral column.

Raphe nuclei
A collection of serotonergic cell bodies in the medial aspect of the reticular formation of the pons and medulla oblongata that distribute axons throughout the brain stem and cortex.

Red nucleus
A collection of cell bodies in the center of the tegmentum of the midbrain that are part of a cerebellar feedback loop (dentato-rubro-olivary loop), as well as a descending rubrospinal tract.

Reflexes
A rapid, involuntary muscular response to a sensory stimulus. For example, tapping the patellar tendon produces a rapid, involuntary knee jerk due to contraction of the quadriceps muscles.

Reticular formation
A large column of poorly defined nuclei in the center of the pons and medulla oblongata that mediate autonomic functions, alertness, and awareness.

Reticulospinal tract
The descending tracts in the anterior spinal cord that carry axons from the pontine and medullary reticular formation to the anterior horn of the spinal cord, mediating autonomic function, arousal, and other reflex actions.

Retina — The layer of the eye that contains the photoreceptive cells and the associated neurons for vision. It has distinct layers, with many neuronal cell bodies and projections.

Retinal detachment — The separation of the retina from the underlying pigment epithelium and choroid of the eye. This can lead to a loss of vision from the affected region.

Rhombencephalon — The caudal end of the developing brain stem (hindbrain) which subsequently becomes the metencephalon (pons and cerebellum) and the myelencephalon (medulla oblongata).

Rinne test — A test for hearing in which a patient is asked to listen to a tuning fork placed outside each ear or on the mastoid process of each ear. This tests the difference between air conductive hearing and bone conductive hearing, respectively, and in normal individuals air conduction hearing should be better.

Romberg test — A patient is asked to stand upright with his feet next to each other and then to close his eyes. Any swaying or falling over is a sign that proprioceptive, vestibular or cerebellar systems may be dysfunctional.

Roof plate — The area of the developing neural tube that is closest to the ectoderm surface and furthest from the notochord.

Rotation test — A vestibular system test in which a patient, with her head tilted forward 30 degrees, is rotated on a spinning stool for approximately 30 seconds. During the rotation and after it has stopped, the patient's eyes are examined for nystagmus. In a normal individual, one direction of nystagmus is observed during the rotation and the opposite direction of nystagmus is observed after the rotation.

Round window — A membrane-lined opening in the temporal bone that communicates between the middle ear and the inner ear. This serves as a pressure relief valve for sound vibrations in the fluid-filled inner ear.

Rubrospinal tract — The descending tract in the spinal cord that carries axons from the red nucleus in the midbrain to the anterior horn of the spinal cord.

Saccule — A space in the membranous labyrinth of the inner ear that contains a vertically-oriented macula for sensing linear acceleration.

Sacral nerves — The five spinal nerves which exit from the first through the fifth fused sacral vertebra.

Sagittal plane — A section of the brain or spinal cord in the anterior to posterior direction and perpendicular to the floor in the upright or anatomical position. It can be in the midline (midsagittal) – producing two equal halves – or it can be lateral to the midline (parasagittal) – producing unequal parts.

Scala media (cochlear duct) — An endolymph-filled spiral tube in the cochlea that is separated from the scala vestibuli by the vestibular membrane and the scala tympani by the basilar membrane.

Scala tympani — A perilymph-filled spiral tube in the cochlea that is separated from the scala media by the basilar membrane.

Scala vestibuli — A perilymph-filled spiral tube in the cochlea that is separated from the scala media by the vestibular membrane.

Schizophrenia — An individual with a cognitive disassociation that involves disrupted thought processes and emotional disturbances.

Schwann cell — The glia cell of the peripheral nervous system that supports and makes the myelin coat for the axons. It is also known as a neurolemmacyte.

Sclera — The thick white outer layer of the eye that is an extension of the dura mater and aids in support and protection of the eye.

Second order neurons — These are sensory neurons in the central nervous system that receive input from first order neurons and project to third order neurons. Most second order neurons decussate and ascend to specific thalamic nuclei.

Semicircular canals — Three half-moon shaped tubes in the temporal bone oriented in three ninety-degree planes (horizontal, vertical, and lateral).

Senile plaques — Amyloid protein and apolipoprotein E complexes that are found in the brains of patients with Alzheimer's disease.

Sensory neglect — The inability to recognize or react to sensory information from one side or one region of the body.

Septum pellucidum — The midsagittal thin layer of tissue that separates the two lateral ventricles just superior to the thalamus.

Sexually dimorphic — Morphologically different structures based on gender.

Shingles — A reactivation in adulthood to the varicella zoster virus that resides in the sensory ganglia, producing pain and inflammation along a specific dermatome.

Sigmoid sinus — A dural venous sinus formed from the transverse sinus and superior petrosal sinus that drains along the lateral wall of the posterior cranial fossa to end at the jugular foramen and the internal jugular vein.

Single photon emission computed tomography (SPECT) — A radiological imaging technique that involves the specific anatomical localization of a radiolabeled compound that was administered to a patient.

Solitary nucleus (gustatory portion) — Second order sensory cell bodies for taste located in the medulla oblongata and caudal pons that project via the central tegmental tract to the thalamus.

Solitary tract — The central processes of pseudounipolar, first order sensory neurons that receive stimulation from taste buds on the tongue and project to the solitary nucleus.

Soma — The cell body of the neuron that contains the nucleus, the Golgi apparatus, and other functional organelles.

Spasticity — The increase in muscle tone and deep tendon muscle reflexes associated with upper motor neuron lesions.

Sphincter pupillae muscle — A circular band of smooth muscle in the medial aspect of the iris which, when parasympathetically contracted, decreases the size of the pupil allowing less light to enter the eye.

Spina bifida — A developmental disorder in the spinal cord due to poor development of the neural tube. It can be found in children whose mothers had inadequate folic acid in their diet.

Spina bifida occulta — A mild variant of spina bifida in which the lumbar vertebral lamina do not fully fuse.

Spinal accessory nerve (XI) — The eleventh cranial nerve arises from cell bodies in the upper cervical spinal cord whose axons join together and ascend through the foramen magnum and then exit through the jugular foramen to innervate two muscles.

Spinal cord — The distal end of the central nervous system made up of 31 spinal segments located in the vertebral column.

Spinal nerve — The combined sensory (posterior roots) and motor (anterior roots) axons from a single segment of the spinal cord.

Spinal nucleus of the trigeminal nerve (V) — Second order sensory cell bodies in the lateral portion of the pons and medulla oblongata that synapse with first order general sensory, pain, and temperature axons from the face, nasal cavity, and throat. The axons from this nucleus ascend through the brain stem in the contralateral trigeminothalamic tract to synapse in the thalamus.

Spinal tract of the trigeminal nerve (V) — First order sensory axons in the lateral portion of the pons and medulla oblongata that carry ipsilateral general sensory, pain, and temperature information from the face, nasal cavity, and throat. The axons in this tract synapse in the spinal nucleus of the trigeminal nerve (V).

Spinocerebellar tracts — Ascending unconscious proprioceptive axons that project ipsilaterally to the cerebellum and are subdivided into posterior and anterior tracts.

Spinocerebellum — The region of the cerebellum that receives input from the spinal cord, including the vermis and intermediate portions.

Spinothalamic tracts — Ascending second order pain and temperature axons that project contralaterally through the spinal cord and brain stem to synapse in the thalamus.

Spiral ganglia — The first order, bipolar, sensory cell bodies for hearing found in the center of the cochlea that send central projections to the cochlear nuclei.

Stapedius muscle — A small skeletal muscle that dampens vibrations in the stapes during loud sounds.

Stapes — The third middle ear ossicle that mechanically transduces sound from the incus to the oval window of the inner ear. The stapedius muscle can modify the vibrations induced at the stapes.

Stellate cells — Interneurons in the molecular layer of the cerebellum.

Stereognosis — The ability to recognize common objects by touch alone.

Straight sinus — A dural venous sinus formed from the inferior sagittal sinus and the great cerebral vein that drains through the tentorium cerebelli into the confluence of the sinuses.

Stria medullaris — A white matter tract on the supero-medial border of the thalamus interconnecting the hypothalamus and the habenula.

Stria terminalis — A white matter tract on the supero-lateral border of the thalamus interconnecting the hypothalamus and the amygdala.

Striatum — The combined nuclei of the caudate and putamen. It receives the majority of input to the basal ganglia.

Stroke — The loss of blood supply to a specific region of the brain or brain stem due to a plaque or clot in the blood vessel supplying the region (ischemia) or due to a rupture in the blood vessel supplying the region (hemorrhage).

Stylomastoid foramen — The opening in the inferior surface of the temporal bone between the styloid process and mastoid process where the facial nerve (VII) exits.

Subarachnoid hemorrhage — A blood clot produced by a break in a cerebral artery that usually flows around the base of the brain and produces a ragged-shaped structure.

Subarachnoid space — The region between and around the arachnoid mater where the cerebrospinal fluid flows.

Subdural hematoma — A blood clot produced by a break in a cerebral vein or dural venous sinus that allows blood to flow into the sulci of the cortex producing a ragged structure.

Subiculum — A subdivision of the hippocampus that contains the majority of cortical output from the hippocampus.

Submandibular ganglion — The postganglionic parasympathetic cell bodies for innervation of the submandibular and sublingual glands. It receives its preganglionic parasympathetic innervation from the chorda tympani and facial nerve (VII).

Substantia nigra — A collection of dopaminergic cell bodies in the anterior portion of the tegmentum of the midbrain just posterior to the cerebral peduncles. The cells contain a high density of melanin, so the region appears black in fresh tissue. The axons project to the striatum of the basal ganglia.

Subthalamic nucleus — A functional part of the basal ganglia which controls motor activity. It is located inferior to the thalamus.

Sulcus — A valley or groove in the cerebral cortex enabling a larger surface area of gray matter.

Superior alternating hemiplegia (Weber's syndrome) — A lesion of the medial portion of the cerebral peduncle and its adjacent oculomotor nerve (III) in the midbrain, producing contralateral motor deficits in the body with ipsilateral deficits in the eye muscles.

Superior cerebellar artery — A branch from the basilar artery that supplies the upper portion of the cerebellum.

Superior cerebellar peduncle — A large white matter tract connecting the cerebellum and the midbrain, composed primarily of efferent fibers from the cerebellum to the vestibular nuclei, red nucleus, and thalamus (for relay to the cortex).

Superior colliculus — A collection of cell bodies in the posterior midbrain (tectum) that act as a specific relay nucleus for vision.

Superior olive (nuclear complex) — A collection of cell bodies located in the central portion of the pons that function in sound localization.

Superior orbital fissure — A gap in the sphenoid bone that allows passage of nerves and blood vessels into and out of the orbit from the middle cranial fossa.

Superior petrosal sinus — A dural venous sinus draining from the cavernous sinus to the sigmoid sinus along the superior border of the petrous ridge of the temporal bone.

Superior sagittal sinus — A dural venous sinus formed at the superior border of the falx cerebri that drains into the confluence of the sinuses.

Superior salivatory nucleus — Preganglionic parasympathetic cell bodies in the caudal pons that provide axons to the ipsilateral pterygopalatine and submandibular ganglia mediating lacrimal secretion (tearing), nasal gland secretions, and salivary secretion from the submandibular and sublingual glands.

Sympathetic nervous system — The subdivision of the autonomic nervous system that responds during activity and stress (fight or flight). It increases heart rate and respiration, while decreasing digestive and renal function.

Syringomyelia — A cyst-like formation in the center of the spinal cord in the vicinity of the central canal.

Syphilitic myelopathy (tabes dorsalis) The loss of the posterior columns in the spinal cord, typically due to a syphilis infection, leading to somatosensory deficits and instability during standing and gait (Romberg's sign).

Taste buds Chemoreceptive cellular structures located on the surface of the tongue.

Tectorial membrane The thick structure in the scala media of the cochlea that rests on the stereocilia of the neuroepithelial receptor cells providing a firm surface for bending the stereocilia during sound reception.

Tectospinal tract The descending tract in the anterior spinal cord that carries visual and auditory information to the cervical portion of the anterior horn of the spinal cord to help coordinate head and neck musculature.

Tectum The region of the midbrain posterior to the cerebral aqueduct, containing the sensory superior and inferior colliculi (corpora quadrigemina).

Tegmentum The region of the midbrain anterior to the cerebral aqueduct containing the red nucleus, substantia nigra, ventral tegmental area, and the cerebral peduncles.

Telencephalon The most rostral portion of the central nervous system composed of the cerebral hemispheres (frontal, parietal, occipital, and temporal cortices), the basal ganglia, parts of the limbic system, and the associated white matter tracts.

Temporal cortex The portion of the brain that is inferior to the frontal and parietal lobes of cortex. It is involved in auditory processing.

Tensor tympani muscle A small skeletal muscle that dampens vibrations in the malleus during loud sounds.

Tentorium cerebelli A double layer of dura mater separating the occipital cortex and the cerebellum. It contains the straight and the transverse dural venous sinuses.

Thalamic pain syndrome (Dejerine-Roussy) A condition with chronic continual pain believed to occur due to a small stroke in the thalamus.

Thalamocortical fibers (radiations) Axonal projections from the thalamus to the cortex that travel in the internal capsule.

Thalamus A bilateral, centrally placed cluster of nuclei in the diencephalon that serve as relay nuclei for virtually all neural signals to the cortex.

Third order neurons These are sensory neurons that receive input from second order neurons and, typically, are found in the thalamus with projections to the cortex.

Third ventricle The midline cerebrospinal fluid-filled space found between the right and left thalamus and hypothalamus in the diencephalon.

Thoracic nerves The twelve spinal nerves which exit below the first through the twelfth thoracic vertebra.

Tonotopic The distribution of pitches (sounds) that are sensed in specific regions of the cochlea and then transmitted through the auditory system in a specific pattern.

Transverse sinus A dural venous sinus formed at the lateral end of the tentorium cerebelli.

Trigeminal (semilunar) ganglion A collection of first order pseudounipolar sensory cell bodies for sensation from the face, orbit, nasal, and oral cavities associated with the trigeminal nerve (V).

Trigeminal nerve (V) The fifth cranial nerve arises from nuclei in the pons and medulla, exits laterally from the pons, passes its associated trigeminal ganglion and subdivides into three branches (ophthalmic, maxillary, and mandibular) which exit out of the skull through the superior orbital fissure, the foramen rotundum, and foramen ovale, respectively. It carries general sensation (touch, pain, and temperature) from the face, nasal, and oral cavities, as well as motor innervation to the muscles of mastication and four other muscles.

Trigeminal neuralgia (tic douloureux) A hypersensitivity of a portion of the trigeminal nerve that produces pain during normal touch or pressure.

Trigeminothalamic tract Second order sensory axons for general sensation, pain, and temperature from the face, nasal cavity, and throat that ascend contralaterally through the brain stem to synapse in the thalamus.

Trochlear nerve (IV) The fourth cranial nerve arises from nuclei in the midbrain, exits superiorly and arches around the midbrain, passes into the cavernous sinus and enters the orbit through the superior orbital fissure. It innervates one ocular muscle: the superior oblique.

Trochlear nucleus The motor cell bodies that contribute to the trochlear nerve (IV) found adjacent to the medial longitudinal fasciculus and the periaqueductal gray in the caudal midbrain.

Two-point discrimination — The distance needed to determine if one or two points are recognized from a closely spaced object, such as the open end of a paper clip. This will normally vary depending on the anatomical region tested, but should be consistent from side to side.

Tympanic cavity — The air-filled middle ear space that contains the three bony ossicles for mechanical transduction of sound from the tympanic membrane to the oval window.

Tympanic membrane — The thin drum-like structure between the outer ear and middle ear that converts sound waves in the air into mechanical vibrations in the ear ossicles.

Ultrasound — A non-invasive, non-radiological imaging technique that uses sound waves to create density images of soft tissue structures. It has limited use in imaging the brain and nervous system due to the interference of the skull.

Unipolar neuron — This is a small unique neuron that has no dendrites and only a single axon, such as the photoreceptor cells.

Unmyelinated axon — A neuronal projection with glial cell support, but without a multi-wrapped myelin coat. It has slower neurotransmission speeds.

Upper motor neurons — The cortical cell bodies and axons that control skeletal muscle function. They originate in the contralateral cortex and descend through the brain stem, decussate in the medulla to continue ipsilaterally in the spinal cord to synapse on lower motor neurons that directly innervate skeletal muscle.

Utricle — A space in the membranous labyrinth of the inner ear that contains a horizontally-oriented macula for sensing linear acceleration.

Vagus nerve (X) — The tenth cranial nerve arises from nuclei in the medulla oblongata, exits laterally from the postolivary sulcus and leaves the skull through the jugular foramen. It supplies the skeletal muscles of the pharynx, larynx, and palate. It also provides parasympathetic innervation to the cardiac muscle and the smooth muscles of the respiratory and digestive system (to the left colic flexure). It also carries general sensation from the larynx, visceral sensation from the lungs and digestive system, as well as taste sensation from the epiglottis.

Varicella zoster — A virus that infects and resides in the sensory ganglia, producing chickenpox in children and shingles in adulthood.

Vascular tunic — The middle layer of the eye, composed of the choroid, iris, lens, and ciliary body. This layer provides nutritional support and excess light absorption for the retina, as well as structures which limit or modify the incoming light waves.

Ventral posterior lateral (VPL) nucleus of the thalamus — Specific thalamic relay nucleus associated with sensory information from the contralateral side of the neck and body (posterior columns, medial lemniscus, spinothalamic tract).

Ventral posterior medial (VPM) nucleus of the thalamus — Specific thalamic relay nucleus associated with sensory information from the contralateral side of the face and head (trigeminal nerve (V)).

Ventral tegmental area — A collection of dopaminergic cell bodies medial to the substantia nigra in the midbrain that are involved in the reward circuit.

Vermis — The midline portion in the cerebellum controlling trunk musculature and some proximal musculature of the extremities.

Vertebral artery — A branch from the subclavian artery that ascends through the transverse foramina of the cervical vertebra, passing medially across the upper surface of the first cervical vertebra (atlas) to join with the vertebral artery from the opposite side, forming the basilar artery.

Vertigo — A form of balance disorientation that can be described as dizziness or feeling that the "room is spinning."

Vestibular apparatus — The semicircular canals, macula, and utricle inside the temporal bone that sense acceleration and gravity.

Vestibular ganglion — The first order bipolar sensory cell bodies for acceleration and gravity found in the temporal bone that send central projections to the vestibular nuclei.

Vestibular membrane — The thin cellular lining that separates the scala vestibule from the scala media in the cochlea.

Vestibular nuclei — Four nuclei (superior, medial, lateral, and inferior) in the lateral aspect of each side of the caudal pons and rostral medulla oblongata that receive ipsilateral first order sensory axons from the vestibular ganglion. The axons from these nuclei project to the spinal cord, brain stem, cerebellum, and cortex.

Vestibulocerebellum The region of the cerebellum that receives input from the vestibular nuclei, notably the flocculonodular lobe of the cerebellum.

Vestibulocochlear nerve (VIII) The eighth cranial nerve arises from the vestibular apparatus and the cochlea in the temporal bone, exits the bone through the internal acoustic meatus and enters the brain stem at the pontomedullary junction, where it ends in the vestibular and cochlear nuclei. It carries balance, spatial, and sound sensations to the brain stem.

Vestibulospinal tract The descending tract in the anterior spinal cord that carries vestibular axons to the anterior horn of the spinal cord, providing balance and spatial information.

Vitreous body A large spherical gelatinous ball that occupies the space posterior to the lens and anterior to the retina in the eye.

Voluntary motor Efferent motor axons that project to skeletal muscle for conscious control of activity.

Weber test A hearing test in which a patient is asked to listen to a tuning fork placed on the center of her head and to distinguish on which side the sound is loudest. In normal individuals, the sound should be the same on both sides.

Wernicke-Korsakoff syndrome A vitamin B1 (thiamine) deficiency that leads to degeneration of the mammillary bodies. It can be found in chronic alcoholics and symptoms can include ataxia, ophthalmoplegia, apathy, and confabulation.

Wernicke's area A region of the posterior superior portion of the left temporal lobe (Brodmann's area 22) that is associated with comprehending speech (comprehension aphasia – Wernicke's aphasia).

White matter The portion of the central nervous system that contains tracts of axons with no neuronal cell bodies.

Index

Essential Clinical Neuroanatomy, First Edition. Thomas H. Champney.
© 2016 John Wiley & Sons, Ltd. Published 2016 by John Wiley & Sons, Ltd.
Companion website: www.wileyessential.com/neuroanatomy

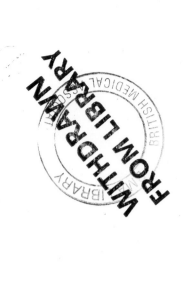